Trace elements in human nutrition and health

World Health Organization
Geneva
1996

WHO Library Cataloguing in Publication Data

Trace elements in human nutrition and health.
  1.Trace elements – metabolism   2.Trace elements – standards
  3.Nutrition   4.Nutritional requirements
  ISBN 92 4 156173 4 (NLM Classification: QU 130)

The World Health Organization welcomes requests for permission to reproduce or translate its publications, in part or in full. Applications and enquiries should be addressed to the Office of Publications, World Health Organization, Geneva, Switzerland, which will be glad to provide the latest information on any changes made to the text, plans for new editions, and reprints and translations already available.

TYPESET IN INDIA
PRINTED IN BELGIUM

93/9811 – Macmillan/Ceuterick – 8000

Contents

Preface

In 1973, a WHO Expert Committee on Trace Elements in Human Nutrition met in Geneva to address questions concerning the essentiality of, requirements for and metabolism of 17 trace elements in humans. The Committee's report (1) recommended ranges of intakes, based on the estimates then available, for population groups consuming diets differing widely in the content and bio-availability of their trace-element constituents. The report also dealt with the toxicity of certain heavy metals, such as cadmium, lead and mercury, by summarizing existing guidelines for safe limits of environmental exposure.

Since 1973, spectacular and far-reaching advances have been made in knowledge relating to the significance of trace elements in human health and disease. Several "new" trace elements have been discovered, and substantial progress has been made in the sophistication of trace-element analysis. In recognition of these developments, the Food and Agriculture Organization of the United Nations (FAO), the International Atomic Energy Agency (IAEA) and the World Health Organization (WHO) considered it appro-priate to convene another expert group to re-evaluate the role of trace elements in human health and nutrition.

To this end, a two-year preparatory process was started in 1988, involving a number of advisory group meetings and small group workshops and the drafting and compilation of individual and working group contributions and reviews. This work culminated in a Joint FAO/IAEA/WHO Expert Consulta-tion on Trace Elements in Human Nutrition, held in Geneva from 18 to 22 June 1990 under the chairmanship of Dr Walter Mertz, Director of the United States Department of Agriculture's Human Nutrition Research Center in Beltsville, Maryland. A list of those contributing to the preparatory process and of participants in the Expert Consultation is given in Annex 1.

During the production of a comprehensive draft report, representing the outcome both of the preparatory work and of the Consultation itself, it was recognized that new data emerging in several key areas were relevant and should also be included. The enormous task of compiling, balancing and editing the final report and incorporating new information as it emerged subsequent to the Consultation was delegated to Professor Colin F. Mills of the Rowett Research Institute, Aberdeen, Scotland. To him the Secretariat would like to extend special thanks.

The final text contains material contributed by numerous experts consulted in different specialized fields, together with the conclusions reached and recommendations made by the Expert Consultation. Its aim is to provide scientists and national authorities worldwide with an up-to-date and authoritative review of trace-element requirements for human health and nutrition, together with guidelines and recommendations that will remain appropriate at least until the turn of the century.

Reference

1. *Trace elements in human nutrition. Report of a WHO Expert Committee.* Geneva, World Health Organization, 1973 (WHO Technical Report Series, No. 532).

Abbreviations used in the text

ASREM	Asian Society for Reference Materials
CV	coefficient of variation
E_{Plmin}^{basal}	basal population requirement for element E
E_{R}^{basal}	basal individual requirement for element E
$E_{Plmin}^{normative}$	normative population requirement for element E
$E_{R}^{normative}$	normative individual requirement for element E
E_{Plmax}^{tox}	upper limit of safe range of population mean intakes of element E
E_{SRI}	safe range of population mean intakes of element E
FAO	Food and Agriculture Organization of the United Nations
GEMS	Global Environmental Monitoring System
IAEA	International Atomic Energy Agency
ICCIDD	International Council for the Control of Iodine Deficiency Disorders
IDD	iodine-deficiency disorder(s)
IU	International Unit(s)
SD	standard deviation
SEM	standard error of the mean
T_3	3,5,3'-triiodothyronine
T_4	3,5,3'5'-tetraiodothyronine; thyroxine
TSH	thyroid-stimulating hormone
UNEP	United Nations Environment Programme
UNICEF	United Nations Children's Fund
WHO	World Health Organization

For full definitions of the abbreviations used for individual and population requirements for trace elements, see Chapter 2. Additional abbreviations used specifically in the context of analytical methodology are explained in Chapter 21.

Technical note

Values in thermochemical kilocalories have been retained in the text when they correspond to the figures given in the cited reference source. The corresponding values in joules can be obtained as follows:

$$1 \text{ cal}_{th} = 4.184 \text{ J}$$

$$1000 \text{ kcal}_{th} = 4.184 \text{ MJ}$$

The results of most sequential calculations preceding the tabulation of data for this report were worked out to three significant figures and finally rounded as appropriate.

1.
Introduction

1.1. Background

The report of the WHO Expert Committee on Trace Elements in Human Nutrition that met in 1973 ended with six important general recommendations for future national and international activities in trace-element nutrition (1). Of these, the first two dealt with the need to obtain reliable information on the trace-element content of foods, especially milk, and to monitor that content in relation to future changes in agricultural and industrial practices. The third recommended that trace-element requirements should be taken into account in food standards and especially in those for formulated foods designed for infants and young children. The next two recommendations were concerned with the need for international centres for the study of trace elements in humans and for international analytical reference laboratories. The final recommendation called for a further review of new findings in trace-element nutrition in order to update the recommended levels of intake.

Every one of these recommendations has since been implemented in some way, thus reflecting the substantial progress in the field of trace-element nutrition, as follows:

- The spectacular advances in trace-element analytical techniques have led to the re-examination of many of the published data for trace elements in foods and body fluids (2). For several elements, the range of ostensibly "normal" values has narrowed, while "normal" values for others have declined by whole orders of magnitude (3). Accuracy of analysis has been improved by the production and certification of a number of biological reference materials in Asia, Europe and North America (4). Because of these developments, the amount and reliability of the data on inorganic elements in foods have markedly improved, and reliable monitoring of concentrations in foods is now possible (5).
- Many formulated foods are now enriched with essential trace elements such as copper, iodine, iron or zinc. Impressive progress has been made towards rationalizing policies with respect to the trace-element content of infant foods and foods for special medical applications and intra-venous alimentation.

1

- With support from national and international organizations, the number of centres with expertise in trace-element research has increased, especially in developing countries, resulting in greater knowledge of requirements and of environmental exposure, and of methods of promoting effective intervention.
- Several international reference laboratories have been established with the support and collaboration of the International Atomic Energy Agency. They are involved in a coordinated research programme aimed at determining the trace-element content of typical national diets around the world.

In addition, several discoveries and numerous refinements in techniques have substantially increased knowledge of the role of trace elements in human health. It is now recognized that trace elements can become limiting not only because of environmental deficiencies, but also because of imbalances in diets that in the past had been accepted as adequate. Such imbalances have been demonstrated in patients maintained on intravenous alimentation, in children during the development of, and even during treatment for, malnutrition, and in infants, children and adolescents consuming locally accepted diets of low trace-element content or bioavailability. Imbalances have also been created when food aid programmes have supplied foods rich in energy and protein but containing inadequate amounts of trace elements to populations in areas affected by famine. Thus, adequacy of micronutrients in the diet must be a concern to all public health authorities.

Since the publication of the 1973 report, it has been realized that both the extent of iodine deficiency and the variety of its pathological consequences have been seriously underestimated. Its significance for public health is clear from evidence that nearly 1600 million people in 118 countries are at risk from iodine-deficiency disorders. Over the same period the discovery of the central role of selenium deficiency in the etiology of Keshan disease in China has greatly stimulated research on human selenium requirements and metabolism. Other permissive etiological factors are known to influence the risks for this disease but have still to be identified. Marginal states of zinc deficiency resulting in retardation of the growth of infants and of preschool and schoolchildren have been identified in several countries. Copper deficiency continues to be reported not only in infants and children undergoing rehabilitation but also in those reared under conditions of social deprivation. Detection of copper and zinc deficiencies is hindered by the relatively low specificity of their clinical features.

Several "new" trace elements have been shown to have essential functions in experimental animals. Although the nutritional essentiality of some of these for humans has yet to be proved, intakes by some human populations are suspected to be less than their probable requirement. Provisional allowances or ranges of intakes have been suggested for some of these elements.

Progress has been made in increasing the understanding of the chemical and physiological factors modifying the bioavailability of trace elements in the diet. This has confirmed early suspicions that such interactions can have a profound influence on the interpretation of data on the dietary intake of some trace elements and the relationship of intake to requirements. There is a particular need to identify situations in which chemical and physiological determinants of bioavailability influence the risks of trace-element-related diseases rather than being of academic interest only.

The period since 1973 has also been notable for the increase in the awareness that anomalies in trace-element supply can influence human health and well-being without necessarily producing diagnostically specific clinical changes. In addition, it is now recognized that the clinical expression of a "latent" deficiency or excess is often contingent on variables such as the enhanced growth achieved during rehabilitation following general malnutrition or challenges such as stress, infection or injury. The fact that the ability of specific populations to tolerate such challenges can be influenced by anomalies in trace-element status emphasizes the need for maintaining intake within tolerable limits.

1.2 Structure and content of the report

The present report uses concepts that differ somewhat from those of the 1973 document and therefore require definition. For the purposes of this report, the definitive feature of a nutritionally significant trace element is either its essential intervention in physiological processes or its potential toxicity when present at low concentrations in tissues, food or drinking-water. Arbitrarily, the term "trace" has been applied to concentrations of element not exceeding 250 μg per g of matrix.

An element is considered essential to an organism when reduction of its exposure below a certain limit results consistently in a reduction in a physiologically important function, or when the element is an integral part of an organic structure performing a vital function in that organism. Proof of essentiality of an element in one animal species does not prove essentiality in another, but the probability of an essential function in any species (including humans) increases with the number of other species in which essentiality has been proved. This definition is not absolute; it depends on what is considered to constitute a "physiologically important function", "consistent" functional impairment, etc.

3

Since the Expert Consultation considered resistance to dental caries to be a physiologically important function, the element fluorine was regarded as essential. It also decided that the enzyme glutathione peroxidase was a "structure" performing a vital function and therefore considered its constituent selenium as essential, even though uncomplicated selenium deficiency has not yet been demonstrated in humans. Not all essential elements as defined in this report are of equal practical importance for public health. Underexposure, overexposure, or both are known to occur under certain environmental conditions for chromium, copper, fluorine, iodine, molybdenum, selenium and zinc. The heavy metals cadmium, mercury and lead and the element fluorine are of great concern because of the excessive concentrations occurring in food chains in many parts of the world. The heavy metals have been studied intensively, and the results of these studies and recommendations of safe intakes are documented in the corresponding volumes of the WHO Environmental Health Criteria Series (6–9). For other elements, such as manganese and the "new" trace elements, there is no evidence at present that abnormally low or high dietary intakes cause substantial nutritional problems in human populations. The essential elements cobalt (in the form of vitamin B_{12}) and iron are not included because they are discussed in a recent FAO publication (10).

The trace elements that were considered by the Expert Consultation have been divided into three groups in the report from the point of view of their nutritional significance in humans, as follows: (1) essential elements; (2) elements which are probably essential; and (3) potentially toxic elements, some of which may nevertheless have some essential functions at low levels. Elements for which there is the clearest evidence that either deficiency or excess causes significant ill-health are considered first within each of these groups. The recommendations made for individual elements are presented in the form of safe ranges of intake for *population groups,* wherever the available data permit. *These ranges do not represent individual requirements but are the limits of adequacy and safety of the* mean *intakes of whole populations.* If the population mean intake falls within these limits, practically all members of that population are considered to have an adequate intake. It is important that the conceptual framework of the recommendations, as presented in Chapter 2, be clearly understood and correctly applied.

At the same time it must be recognized that the quality of the databases to which the conceptual approach was applied varies substantially among the individual elements because of the vast differences in knowledge of dietary intakes, metabolism and requirements. The impressive data relating different levels of intake to deficiency, adequacy and toxicity of selenium, for example, differ markedly from the indirect and often fragmentary evidence for other trace elements. Homoeostasis is maintained by different means for different elements

4

and the mechanisms regulating absorption or excretion in response to changes in nutritional status are poorly quantified. Yet these mechanisms, together with dietary interactions that affect biological availability, have a profound effect on dietary requirements. Whenever a lack of exact data made a strictly statistical derivation of requirements impossible, they had to be based more on personal judgement, common sense and consensus after intensive discussion. Any conclusions resulting from that approach are clearly indicated in the individual chapters.

Other sections of the report deal with topics particularly relevant to an understanding of the causes of, and the factors governing, responses to trace-element deficiency or excess. They cover subjects such as the physiological variables modifying requirements and tolerance, as well as bioavailability phenomena and analytical procedures, and should assist in the task of identifying circumstances likely to increase the risks of development of trace-element-related diseases.

The final chapter presents the recommendations of the Expert Consultation for future activities. Only some of them relate to the research needed to fill important gaps in knowledge and in the ability to diagnose marginal states of trace-element nutrition, the remainder being intended to increase the awareness of the great potential health benefits of intervention programmes for whole populations in which trace-element deficiencies, environmental or dietary, have been diagnosed. The conquest of iodine-deficiency disorders in many countries (11) and of Keshan disease in China (12) are examples of what can be achieved.

It is hoped that this report will offer more reliable criteria with which to assess the possibility that the dietary habits of specific communities may have adverse effects on health attributable to the deficiency or excess of a specific trace element. Used in conjunction with other criteria, biochemical, environmental and socioeconomic, the guidelines offered here may not only serve as a means of assessing probable trace-element status but also contribute to the more effective diagnosis and control of such problems.

References

1. *Trace-elements in human nutrition. Report of a WHO Expert Committee.* Geneva, World Health Organization, 1973 (WHO Technical Report Series, No. 532).
2. Versiek J, Cornelis R. Normal levels of trace elements in human blood plasma and serum. *Analytica chimica acta*, 1980, **116**: 217–254.
3. Smith Jr, JC et al. Evaluation of published data pertaining to mineral composition of human tissue. *Federation proceedings*, 1981, **40**: 2120–2125.
4. Wolf WR, ed. *Biological reference materials.* New York, John Wiley, 1985: 425.
5. *Minor and trace elements in breast milk. Report of a Joint WHO/IAEA Collaborative Study.* Geneva, World Health Organization, 1989.

6. *Lead—environmental aspects*. Geneva, World Health Organization, 1989 (Environmental Health Criteria 85).

7. *Mercury—environmental aspects*. Geneva, World Health Organization, 1989 (Environmental Health Criteria 86).

8. *Methylmercury*. Geneva, World Health Organization, 1990 (Environmental Health Criteria 101).

9. *Cadmium*. Geneva, World Health Organization, 1992 (Environmental Health Criteria 134).

10. *Requirements of vitamin A, iron, folate and vitamin B_{12}. Report of a Joint FAO/WHO Expert Consultation*. Rome, Food and Agriculture Organization of the United Nations, 1988 (FAO Food and Nutrition Series, No. 23).

11. Hetzel BS. Iodine deficiency disorders. *Lancet*, 1988, **i**: 1386–1387.

12. Keshan Disease Research Group. Observations on effect of sodium selenite in prevention of Keshan Disease. *Chinese medical journal*, 1979, **92**: 471–476.

2.

Trace-element requirements and safe ranges of population mean intakes

The requirement estimates in this report are expressed in a way that differs from, but is consistent with, those found in earlier reports. In this chapter, the derivation of requirement estimates and of the safe range of population mean intakes is described and examples of two modes of application are presented. (For further details, see Annex 2.)

In earlier reports, the emphasis was on the estimation of the level of nutrient intake deemed "safe" for the randomly selected individual; few individuals would be expected to have requirements exceeding this level. Of necessity, the *recommended intake* (1, 2) or *safe level of intake* (3–5) exceeded the actual requirements of almost all individuals (6). The application of such estimates to population data was generally a source of confusion. In a recent report (7) a WHO Study Group considered the level of group mean intake that would offer assurance of a low prevalence of inadequate intakes within the group. The change in focus from the individual to the group or population was facilitated by an in-depth exploration of the concepts involved and relationships between distributions of intakes and requirements (8). Following the lead of the earlier report on trace-element requirements (9), recent reports have also directed attention towards the estimation of the upper limit of "safe" intakes either for the individual (4, 5) or for the population group (7). Recent reports on human nutrient requirements have paid greater attention to the question of "requirement for what?" As a result, two levels of requirement, namely a basal requirement level and a normative requirement level, have emerged (5). The present report continues this conceptual development, recognizing that the newer modes of expression have unique advantages for many areas of current application. A direct comparison of the two types of estimates is presented in Table A1 of Annex 2.

2.1 Definitions

The definitions used in the present report, except where new terms are introduced, are consistent with usage in previous FAO/WHO reports. Unless otherwise qualified, the terms *requirement, basal requirement* and *normative requirement* (see below) relate to the needs of individuals.

7

2.1.1 Definitions relating to the needs of individuals

Requirement. This is the lowest continuing level of nutrient intake that, at a specified efficiency of utilization, will maintain the defined level of nutriture in the individual. Where appropriate, the *requirement* for an element E will be given the symbol E_R.

Basal requirement. This refers to the intake needed to prevent pathologically relevant and clinically detectable signs of impaired function attributable to inadequacy of the nutrient. Where appropriate, *basal requirement* will be given the symbol E_R^{basal}.

Normative requirement. This refers to the level of intake that serves to maintain a level of tissue storage or other reserve that is judged by the Expert Consultation to be desirable. Where appropriate, *normative requirement* will be given the symbol $E_R^{normative}$.

The essential difference between the *basal requirement* and the *normative requirement* is that the latter usually facilitates the maintenance of a desirable level of tissue stores. For most trace elements discussed in this report, metabolic and tissue-composition studies indicate the existence of discrete stores which, by undergoing depletion at times of reduced intake or high demand, can provide protection for a certain period against the development of pathological responses to trace-element deficiency. Since higher levels of intake are needed to maintain these reserves the *normative requirement* is necessarily higher than the *basal requirement*.

In the specific case of zinc (see Chapter 5), the concept of a normative "reserve" appears to be inappropriate and its physiological role is replaced by a physiological capacity to reduce body losses of zinc if intake is reduced and status threatened. At the *basal requirement* level, the ability to increase the efficiency of zinc retention will have been fully exploited. As zinc intake approaches the *normative requirement*, this potential to utilize zinc with greater efficiency has no longer to be exploited and this gives the subject a normative reserve capacity to adapt to transient decreases in zinc intake. In discussing zinc requirements (Chapter 5), the term *physiological requirement* is therefore used to describe the amounts of zinc that must be absorbed (in contrast to the definitions given above that refer to amounts present in the diet as ingested).

For all the elements discussed in this report, no demonstrable association between function and intake exists once the basal requirement has been met. It is emphasized that the difference between intakes meeting the *basal requirement* and the *normative requirement* lies only in the ability of the latter to promote responses which, although differing in mechanisms, provide protection against future adverse conditions such as a reduction in trace-element intake or an increase in need. The desirable magnitude of these reserves is often a matter of judgement, and hence has been called the *normative requirement* (5).

Unless otherwise stated, all requirement estimates in this report are presented as the quantity of the element that must be present in the daily diet, as consumed, to meet the basal or normative requirement. The estimates will have been adjusted to take into account the nature of the diet and the dietary factors that affect the ability of the body to release and absorb the element. As discussed in Annex 2, "daily intake" is defined as the individual's average intake persisting over moderate periods of time without necessarily being present in those amounts each day. The Expert Consultation specifically dissociated itself from any notion of an "optimal" intake level for the individual.

Individuals differ in their requirements, even though they may have the same general characteristic (e.g. age, sex, physiological state, body size). One may therefore speak of the *average requirement* of a group of individuals (e.g. young

Figure 2.1. Distribution of requirements among individuals, showing the average requirement and the recommended or safe level of intake as presented in earlier reports (1–5)

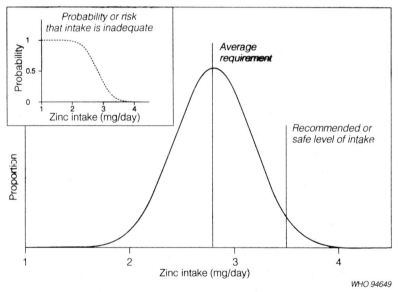

WHO 94649

The diagram shows the basal zinc requirements of young adult men consuming a diet in which 35% of the zinc is available for absorption. For the purpose of this and other figures, the coefficient of variation (CV) of individual requirements has been taken as 12.5% although no specific estimate is offered in this report. The insert shows the probability or "risk" that a given level of usual intake will be inadequate to meet the actual requirement of a randomly selected individual (4).

adult men) or of the level that marks a point in the upper tail of the requirement distribution, the level previously identified as the *recommended or safe level of intake (1–5)* (see Fig. 2.1). Except where specifically indicated, the estimates refer to the maintenance of a defined level of nutritional status in individuals already in that state. They refer to healthy individuals, and the estimated requirements may be altered by disease or other conditions (see Chapter 23).

2.1.2 Definitions relating to population group mean intakes

In this report, the term "population" or "population group" is used to refer to a group, usually large, that is homogeneous in terms of age, sex and other characteristics believed to affect requirements. The term "population" is not used in its usual sense to mean a collection of individuals reflecting the demographic structure of the people living in a country or region. (See Annex 2 for further discussion.)

As previously noted, following the lead of an earlier WHO report (7), the present report offers estimates of ranges of group mean intakes that would suffice to ensure a low prevalence of individuals at risk of either inadequate or excessive intakes. Such estimates are referred to as the *safe range of population mean intakes,* as defined below.

> *Safe range of population mean intakes.* This term refers to the range of population group mean intakes deemed adequate to sustain existing nurtiture in healthy population groups. If the mean intake of such groups is maintained in the safe range over long periods of time, it is judged unlikely that there will be evidence of either inadequacy or excess of intake in more than a very small proportion of the individuals (low population group risk). For this purpose, population groups are considered to be relatively homogeneous in terms of age and sex. Where appropriate, the *safe range of population mean intakes* of an element (E) will be given the symbol E_{SRI}.

Increasing the population group mean intake (PI) decreases the proportion of individuals whose intakes fall below their own normative requirements; it decreases the likelihood of depletion (see Fig. A2 in Annex 2). Further increases in group mean intake (shifting the whole distribution of intakes upward) will ultimately increase the proportion of individuals with intakes above safe levels and thus approaching the toxicity threshold. The safe range of population mean intakes (E_{SRI}) has, as a lower limit, the lowest population mean intake ($E_{PImin}^{normative}$) at which the population risks of depletion remain acceptable when judged by *normative* criteria (see above). The upper limit of the safe range of population mean intakes is defined, correspondingly, by the maximum population group mean intake E_{PImax}^{tox} at which the risks of toxicity remain tolerable.

Both limits reflect *normative* judgements; between these limits, risks of inadequacy or excess are acceptably low and the distributions of intakes are deemed safe. There is no recognized "optimal" level. This concept is shown graphically in Fig. 2.2.

For both planning and assessment purposes, it is also useful to identify the lowest population mean intake that is still accompanied by an acceptable risk of functional impairment attributable to dietary deficiency of the element concerned. This intake will satisfy the *basal* requirements of all but a very small proportion of individuals. As appropriate, it will be given, for an element E, the symbol E_{PImin}^{basal}. The population risk (expected prevalence) of functional impairments from such intakes will remain low even though the group mean intake falls below the normative safe range of intakes $(E_{SRI}^{normative})$. As the group mean intake falls below E_{PImin}^{basal}, the prevalence of individuals expected to show

Figure 2.2. The concept of the safe range of population mean intakes

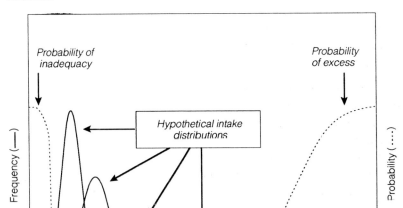

WHO 94650

The diagram shows the risk curves for the probability of inadequacy of intake and of excess of intake (risk to individual), together with a series of intake distributions, all of which would be associated with a low prevalence of effects of either inadequate or excess intake. All these intake distributions would be characterized as falling within the *safe range of population mean intakes*. The diagram is based on the zinc intakes of young adult men consuming a diet of moderate zinc availability.

demonstrable signs of functional impairments will gradually increase (see Fig. A2 in Annex 2).

2.2 Derivation of estimates

In estimating human nutrient requirements, the Expert Consultation considered evidence derived from both experimental and epidemiological (population) studies. In each case, consistency of requirement estimates with both types of evidence was a major consideration. Animal studies were examined primarily to gain further understanding of the utilization of the element so that human studies might be more correctly interpreted. The specific evidence, and the assessment and interpretation of that evidence, are presented in the chapters that follow. The derivation of estimates of the safe range of population mean intakes and of the lower limits of both basal and normative group mean intakes are discussed below and illustrated in the accompanying figures, all of which examples are based on the zinc requirements of young adult men consuming a diet of moderate zinc availability (35% at the level of the basal requirement and 30% at that of the normative requirement—see Chapter 5, Table 5.6).

The usual first step was the estimation of the average individual *basal requirement* of the element (for specified age and sex groups). For zinc, the first level of estimation, based on a factorial model, was the basal *physiological requirement* for absorbed zinc (1 mg/day for the adult male; Chapter 5, Table 5.3); from this an estimate of the dietary zinc intake required to supply 1 mg of absorbed element (in this example, $Zn_R^{basal} = 2.8$ mg/day) was derived, taking into account the fraction absorbed from the diet (35% for a moderate-availability diet at the level of the basal requirement).[1] The next step was to determine the distribution of usual intakes that would meet the condition that very few individuals would be expected to have intakes below their own basal requirements. Based on the empirical relationships developed in a previous report (9), this condition is approximated when the proportion of individuals with intakes below the average basal requirement is 2–3%. Given an estimate of the variability of the usual intakes within the population group, the position of the population intake distribution and, hence, the mean population intake that satisfies basal needs were estimated. For zinc, it was considered that a typical intake distribution would have a coefficient of variation (CV) of 25% and that it could be assumed to approximate normality (see Annex 2 for further discussion

---

[1] In the case of selenium (see Chapter 6), the primary epidemiological data available for examination related to the population mean intake that satisfied basal requirements. The average basal requirement was then inferred from that base by applying parallel logic.

of this assumption). In this way, the lower limit of the population mean intakes satisfying basal needs (Zn_{Plmin}^{basal}) was set at 5.7 mg/day (Chapter 5, Table 5.7). This is illustrated in Fig. 2.3.

The lowest population mean intake sufficient to meet normative needs is estimated (see Fig. 2.4) by means of an approach similar to that described above. From an estimate of the normative physiological requirement (1.4 mg/day) and an estimated availability of 30%, $Zn_R^{normative}$ is found to be 4.7 mg/day, and from this, again assuming a 25% CV for usual intake, $Zn_{Plmin}^{normative}$ is estimated to be 9.4 mg/day.

The upper normative limit for population mean intakes was established in the same way, as illustrated in Fig. 2.5. As discussed in Chapter 9, an upper limit for the population mean intake was established on the basis of evidence relating to undesirable interactions between zinc and other elements. The intake level estimated to represent an average threshold for toxic effects was taken as

Figure 2.3. Derivation of the lower limit of the population mean intake satisfying basal needs of zinc for adult men (Zn_{Plmin}^{basal})

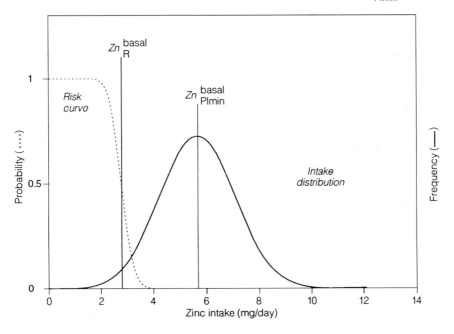

WHO 94651

The diagram shows the mean basal requirement (Zn_R^{basal}) and the distribution of usual intakes meeting the condition that only 2–3% of individuals would have intakes below Zn_R^{basal}. The mean of this distribution is Zn_{Plmin}^{basal}.

Figure 2.4. Derivation of the lower limit of the population mean intake satisfying normative needs of zinc for adult men ($Zn_{PImin}^{normative}$)

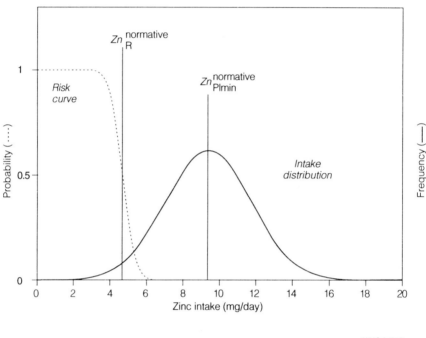

WHO 94652

The diagram shows the mean normative requirement ($Zn_R^{normative}$) and the distribution of usual intakes meeting the condition that only 2–3% of individuals would have intakes below $Zn_R^{normative}$. The mean of this distribution is $Zn_{PImin}^{normative}$.

60 mg/day. On the assumption, once again, of a 25% variability of usual intake, the highest population mean intake that would be associated with a low (2–3%) prevalence of intakes above the 60 mg/day cut-off (Zn_{PImax}^{tox}) would be approximately 40 mg/day.

Given estimates of the lower and upper limits of acceptable population mean intakes, the safe range of population mean intakes, Zn_{SRI}, is defined as shown in Fig. 2.6. Fig. 2.2 shows the same range of population distributions, but in that figure, risk curves were included to demonstrate that, as the distributions shift beyond the safe range, the *risk* of inadequacy or of excess increases. The definition of the safe range remains a probability assessment, not a binary statement of "adequate" or "inadequate"; this must be recognized when observed intakes are assessed. The limits of the safe range mark the beginnings of concern about the prevalence of inappropriate (too low or too high) intakes in the population group. (See Annex 2 for additional discussion.)

14

Figure 2.5. Derivation of the upper limit of the population mean intake avoiding zinc toxicity as judged by normative criteria, for adult men (Zn$^{tox}_{Plmax}$)

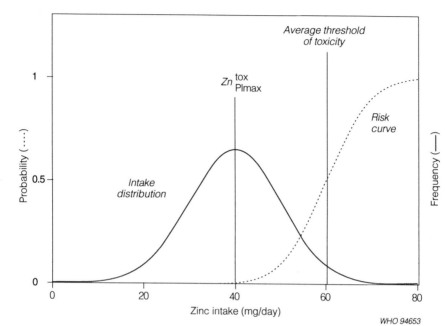

The diagram shows the estimates of the mean threshold for deleterious effects and the distribution of usual intakes meeting the condition that only 2–3% of individuals would have intakes above this level. The mean of this distribution is Zn$^{tox}_{Plmax}$. It is accepted that there is individual variability in the level at which detrimental effects are seen, but this variability has *not* been defined. For illustrative purposes, a CV of 12.5% was assumed in drawing the risk curve.

2.3 Application and interpretation of requirement estimates

Estimates of human nutrient requirements find many applications. No single numerical descriptor of requirements can serve all applications (*10*). Rather, approaches to specific applications should be derived from a consideration of the concepts underlying published requirement estimates (*4*). Two types of application, one prescriptive and the other diagnostic, both applicable to populations, but not to individuals, are described below.

2.3.1 Prescriptive application—food and nutrition planning

Estimates of human nutrient requirements are frequently used in the planning of diets for groups or populations. The safe range of population mean intakes

Figure 2.6. Safe range of population mean intakes of zinc for adult men

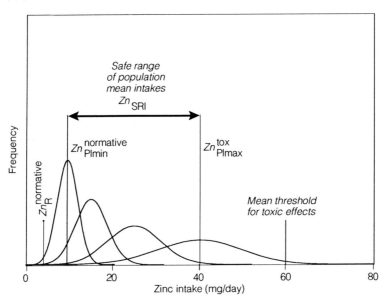

WHO 94654

It is assumed that 30% of the zinc in the diet is available for absorption and that the CV of usual intakes is 25%. All intake distributions with mean intakes in the safe range would be deemed satisfactory. The average individual normative requirement and the mean threshold for toxic effects are also shown for information purposes.

(Fig. 2.6) is directly applicable for this purpose; the goal should be to ensure food supplies and intake patterns such that group mean intakes fall within the safe range. Since this report is concerned with safe ranges of mean intakes for groups of specified age, sex and physiological characteristics, it follows that, for planning purposes, total populations should be subdivided into the corresponding strata.

Given that population groups defined by social, economic and other descriptors may differ in their typical intakes of nutrients, the planner may wish to stratify the population by such characteristics as well as by their physiological characteristics, when planning food supplies. The nature of the diet consumed, or expected to be consumed, in so far as it may affect nutrient utilization, must be considered and the appropriate safe ranges of population mean intakes selected. If serious constraints on meeting normative goals exist in a particular setting, the planner might consider it a matter of high priority to meet at least the basal needs of the group concerned (Fig. 2.3).

Two important limitations to this approach to the application of require- ment estimates warrant emphasis. The first is the fact that such estimates, and hence planning goals, are based on the *maintenance of health in healthy individuals*. With a nutrient-depleted population, in contrast, it may be necessary to consider approaches that remedy existing deficiencies before maintenance goals can be established. If the utilization of, or need for, a nutrient is affected by disease, then the lower limit of the safe range of population mean intakes may be an underestimate of the desirable goal for population mean intakes. It is also possible that, in some clinical conditions, sensitivity to high intakes of certain elements may increase, so that the upper limit of the safe range might then have to be reconsidered.

An example of a situation requiring specific modification of the requirement estimates might be found in nutritional rehabilitation programmes. If such programmes are designed in such a way that significant growth response in previously undernourished children is expected, it can be assumed that the zinc requirements to support accelerated growth will be greater than those for the maintenance of normal children of the same sex and age (see discussion in Chapter 5). Obviously the programme manager must take this into account in planning the dietary supplies for the programme.

The second important limitation to the approach adopted by the Expert Consultation is that the recommendations made in this report apply essentially to large groups. While, with some reservations (see Annex 2), they are also applicable to smaller groups with clearly defined characteristics, the Expert Consultation stressed the need to include adequate numbers of individuals in studies of dietary intakes of trace elements. This view is emphasized in Chapter 22, which gives detailed consideration to the results of a wide range of dietary surveys that differ greatly in scale.

2.3.2 Diagnostic application—assessment of observed intakes

Assessment of dietary intake can never provide an assessment of nutritional health (the state consequent on the ingestion and utilization of nutrients). It can, however, provide valuable guidance as to whether or not existing intakes are *likely* to be adequate to maintain health in healthy individuals. Two distinct approaches to diagnostic assessment are briefly described below.

In the first, *only population mean intake estimates are available for consideration*. Fig. 2.7 (for which zinc has been used as an example) shows a series of such estimates superimposed upon the estimated safe range of intakes. All groups marked with an asterisk would be considered to be at low risk of either inadequacy or excess. They should not be a cause of concern (with regard to zinc intake) to the public health authorities. The population group with a

Figure 2.7. Assessment of observed intakes—only population mean intake available

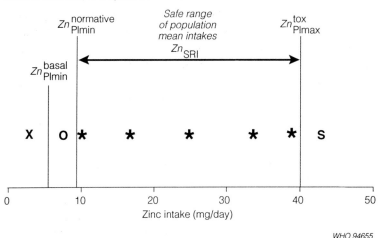

WHO 94655

The diagram shows the limits of the safe range of intakes and Zn_{Plmin}^{basal}, as well as points representing a range of population group mean intakes. The group means marked by an asterisk would include very few individuals with either inadequate or excessive intake and hence are not of concern. The other groups represent varying degrees of risk and hence of concern (see text for discussion).

mean intake marked with O reflects a situation in which a higher than desirable proportion of individuals may be in a compromised state of zinc nutriture, or at least one with a reduced adaptive capacity. As the mean intake falls below Zn_{Plmin}^{basal} (e.g. point "X" in Fig. 2.7), functional signs of zinc inadequacy may be present in a small but significant proportion of individuals, who have intakes below their own basal requirements. Concern should therefore increase, and it might be appropriate to take steps to investigate this potential problem. As the group mean intake falls even further, both the level of concern and the priority for action should increase (see Fig. A2, Annex 2, for the relationship between the population mean intake and the expected prevalence of inadequate intakes). A similar rationale and response apply to high population mean intakes. If, for example, the group mean intake were at the point designated "S" in Fig. 2.7, some individuals might be exposed to detrimentally high levels of zinc intake (though they would not necessarily exhibit functional effects of such exposure). Since the high intakes have no recognized advantage, the potential detrimental effects are a matter of concern.

In the second approach, *the distribution of usual intakes of individuals is known,* and further refinement of the assessment approach is possible and is strongly preferred. The proportion of individuals in a group or population with usual intakes below the average requirement (or above the toxic threshold) for that class of individual provides a crude estimate of the prevalence of inadequate (or excessive) intakes (9). This is illustrated in Fig. 2.8. A group's distribution curve of usual intakes is shown together with vertical lines indicating the estimated mean *basal* and *normative* requirements. The inserts show the lower tail of this distribution. The area of the dark shaded portions, as a proportion of the area under the entire distribution curve, represents the estimated prevalence of individuals with inadequate intakes. In this example, about 15% of the men would have intakes below their own normative

Figure 2.8. Assessment of observed intakes—estimated distribution of usual intakes available

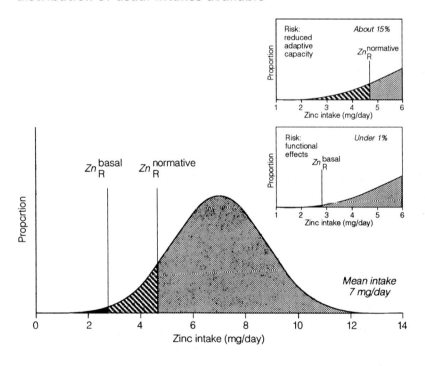

WHO 94656

The diagram shows a hypothetical distribution of usual zinc intakes for a group of adult men consuming a moderate-availability diet, together with the average *basal* and *normative requirements* for this class of individual. The areas in the tail of the curve beyond these lines (see dark shaded areas in insets) represent the proportion of individuals expected to have intakes below their own *basal* or *normative requirements*. These areas can be estimated by statistical methods or can be obtained by performing actual counts of individuals falling below the cut-offs. Note, however, that the approach does not identify the affected individuals, only the proportion affected.

requirements and would be expected to have reduced adaptive capacity. However, fewer than 1% would be expected to have intakes below their own basal requirements and possibly functional impairments attributable to zinc deficiency.

This more refined approach to assessment is preferred when actual intake distributions are available since it does not depend on the validity of the assumptions about the nature of the intake distribution (e.g. the variability may be larger or smaller than that assumed in the derivation of the safe range of population mean intakes, or the intake distribution may be skewed). However, it is critically important to examine the distribution of *usual* intakes rather than assume that the distribution is normal; otherwise estimates of the prevalence of low or high intakes may be significantly distorted (see Annex 2). While the approach provides an estimate of the proportion of individuals with inadequate or excessive intakes, it *cannot* identify which particular individuals are affected.

The example shown in Fig. 2.8 also suggests the desirability of performing a dual assessment using estimates of both the *basal* and the *normative requirement*. This offers much more information about the nature and severity of problems, and hence about the urgency for action, for the guidance of public health planners. More information is required if the second mode of assessment is to be used than can be obtained by merely examining the population mean intakes. The first type of assessment might therefore well be the simpler of the two; however, if that assessment suggests that a problem may exist, further dietary, biochemical and clinical studies may be needed before a high priority for action can be assigned.

References

1. *Joint FAO/WHO Expert Committee on Nutrition. Eighth Report.* Geneva, World Health Organization, 1971 (WHO Technical Report Series, No. 477).
2. *Requirements of ascorbic acid, vitamin D, vitamin B_{12}, folate and iron. Report of a Joint FAO/WHO Expert Group.* Geneva, World Health Organization, 1970 (WHO Technical Report Series, No. 452).
3. *Energy and protein requirements. Report of a Joint FAO/WHO Ad Hoc Expert Committee.* Geneva, World Health Organization, 1973 (WHO Technical Report Series, No. 522).
4. *Energy and protein requirements, Report of a Joint FAO/WHO/UNU Expert Consultation.* Geneva, World Health Organization, 1985 (WHO Technical Report Series, No. 724).
5. *Requirements of vitamin A, iron, folate and vitamin B_{12}. Report of a Joint FAO/WHO Expert Consultation.* Rome, Food and Agriculture Organization of the United Nations, 1988 (FAO Food and Nutrition Series, No. 23).
6. Department of Health and Social Security. *Recommended intakes of nutrients for the United Kingdom,* London, HMSO, 1969.

7. *Diet, nutrition and the prevention of chronic diseases. Report of a WHO Study Group.* Geneva, World Health Organization, 1990 (WHO Technical Report Series, No. 797).

8. National Research Council Subcommittee on Criteria for Dietary Evaluation. *Nutrient adequacy: assessment using food consumption surveys.* Washington, DC, National Academy Press, 1986.

9. *Trace elements in human nutrition. Report of a WHO Expert Committee.* Geneva, World Health Organization, 1973 (WHO Technical Report Series, No. 532).

10. Beaton GH. Criteria of an adequate diet. In: Shils ME, Olsen JA, Shike M, eds. *Modern nutrition in health and disease*, 8th ed. New York, Lea & Febiger, 1993.

3.
Trace-element bioavailability and interactions

Factors influencing trace-element bioavailability often dominate relationships between total element supply and the extent to which this remains within the limits required to maintain health. This chapter deals with the influence of physiological and dietary variables that affect element utilization and must therefore be taken into account when comparing data on dietary intakes with estimates of requirement or tolerance. The term "bioavailability" is used in this report to describe the effects of any process, physicochemical or physiological, which influences the fraction of an ingested trace element ultimately presented to tissues in forms that can be used to meet functional demands. Use of the term in this context is not confined to digestive or absorptive phenomena; processes which modify the systemic utilization of elements after their absorption are included.

Such an approach takes account of the fact that the supply to tissues of specific trace elements in forms that can be used for functional purposes is governed by a wide range of variables. They include: (i) the physicochemical characteristics of trace-element sources in the diet; (ii) the biochemical inter-actions of these elements with synergists or antagonists either in the gut lumen or in tissues; and (iii) physiological variables which, in response to changing relationships between element supply and demand, influence the efficiency of element absorption, storage or incorporation into functional sites.

The discussion of trace-element bioavailability and interactions in this report concentrates on aspects particularly relevant to trace-element nutrition in humans. Relationships revealed by investigations on experimental animals are considered only when there are good reasons to believe that they are relevant to humans. Others have been reviewed elsewhere (1, 2). The influence of genetic abnormalities and of non-nutritional diseases on trace-element utilization is not considered.

The principal variables influencing trace-element bioavailability and utilization are broadly summarized in Table 3.1. The interactions between them are frequently complex and thus it is often difficult to predict the quantitative significance of each. Although experimental studies of such quantitative relationships are making progress, it is unrealistic to expect that the detailed

22

compositional data needed to define the dietary content of synergists or antagonists of the utilization of most nutritionally important trace elements will become available for the wide variety of diets in common use. Instead, it is suggested that a general understanding of the mechanisms of action of factors governing bioavailability can help with the identification of the principal dietary regimens and physiological states likely to modify the risks of trace-element deficiency or excess. This will permit more effective anticipation of the influence of dietary, environmental and other variables on such risks.

3.1 Physiological variables influencing trace-element utilization

3.1.1 Age-related changes

A wide range of studies on experimental animals indicate that the "immature" gut of the newborn lacks the ability to achieve homoeostatic regulation of the

Table 3.1. Variables influencing trace-element bioavailability and utilization

A. Intrinsic (physiological) variables

1. *Absorptive processes*
   Development changes:
   Infancy: immediate postnatal absorption poorly regulated (e.g. of chromium, iron, zinc and probably of lead) until homoeostatic regulatory mechanisms become established with increasing gut maturity.
   Senility: probable decline in efficiency of absorption of copper and zinc.

   Homoeostatic regulation:
   — adaptation to low trace-element status or high demand (e.g. during pregnancy) by modifying activity/concentration of receptors involved in uptake from gastrointestinal tract (applicable to chromium, copper, manganese, zinc, probably not to fluorine, iodine, lead, selenium);
   — relationship of intraluminal soluble content of element to proportional saturation of receptors involved in absorption (marked influence on zinc utilization).

2. *Metabolic/functional interactions*
   Interdependence of elements in processes involved in storage and metabolism (e.g. copper and iron in catecholamine metabolism; selenium in iodine utilization; zinc in protein synthesis/degradation).
   Metabolic interrelationships enhancing element loss or reducing mobility of stored element (e.g. tissue anabolism sequestering zinc; physical activity promoting chromium loss; tissue injury promoting zinc loss).
   Metabolic interrelationships enhancing release of stored element (e.g. low calcium promoting skeletal zinc release; tissue catabolism promoting zinc redistribution).

23

Table 3.1 (continued)

B. Extrinsic (dietary) variables

Solubility and molecular dimensions of trace-element-bearing species within food, digesta and gut lumen influencing mucosal uptake (e.g. non-available iron oxalates, copper sulfides, trace-element silicates; zinc, iron and lead phytates associated with calcium).

Synergists enhancing mobility of element:
— enhancing absorption (e.g. citrate, histidine, enhancing zinc absorption; ascorbate modifying iron/copper antagonism);
— maintaining systemic transport and mobility of some elements (e.g. transferrins, albumins and other plasma ligands).

Antagonists limiting mobility of element:
— decreasing gastrointestinal lumen solubility of element (e.g. calcium/zinc/phytate, copper/sulfides);
— competing with element for receptors involved in absorption, transport, storage or function (e.g. cadmium/zinc, zinc/copper antagonism);
— mechanisms unknown (e.g. iron/copper, iron/zinc antagonism).

---

uptake of several essential elements. Discrimination against toxic elements is absent or poorly developed (for review, see reference 3). For example, it is known that absorption of cadmium, copper, iron and lead can decline by as much as 80% during the first few days of life of the rat. Absorption of these elements in the form of metal–protein complexes by pinocytosis within the intestinal mucosa may well account for the fact that, unlike what happens in later stages of development, the efficiencies of absorption of copper, zinc and other trace metals appear to be unrelated to the existing tissue status of these elements in the young animal. In the light of such evidence from experimental animals of an enhanced capacity for metal uptake by the immature gut, it is surprising that no corresponding studies have been undertaken on human infants. Recent studies (4) indicate, however, that the extent of passive absorption of low molecular weight solutes changes rapidly after birth. Infants offered maternal milk exhibit a marked decline in intestinal permeability during the first 6 days after birth, whereas those offered cow's milk formulae show no such decline. Changes in trace-metal absorption during this period have yet to be investigated with sufficiently sensitive techniques. In studies with older infants (5), however, absorption of copper and of iron at 1 month of age differed greatly between individuals; absorption of iron tended to decrease during the first 3 months while that of copper, manganese and zinc remained relatively constant. Investigations on younger infants are desirable in view of evidence from other species that, at this stage of early development, uptake of a number of essential or toxic trace elements can be 10–40 times greater than after "gut closure" (for review, see reference 3).

In contrast, the efficiency of intestinal uptake of a number of trace elements declines in the elderly, even in those in normal health (6). Turnlund et al. (7) and King et al. (8) have reported on a comprehensive study in which men aged between 65 and 74 years absorbed 17% of dietary zinc in contrast to the 33% absorbed by younger male subjects (22–30 years) when the diet provided 15 mg of zinc/day. From diets with a more typical content of zinc (10 mg/day), an elderly person may absorb as little as 1.5 mg/day (8). Although other reports suggest that a negative copper balance may be common in the elderly (6), it is not yet clear whether this results from a lower efficiency of copper absorption. Present indications are that the physiological significance of the phenomenon is less than it is for zinc. The efficiency of absorption of orally administered chromium was not significantly different for elderly subjects (9, 10), nor was that of selenium.

3.1.2 Influence of trace-element intake and status

The inverse relationship between pre-existing trace-element status and the efficiency of absorption of specific elements was first demonstrated comprehensively in studies of iron utilization. The implications of this relationship for the interpretation and application of data on the potential biological availability of iron sources are well recognized (11). Thus, the definition of iron stores or direct monitoring of physiological responses to a standard source of iron is now regarded as an essential feature of most investigations of iron bioavailability from foods. Until recently, the need to consider such relationships was less widely recognized for other essential trace elements. This situation is now changing.

The efficiency of zinc absorption is related inversely to both the current intake of zinc and the existing zinc status (12, 13; see also Figs. 5.1 and 5.2 on pp. 89 and 90). It was shown by the use of vascularly perfused intestinal preparations that the efficiency of zinc absorption and transfer to the vascular system in rats previously depleted of zinc was approximately twice that of normal rats over a wide range of intakes. Uptake and retention of orally administered zinc can range between 95% and 5% of intake depending on pre-existing zinc status. That similar relationships govern zinc uptake by humans is becoming clear. Jackson (14), studying stable isotope zinc metabolism in a subject previously given 7, 15 and 30 mg of zinc/day, found that zinc absorption was 47, 32 and 21% respectively. Thus a four-fold higher zinc intake resulted in only a doubling of the absolute amount of zinc absorbed. Corresponding evidence of inverse relationships between zinc status or supply and zinc absorption has been provided from other work (*8, 15, 16*) and is taken into account in the estimates of zinc requirements given later in Chapter 5.

Copper absorption is also inversely related to copper intake or status (*17*), and this may account for much of the intraexperimental variability in studies of copper absorption; values ranging from 25% to 60% efficiency of absorption of administered copper have been common (for review, see reference *18*). Another report (*17*) summarizes data from subjects with copper intakes ranging from 1.4 mg/day to 3.3 mg/day for which the respective absorptive efficiencies were between 41% and 26%, and absolute absorption of copper ranged from 0.59 to 0.84 mg/day. However, quantitative data on such relationships are insufficient, as yet, for it to be possible to allow for their effect when estimating copper requirements.

Chromium absorptive efficiency is also inversely related to previous dietary intake of chromium. It was reported (*9*) that 0.5% of a dose of 40 μg of chromium was absorbed by subjects receiving 40 μg/day as compared with 2% when intake was 10 μg of chromium/day. Above intakes of chromium of 40 μg/day, efficiency of absorption remained virtually constant at 0.4%, homoeostasis being achieved by increased urinary output. Although the efficiency of selenium absorption is influenced by the chemical species of the element ingested, there is no convincing evidence that existing status influences absorption (for review, see reference *19*). Absorption of iodine also appears to be independent of existing status.

The data from which it can be inferred that the efficiency of trace-element utilization is inversely related to status or dose are rarely adequate to determine whether this fluctuating relationship predominantly reflects an adaptive change in the net activity of element absorption or a compensatory change in endogenous losses. However, it is already evident that, as for iron, the absorption of copper, zinc and possibly of chromium is influenced by pre-existing status. This has the following implications:

- The increases in absorptive efficiency evident in deficient subjects or induced if element intake is low represent a compensatory mechanism. This cannot be ignored when endeavouring to establish basal dietary requirements by "factorial" techniques rather than by monitoring relationships between physiological performance and element intake. If, for example, studies on *normal* subjects indicate that the bioavailability of zinc from a diet is 20%, this result does not reveal that such subjects could well respond to a reduced supply of potentially absorbable zinc by increasing their efficiency of zinc absorption to 30% or more. Figures for basal dietary requirements derived by factorial techniques which ignore this compensatory capacity when supply declines have frequently been overestimates.

- Ideally, experimental estimates of bioavailability should be derived from data obtained with subjects of defined trace-element status. Such status could be defined on the basis of accepted indices of element storage, characterized from measurements of endogenous loss where this is known to relate to status, or based on biochemical criteria of functional normality. Only if such indices of status are provided is it feasible to assess the relevance of the bioavailability data obtained to situations where trace-element supply is declining to levels barely adequate to meet *basal* or *normative* requirements.

Certain variables governing bioavailability act solely through the physicochemical reactions occurring during food processing or digestion to reduce the intraluminal concentration of trace-element-bearing species potentially available for absorption. Prediction equations describing their effects on the requirements of some non-human species for copper and zinc have been developed, but, as indicated later, further work is needed to establish their value

Figure 3.1. Zinc absorption by human adults from aqueous solutions of zinc (●) or from single meals from which zinc is moderately available (▲) (category B, Table 5.5)

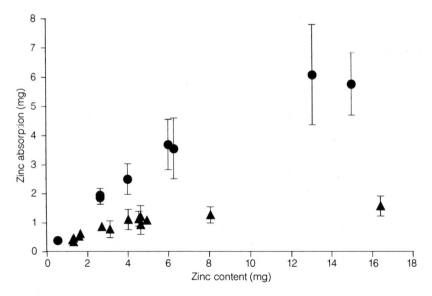

WHO 94657

Bars represent SDs (B. Sandström, personal communication, 1992).

in predicting trace-element bioavailability from human diets. Despite this lack of quantitative information, it is reasonable to anticipate that such processes account for the frequently much greater efficiency with which some elements are absorbed from liquid supplements or feeds than from solid diets—a phenomenon clearly illustrated for zinc in Fig. 3.1 (B. Sandström, personal communication 1992).

Evidence of an atypically high absorptive efficiency can frequently be regarded as a diagnostically valuable index of impending deficiency in situations where functional criteria of deficiency are not available or clinical signs lack diagnostic specificity. The fact that such responses indicate an adaptation initiated by the physiological "sensing" of imminent deficienc could well be accorded greater emphasis in the future search for diagnostic criteria of deficiency. Such adaptation is not ubiquitous, however. Thus there are no indications that selenium deficiency increases the fractional efficiency of selenium utilization from the gut (20), and the absorption of soluble iodides and molybdates appears not to be influenced by the pre-existing tissue status of these elements.

3.2 Metabolic and functional aspects of bioavailability

3.2.1 Multielement interactions involving iron

Iron is involved in an extensive series of interactions which modify the utilization or metabolism of both essential and potentially toxic trace elements. Evidence of virtually all such iron-related interactions was initially confined to data from experiments involving laboratory rodents but, with time, many have been found to have human relevance.

Evidence that the severity of copper-deficiency anaemia in rats could be ameliorated by increases in iron intake (for review, see reference 21) was the first indication of a metabolic interaction between these two elements. Later work showed that severe copper-deficiency anaemia in infants was partially responsive to iron therapy. The striking claim that supplementary iron rectifies growth failure in copper-deficient rats (22) has yet to be verified for humans.

Nutritional deficiency of copper is usually accompanied by a marked decline in plasma caeruloplasmin activity and an associated inhibition of iron release from the liver and other tissues. These changes reflect the suggested role of caeruloplasmin as a ferroxidase (23). Tissue deposition of ferritin, and later of haemosiderin, accompanying a decline in plasma iron is a well established feature of severe copper deficiency in most species. Changes in plasma iron have been noted in copper-deficient infants, but the extent to which ferritin mobilization is influenced in infants is not known.

Although concurrent deficiencies of iron and copper are known to occur in some socially deprived communities whose infants are offered unfortified cow's milk and other low-copper foods, evidence of mutually interactive responses to iron and copper supplements has not been sought.

Defects in catecholamine metabolism typified by reduced noradrenaline concentrations exist in a range of tissues in copper-deficient subjects. They arise from the interruption of both copper-dependent and iron-dependent steps in synthetic pathways involved in noradrenaline synthesis from tyrosine via dopa. This mutual involvement could well account for the confusing inconsistency of the evidence of deranged catecholamine metabolism induced by copper deficiency in humans and other species. Responses to copper depletion may well be influenced by differences in the iron status of individuals. It should also be noted that indications of anomalous metabolism of enkephalins and endorphins in copper-deficient human subjects (24) are similar to those reported to accompany the early stages of iron deficiency.

3.2.2 Tissue anabolism/catabolism and utilization of tissue zinc

The systemic availability of tissue zinc is profoundly influenced by the balance of anabolic and catabolic processes governing the turnover of soft tissues and the skeleton. The important influence of this relationship on pathological responses to a low zinc status in infants and during pregnancy has been reviewed by Golden et al. (25, 26). Their demonstration that clinical manifestations of zinc deficiency can be "switched" on or off by dietary manipulations which stimulate or retard growth has been fully confirmed and must be taken into account whenever estimates of zinc intake and basal requirements are used in a diagnostic context. The implication that the mobilization of tissue stores of zinc can be governed by nutritional and other factors influencing tissue turnover has important implications for the definition of normative requirements for zinc. The adequacy of protein and energy intakes may well be the primary determinant of such release and of the unsatisfied demands of growing tissues for zinc that provoke the pathological signs of zinc deficiency. The important influence of catch-up growth on zinc requirements during rehabilitation is considered in Chapter 5. Studies on non-human species also suggest that skeletal zinc can be redistributed and utilized if skeletal resorption is induced by a low calcium intake. The influence of calcium status on the systemic metabolism of zinc in humans has not been investigated.

3.2.3 Selenium status and iodine utilization

Early interest in the biochemical role of selenium centred exclusively on its action as a constituent of the "antioxidant" enzyme, glutathione peroxidase.

However, recent studies show that iodine and selenium metabolism are interrelated in the conversion of thyroxine to 3,5,3′-triiodothyronine (T$_3$) by a selenium-containing deiodinase enzyme. The effects of iodine deficiency in rats on thyroid weight, thyroid-stimulating hormone and T$_3$ in plasma are strongly exacerbated if dietary selenium is also low (27, 28). While the pathological implications of this interaction in humans have yet to be resolved, it is clear from a recent study in Zaire that human responses to iodine deficiency are also accentuated if selenium status is low (29).

3.2.4 Other functional interactions

There are clear indications from studies with rats and chicks that the development of copper deficiency adversely affects the utilization of selenium. Although copper deficiency has little or no effect on tissue selenium concentrations, its use for the synthesis of the selenoenzyme glutathione peroxidase is impaired. The mechanisms of this copper-dependent interrelationship are not known, nor is it known whether the defect arises in copper-deficient humans.

3.3 Interactions limiting element mobility

3.3.1 Interactions involving dietary phytate and other inositol phosphates

Evidence that staple dietary constituents such as cereal grains and pulses rich in phytate (inositol hexaphosphate) are potentially antagonistic to the utilization of zinc and iron first emerged 20–30 years ago (30, 31). Since then, experimental work with a variety of species offered relatively simple, chemically defined diets to which soluble phytate had been added has often suggested that antagonistic potency should be predictable from a knowledge of dietary phytate content. However, progress towards this objective has been delayed by oversimplistic views as to the mechanism of action of phytate as an iron and zinc antagonist. For example, it is evident that the antagonism is not attributable merely to the formation of iron or zinc phytate, since the metals of either phytate complex can be used physiologically when they are given as dietary supplements. In contrast, *dietary* interactions involving phytate can inhibit utilization of either element and suggest that more complex mechanisms are involved (32, 33).

In many recent studies, attempts have been made to define the action of variables that modify the potency of phytate as a trace-element antagonist in humans. From evidence that phytate/zinc (molar) ratios in excess of 15 depressed the growth rate of rats, it has been suggested that similar quantitative relationships might apply to humans. Initially accepted, this proposal has been modified in the face of evidence that the zinc of zinc phytate is readily available (*34, 35*) and that dietary calcium is an important potentiator of the phytate antagonism, apparently because of the formation of insoluble calcium-zinc phytates during digestion. Prediction of zinc availability on the basis of the estimation of the phytate/zinc ratio is unquestionably feasible for non-ruminant farm animals and laboratory animals maintained on relatively high-calcium ($> 0.5\%$) diets. Its predictive value for human subjects with typically lower intakes of calcium has yet to be established.

To take account of this additional factor, the validity of predictions of the inhibitory potency of phytate based on the estimation of the ratio Ca × phytate/Zn (mmol/1000 kcal) is being investigated retrospectively from data derived from human studies in which phytate-containing diets either reduced zinc absorption or produced a negative zinc balance (*36–40*). From this it appears probable that diets with a Ca × phytate/Zn ratio greater than about 150 mmol/1000 kcal might be expected to reduce zinc utilization.

Constructive reviews of the merits and limitations of attempts to predict zinc availability from phytate/zinc ratios or Ca × phytate/Zn ratios have suggested (*35, 41*) that zinc absorption might be reduced by 25% if the Ca × phytate/Zn ratios exceed 140 mmol/1000 kcal for soya bread meals, 110 for cereal meals and 350 for soya-based meat substitute meals. In addition, Morris & Ellis (*35*) found negative zinc balances in adult men given diets for which the Ca × phytate/Zn ratios were 120 or 175 mmol/1000 kcal.

While the Ca × phytate/Zn ratio may have had reasonable predictive value for the relatively simple diets used in animal studies, its value for predicting available zinc from more complex human diets has yet to be established.

Sandström, Kivisto & Cederblad (*42*), suggest that, except for situations where calcium supplements are taken (or probably when geophagia is practised with calcareous soils—see section 23.4) and phytate-rich diets are consumed, there is little practical advantage in considering the modifying influence of calcium on the phytate/zinc relationship. For cereal-based meals offered with 200 g of milk, a particularly close inverse relationship was consistently observed between phytic acid intake (x; μmol) and zinc absorption (y; %), as follows:

$$y = 38 - 8.5 \ln x,$$

with a significant decline in zinc absorption when phytate/zinc ratios exceeded 5 (*42*). For soya-protein-containing meals, zinc absorption could be related to the phytate/zinc molar ratio when animal protein content was low and calcium content high. Such relationships did not hold for meals with a high protein content. Other constituents of the diet also influence the predictive value of such ratios. Thus interactions involving milk or other protein sources may be responsible for conflicting views on the advantages of including calcium in prediction equations. It has been emphasized (43) that both the nature and the content of dietary protein modify the influence of high dietary phytate levels on the content of absorbable zinc. A fall in the fractional absorbability of zinc from a legume-based diet when milk was added was tentatively attributed to the increase in dietary calcium that resulted. However, the decrease in zinc availability was largely offset by the substantial contribution of milk to the total dietary zinc content. Although relatively small quantities of other animal proteins significantly improved zinc utilization from such a phytate-rich diet, a recent re-examination of the data from these studies suggests that a residual influence of calcium in potentiating the inhibitory effect of phytate on zinc absorption may still remain. Further details of such relationships are needed if any adverse affects on zinc supply arising from calcium fortification of diets or from the practice of geophagia in some communities are to be prevented.

In practice, there is little to choose between the zinc/phytate ratio and the $Ca \times phytate/Zn$ ratio as predictive indices (42, 43). Both suffer from the problem that additional unidentified variables influence the relationships between the absolute value of the ratio and the absorbability of dietary zinc. Either might be suitable for use in comparing the zinc availability of diets differing markedly in the nature of their protein source, and they could also be useful for predicting the effect of modifications to, say, a cereal-based diet, a soya-protein-based diet or other legume-protein-based diets. Provisionally, however, it appears reasonable to suggest that, if the phytate/zinc molar ratio of a diet is greater than 15 or the $Ca \times phytate/Zn$ ratio is greater than 150 mmol/1000 kcal, the content of available zinc in the diet is then likely to be low.

There are indications that this criterion of zinc availability may be more generally applicable to milk-substitute diets for infants than to the more complex conventional diets of adults.

Evidence that only the hexa- and pentaphosphorylated forms of "phytate" inhibit zinc utilization (44, 45, 46) suggests the possibility that the erroneous inclusion of less highly phosphorylated derivatives in previous analyses for "phytate" has led to overemphasis of the significance of this potential antagonist to zinc nutrition in humans. Exogenous phytases, either activated during digestion or denatured during food processing, certainly modify the extent to which "phytate" from foods influences both iron and zinc utilization (37). The practice in many rural communities of fermenting staple vegetable crops before they are consumed undoubtedly promotes extensive enzymic degradation of intrinsic phytate and affords significant protection against the development of zinc deficiency in such groups (40).

Extrusion cooking of brans, by destroying food phytases, decreases the intestinal degradation of inositol hexa- and pentaphosphates to their tetra- and lower derivatives (*47*). Studies on rats (*46*) and humans (*45*) indicate that progressive dephosphorylation of phytate decreases its inhibitory potency as a zinc antagonist. Both for iron and for zinc there is now evidence that the tetra- or less phosphorylated analogues (which, when determined by non-discriminatory analyses, are merely reported as "phytate") have little influence on iron or zinc availability.

It is likely that the practical nutritional significance of processing techniques which, by denaturing intrinsic phytase activity, virtually protect the hexa- and pentaphosphoinositols responsible for zinc binding can also be modified by other dietary constituents. Thus the failure in one study (*48*) to reproduce the inhibitory effect of extrusion cooking on zinc utilization (*49, 50*) probably reflects the fact that liquid milk was offered with the extruded cereal sources of phytate. Both the inhibitory effects of milk (*51*) and those of the products of protein digestion (*33*) on the experimental laboratory precipitability of zinc phytate and zinc calcium phytate are likely to be relevant to conditions during digestion. Such interactions may well modify the nutritional significance of the phytate/zinc or Ca × phytate/Zn ratios.

3.3.2 Influence of phytate/protein interactions on zinc availability

Processing conditions during the isolation of phytate-rich foods such as soya protein can have a marked influence on the potency of phytate as a zinc inhibitor (*52*). The formation of protein/phytate/mineral complexes during processing at a neutral pH favours the persistence of stable zinc complexes during subsequent digestion. In contrast, acid-precipitated soya protein isolates retain zinc in a highly available form. The potential reactivity of the phytate-containing product must also influence the availability of zinc added to fortify the diet. Thus it has been claimed (*53*) that the availability to rats of intrinsic zinc from diets based on soya protein isolates is much less than that of extrinsic zinc. Even so, the availability of intrinsic zinc from phytate-containing foods is influenced by processing. Thus, in addition to pH-dependent effects (*52*), exclusion of water from peptide- or protein-associated phytate/mineral complexes could yield derivatives poorly digestible in the gastrointestinal tract, from which zinc is relatively unavailable (*54*). Thus the fact that, in rats, zinc retention from defatted soya flour and from acid-precipitated and neutral soya protein concentrates was 75%, 18% and 52%, respectively, reflects the protein digestibility of these products.

3.3.3 Interactions of phytate with other metals

The calcium-phytate complex has a strong affinity for both lead and cadmium (*33*). Studies of the biological implications of this interaction (*55*) demonstrate that, if dietary calcium exceeds 0.6%, phytate inhibits lead retention by rats by up to 80%. Preliminary studies suggest that diets high in both phytate and calcium also restrict lead retention by humans (55).

Inhibition of iron absorption by phytate is related to the extent of metal saturation of the iron-phytate complexes present in food or digesta. Iron from monoferric phytate is readily utilized (56). However, soluble phytate (as little as 2 mg per meal) significantly inhibited iron absorption (57) and, although 25 mg of phytate reduced iron absorption by 70%, this effect was entirely eliminated by concurrent administration of 100 mg of ascorbic acid. The influence of dietary calcium on the potency of phytate as an iron antagonist does not appear to have been studied.

Although dietary phytate restricts the absorption of both copper and manganese by rats, there is no evidence that such effects are significant in human nutrition (58).

3.3.4 Iron-related antagonistic interactions

Studies on many species indicate that high intakes of iron can interfere with the utilization of other essential trace elements. However, the results of such studies are frequently in disagreement with one another with respect to both the magnitude of the "iron effect", if any, and its practical relevance for human nutrition (59–64).

Interactions induced by high intakes of iron appear to be potentiated by increasing intakes of ascorbate. However, one human study suggests that this may not apply if the diet is high in phytate (57). The adverse effects of zinc on iron absorption induced by an iron:zinc ratio of 2:1 are aggravated by decreases in dietary ascorbate when the dietary phytate content is high. Such results suggest that these antagonisms may depend not on total iron but on the proportion of iron present in oxidized or reduced forms. Other evidence that the form of iron is important is the finding that haem iron in the diet inhibits neither the absorption nor the systemic utilization of zinc by humans (62, 63). Iron-dependent interactions and antagonisms are much more clearly evident when iron and other elements (e.g. copper or zinc) are administered in solution or in discrete doses rather than as supplements dispersed in solid diets (65). Under such circumstances, the existing iron status of the subject appears to have far less influence on the antagonistic potency of iron.

In infants given ascorbate-fortified formula milk for up to 20 weeks after birth, supplements of iron providing > 6 mg/day restricted the utilization of copper for the synthesis of the copper-dependent enzyme superoxide dismutase in erythrocytes (66).

A mild iron deficiency trebled the absorption of cadmium in subjects with normal blood haemoglobin but low serum ferritin. Evidence of the effects of mild iron deficiency on the absorption of lead by human subjects is conflicting. One study showed that reducing iron status increased the absorption of carrier-free lead-203 from 20% to 47% (*67*). Variables other than the iron/lead ratio must influence this interaction (*68*). For example, it is strongly suspected that absorption of both iron and lead is inversely related to dietary phytate and calcium (*33, 55*). From none of the reports referred to above is it possible to define the full influence of phytic acid and calcium on the iron/lead relationship.

Low dietary iron also enhances the absorption and retention of cadmium, cobalt, manganese and zinc by experimental animals (*69*). Although much less is known about such interactions in humans, it is important to bear in mind the possibility that a low iron status may well increase sensitivity to potentially toxic concentrations of such metals.

Also relevant is the finding that the increased absorption of lead when a low iron status is achieved by dietary depletion is not reproducible if iron depletion is an experimental consequence of blood loss (e.g. from phlebotomy) (*70*). The influence of differences in iron status resulting from intestinal blood loss (e.g. from parasitism) on the efficiencies of absorption of cadmium and lead has not been investigated.

Studies on both rats and humans suggest that the magnitude of the antagonistic relationship between iron and zinc is substantially greater if a critical minimum level of these two elements in the ingesta is exceeded (*48, 71*). In adult humans, it appears that iron restricts zinc utilization most effectively if the total ionic load of iron plus zinc in the ingesta exceeds 25 mg (*72*).

The depressive effects of high copper levels on iron utilization have been well established from studies on experimental animals; their human significance is questionable (*62*), and the effects of high zinc levels are probably more important. Thus, zinc at a dose of 50 mg/day depressed copper utilization by women as judged by a decline in their erythrocyte superoxide dismutase and interfered with their metabolism of iron, as shown by depressed serum ferritin, blood haemoglobin and haematocrit. Concurrent administration of 50 mg of iron with the zinc eliminated all effects on serum ferritin. Doses as small as 25 mg of zinc/day are sufficient to depress the iron status of menstruating women (*73*) and the copper status of men (*74*). Conversely iron therapy depresses the zinc status of pregnant women (*61*).

Nutritionally realistic variations in dietary concentrations of cadmium, iron, manganese and molybdenum do not significantly affect the utilization of selenium by rats (*75*).

3.3.5 Other factors influencing element mobility and utilization

Interactions influencing the intraluminal release and mucosal uptake of elements such as copper, iron and zinc by infants (*76, 77*) appear to be responsible for significant differences in the bioavailability of these elements from maternal milk, cow's milk and milk- and soya-based formulae. Controversies as to the nature of the factors resulting in the bioavailability of zinc being lower in cow's milk than in human milk have been reviewed elsewhere (*78*). It has been suggested that homologous milk lactoferrin may act as a ligand facilitating the absorption of iron (*78*) and zinc (*79*). Both milk copper, bound variously to albumin, casein, citrate and an unidentified lipid-associated constituent, and the copper of bovine casein-based formulae are more readily utilized by infants than copper from soya-based formulae (*5*).

There are indications that colloidal calcium phosphates within the bovine casein micelle may sequester a fraction of milk zinc in a form that is unavailable to young infants, and that removal of these colloids improves zinc bioavailability (*80*).

The physical occlusion of elements within the clotted milk proteins in the stomach, where they will be digested at different rates depending on their source (homologous or heterologous milks), is a further possible cause of differences in the bioavailability of some trace metals from infant formulae (*81, 82*). These differences, like the depressive effects of soya-derived phytate on iron and zinc utilization, are consistent and undesirable attributes of milk substitutes, the effects of which on the availability of copper, iron and zinc to infants need to be more precisely determined.

Differences between foods in the bioavailability of the selenium they contain are not yet explicable. The results of studies on human subjects agree with those from studies on rats in showing that wheat selenium is the most biologically active (*19, 20*). Selenium from meats is probably utilized more readily than that from fish and much more than that from fungi. However, it appears improbable that differences in selenium bioavailability have a significant influence on the distribution or severity of selenium-responsive disorders in humans.

3.3.6 Other extrinsic variables influencing bioavailability

Antagonists of the utilization of iodine for thyroid hormone synthesis have a dominant influence on the world distribution of goitre. According to Matovinovic (*83*), "... iodine deficiency in some areas is only the *permissive* factor ..." and "the natural goitrogens are probably the dominant cause of goitre in some localities where iodine intake is abundant." The association of low iodine with a high goitrogen intake is probably responsible for both widespread goitre and myxoedematous endemic cretinism in some developing countries.

Broadly, two types of goitrogenic activity can be distinguished, the effects of only one of which can be ameliorated by increasing iodine intake. Thus, the degradation of the glucosinolate conjugates of cruciferous vegetables, such as cabbage, rape and mustards, yields a variety of alkyl isothiocyanates and vinylthiooxazalidones which inhibit iodination and the condensation of thyroid-hormone precursors. Their action cannot be eliminated by dietary fortification with iodine.

In contrast, the goitrogenic activity of endogenous or exogenous thiocyanates arises from the competitive inhibition of iodine trapping and from the acceleration of tissue iodine depletion. The physiological effects of the thiocyanates, which include reduced transplacental and mammary transfer of iodine, are ameliorated by increasing iodine intake. The thiocyanates implicated in iodine-deficiency diseases are derived, typically, from the degradation during processing of vegetable foods rich in cyanogenic glucosides such as the linamarin of cassava. The action of the intrinsic enzyme linamarinase yields cyanide, traces of which remaining after the pulverized food has been washed are "detoxified" to thiocyanate by the enzyme thiosulfate sulfurtransferase (rhodanese) of liver and kidney.

The intervention of selenium in the functional metabolism of iodine (84) during the synthesis of T_3 is considered in sections 4.5 and 6.2.1. It is probable that, in addition to the goitrogens, selenium deficiency may modify both the geographical distribution and the pathological manifestations of iodine-deficiency diseases. Although at present it is not possible to define quantitatively the etiological relationships between iodine and its antagonists, it is imperative that efforts should be made to define more clearly those geochemical and social factors influencing both the intake of iodine and the factors which modify its physiological utilization.

Although elevated intakes of ascorbate have been shown to depress copper utilization by experimental animals, its effects on human utilization of copper have yet to be elucidated (17, 85, 86). High calcium and phosphorus intakes (2 g of calcium or 2 g of phosphorus/day) increase the faecal output of copper by up to 15% (87). The possibility that elevated intakes of molybdenum may restrict copper utilization (88) is discussed in Chapter 7.

3.4 Conclusions and nutritional implications

Trace-element bioavailability is influenced by a complex matrix of interacting variables, some physiological, some reflecting the intrinsic composition of foods from which the diet is composed. While it would be highly desirable to be able to predict quantitatively the effects of such variables on availability, the necessary investigations have only recently been started. However, it must also be appreciated that the analytical task of defining the pattern of trace-element antagonists and promoters in typical diets will be substantial. Except under special circumstances, it is unreasonable to expect that such data can be provided as a matter of routine for the wide variety of diets in common use. It is for this reason that, in this chapter, the diverse nature and the mechanisms of action of the factors governing element utilization have been emphasized.

Our inability in most instances to describe such relationships quantitatively implies that the information provided must be used subjectively. Its greatest relevance will be in situations where it is suspected that anomalies in dietary composition or ill-defined physiological or environmental factors have initiated trace-element-related pathological changes, even though trace-element intake appears to be within the limits proposed in subsequent chapters. *Appreciation of the modifying action of factors likely to influence availability should serve to warn the reader against the inflexible application of tabulated data on trace-element requirements when endeavouring to interpret dietary analyses in a diagnostic context.* However, considerations of trace-element supply, probable availability and requirement may well narrow the field of enquiry and suggest appropriate additional approaches to the detection of trace-element deficiency or excess.

As already mentioned, the variables likely to influence trace-element bioavailability and utilization in human subjects are summarized in Table 3.1, which covers only those that are known or strongly suspected to be nutritionally relevant; many other factors have been identified in studies on experimental animals, but their practical relevance remains uncertain. Table 3.2 lists some of the antagonists restricting and synergists promoting the absorption, utilization or retention of trace elements in humans.

In what follows, a brief account is given of those aspects of trace-element bioavailability or metabolic interactions that should be taken into particular account when considering relationships between dietary trace-element data and estimates of the lower and upper tolerable intakes of individuals or population groups.

3.4.1 Copper

Although most reported instances of copper deficiency have been attributed specifically to an inadequate copper intake, it is likely that susceptibility to this deficiency may be aggravated by overenthusiastic and excessive chronic administration of iron or zinc supplements. Evidence of a decline in copper status or a decrease in copper absorption has been provided by both experimental studies

Table 3.2. Antagonists restricting and synergists promoting absorption, utilization or retention of trace elements in humans[a]

Element	Antagonists restricting absorption, utilization or retention	Synergists promoting absorption, utilization or retention
Zinc	Phytate with high calcium intake	Low calcium intake, animal proteins
	High iron intake	Homologous milk (infants only)
	Heterologous milks (infants only)	[Late pregnancy; lactation]
	[High zinc status; aging]	[Low zinc status]
Copper	High iron, high zinc intakes	High protein intake
	[High copper status]	[Late pregnancy; lactation?]
	High molybdenum with high sulfur intake?	[Low copper status]
Iodine	Elevated goitrogen intake	—
	[Low selenium status?]	—
Selenium	Elevated heavy-metal intake?	—
Chromium	Oxalates, high iron intake	[Low chromium status]
	[High chromium status]	
Manganese	High calcium intake (infant formulae)	—
	[High manganese status]	—
Cadmium	High calcium intake	Low iron intake, low calcium intake
Lead	Phylate with high calcium intake	Low iron, low calcium and phosphorus intakes

[a] Evidence from experimental animal studies considered probably relevant to humans is indicated by a question mark; physiological variables influencing efficiency of utilization are enclosed in square brackets.

and case histories of the effects of prolonged iron administration in both infants and adults.

3.4.2 Iodine

Although the inhibitory effects of vegetable goitrogens have been established beyond doubt, relationships between goitrogen dose, the potentiation or amelioration of goitrogen activity by food processing, and the influence of these variables on iodine requirement have not been adequately quantified. Their effects should be prevented by modest increases (+ 50%) in the provision of iodine if crops rich in goitrogens are staple dietary constituents.

Recent but unequivocal evidence suggests that the effective utilization of iodine depends on a selenium-containing enzyme and thus on an adequate selenium status. It is therefore possible that both the geographical distribution and the severity and pathological manifestations of iodine deficiency could be modified by concurrent regional anomalies in dietary iodine and selenium caused by soil and geochemical factors that limit the supply of both elements. Geochemical data suggest that such areas may not be uncommon.

3.4.3 Lead and cadmium

Diets low in calcium promote significant increases in the absorption and retention of both lead and cadmium. High-calcium, high-phytate diets appear to restrict lead uptake. There are clear indications that iron deficiency promotes cadmium retention and may thus decrease the tolerance of high environmental or dietary cadmium concentrations. Evidence from a variety of experiments on animals suggests that iron deficiency also promotes lead uptake and retention; the evidence for humans is conflicting, but in some studies substantial increases in lead uptake are said to have occurred when dietary iron and iron status were low.

3.4.4 Selenium

The etiology of the selenium-responsive cardiomyopathy of Keshan disease in China strongly suggests that selenium deficiency is not the sole pathogenic factor. Studies on many non-human animal species clearly indicate that close metabolic relationships exist between selenium and vitamin E, with both acting as antioxidants to restrict tissue damage from oxidative reactions. Deficiencies of both are involved in the etiology of cardiac and skeletal muscular dystrophy and in nutritional hepatic necrosis, and both are active therapeutically against such disorders. After long periods of uncertainty as to whether selenium deficiency is the only nutritional anomaly involved in Keshan disease, very recent evidence suggests that the vitamin E status of subjects at risk might also be lower than normal, judging from plasma vitamin E data. It remains to be determined whether, as with many selenium-responsive syndromes in other species, susceptibility to Keshan disease involves concurrent deficiencies of vitamin E and selenium even though, as with animal syndromes, selenium administration alone can be therapeutically effective.

3.4.5 Zinc

Sensitivity to phytate as an antagonist of zinc is likely to be significant only when diets are based predominantly on unrefined cereals or on pulses (or on their crude protein or fibre fractions) and when calcium intake is also high. Typical vegan diets, although phytate-rich, are usually low in calcium and thus low zinc availability is unlikely unless calcium supplements are given, lime is added as a "conditioner" during food processing or geophagia is practised with calcareous soils. In contrast, elevation of calcium intake by increasing consumption of milk appears not to be attended by potentiation of the inhibitory effect of phytate. Milk, and probably other animal sources of protein, appear to promote zinc release from its phytate complex and also provide intrinsic zinc in a highly available form (see Chapter 5).

Infants appear particularly sensitive to phytate if it is consumed as a constituent of vegetable protein isolates in infant formulae. In addition, infants, but not apparently adults, exhibit a lower capacity to utilize zinc from heterologous milk that from maternal milk. All the above variables should be considered when selecting appropriate "availability factors" to interpret the data for safe ranges of intake for zinc given in Chapter 5.

Chronic provision of iron supplements, especially in aqueous form, can promote a nutritionally significant decline in zinc status both in infants and in adults as a consequence of the induction of an iron/zinc imbalance.

Fermentation (e.g. leavening of bread) during the processing of foods will, by its enzymatic degradation of phytate, eliminate the risks that would otherwise be associated with excessive reliance upon high phytate regimens.

Factors such as those mentioned above which modify zinc availability should be taken into particular account in estimating the zinc requirement of infants and adolescents during phases of rapid growth, at which time sensitivity to a suboptimal zinc supply is at a maximum.

References

1. Mills CF. Dietary interactions involving the trace elements. *Annual review of nutrition*, 1985, 5: 173–193.
2. Bremner I. Mechanisms and nutritional importance of trace element interactions. In: Hurley LS et al., eds. *Trace elements in man and animals—TEMA 6*, New York, Plenum Press, 1988: 303–307.
3. Mills CF, Davies NT. Perinatal changes in the absorption of trace elements. In: Elliott K, Whelan J eds. *Development of mammalian absorptive processes*. Amsterdam, Excerpta Medica, 1979: 247–266.
4. Weaver LT et al. Milk feeding and changes in intestinal permeability and morphology in the newborn. *Journal of pediatric gastroenterology and nutrition*, 1987, 6: 351–358.

5. Miller C. *A study of the influences on mineral homeostasis in infants fed synthetic milk formulae* [PhD thesis]. Aberdeen University Medical School, 1987.

6. Buncker VW et al. Assessment of zinc and copper status of elderly people using metabolic balance studies and measurements of leucocyte concentrations. *American journal of clinical nutrition*, 1984, **40**: 1096–1102.

7. Turnland J et al. Stable isotope studies in young and elderly men. *Journal of nutrition*, 1986, **116**: 1239–1247.

8. King JC, Turnland JR. Human zinc requirements. In: Mills CF ed. *Zinc in human biology*. London, Springer, 1989: 335–350.

9. Anderson RH, Kozlowsky AS. Chromium intake, absorption and excretion of subjects consuming self-selected diets. *American journal of clinical nutrition*, 1985, **41**: 1177–1183.

10. Doisy RJ et al. Chromium metabolism in man and biochemical effects. In: Prasad AS, Oberleas D eds. *Trace elements in human health and disease*, Vol. 2. New York, Academic Press, 1976: 79–104.

11. Layrisse M et al. Food iron absorption; a comparison of vegetable and animal foods. *Blood*, 1969, **33**: 430–433.

12. Steel L, Cousins RJ. Kinetics of zinc absorption by luminally and vascularly perfused rate intestine, *American journal of physiology*, 1985, **248**: G46–53.

13. Coppen DE, Davies NT. Studies on the effects of dietary zinc dose on ^{65}Zn absorption *in vivo* and on the effects of Zn status on ^{65}Zn absorption and body loss in young rats. *British journal of nutrition*, 1987, **57**: 35–44.

14. Jackson MJ et al. Zinc homeostasis in man: studies using a new stable isotope-dilution technique. *British journal of nutrition*, 1984, **51**: 199–208.

15. Baer MT, King JC. Tissue zinc levels and zinc excretion during experimental zinc depletion of young men. *American journal of clinical nutrition*, 1984, **39**: 556–570.

16. Wada L, Turnlund JR, King JC. Zinc utilisation in young men fed adequate and low zinc intakes. *Journal of nutrition*, 1985, **115**: 1345–1354.

17. Turnland JR. Copper nutriture, bioavailability and the influence of dietary factors. *Journal of the American Dietetic Association*, 1988, **88**: 303–308.

18. Mason KE. A conspectus of research on copper metabolism and requirements of man. *Journal of nutrition*, 1979, **109**: 1979–2066.

19. Levander OA. Selenium. In: Mertz W, ed. *Trace elements in human and animal nutrition*, 5th ed., Vol 2. Orlando, Academic Press, 1986: 209–275.

20. Levander OA et al. Bioavailability of Se to Finnish men as assessed by platelet GSH-Px activity and other blood parameters. *American journal of clinical nutrition*, 1983, **37**: 887–897.

21. Hill CH. Interactions among trace elements. In: Prasad AS, ed. *Essential and toxic elements in human health and disease*. New York, Alan R. Liss, 1988: 491–500.

22. Weisenberg E, Halbreich A, Mager J. Biochemical lesions in copper deficient rats caused by secondary iron deficiency. *Biochemical journal*, 1980, **188**: 633–641.

23. Frieden E. Caeruloplasmin: a multifunctional metalloprotein of vertebrate plasma. In: Evered D, Lawrenson G, eds. *Biological roles of copper*. Amsterdam, Excerpta Medica, 1980: 93–124.

24. Bhathena SJ et al. Decreased plasma enkephalins in copper deficiency in man. *American journal of clinical nutrition*, 1986, **43**: 42–46.
25. Golden MHN. The diagnosis of zinc deficiency. In: Mills CF, ed. *Zinc in human biology*. London, Springer, 1989: 323–333.
26. Golden BE, Golden MHN. Plasma zinc, rate of weight gain and the energy cost of tissue deposition in children recovering from severe malnutrition on a cows' milk or soya protein based diet. *American journal of clinical nutrition*, 1981, **34**: 892–899.
27. Arthur JR, Beckett GJ. Selenium deficiency and thyroid hormone metabolism. In: Wendel A, ed. *Selenium in biology and medicine*. Heidelberg, Springer-Verlag, 1989: 90–95.
28. Arthur JR et al. The effects of selenium depletion and repletion on metabolism of thyroid hormones in the rat. *Journal of inorganic biochemistry*, 1989, **39**: 101–108.
29. Vanderpas J et al. Iodine and selenium deficiency associated with cretinism in Northern Zaire. *American journal of clinical nutrition*, 1990, **52**: 1087–1093.
30. McCance RA, Edgecombe CN, Widdowson EM. Phytic acid and iron absorption. *Lancet*, 1943, **ii**: 126–128.
31. Oberleas D, Muhrer ME, O'Dell BL. Dietary metal complexing agents and zinc availability in the rat. *Journal of nutrition*, 1966, **90**: 56–62.
32. Cheryan M. Phytic acid and interactions in food systems. *CRC critical reviews of food science and nutrition*, 1980, **13**: 297–335.
33. Wise A. Dietary factors determining the biological activity of phytate. *Nutrition abstracts & reviews, reviews of clinical nutrition*, 1983, **53**: 791–806.
34. Mills CF. Interactions involving inorganic nutrients. In: Taylor TG, Jenkins NK, eds. *Proceedings of the 13th International Congress on Nutrition*. London, John Libbey, 1985: 532–536.
35. Morris ER, Ellis R. Usefulness of the dietary phytic acid/zinc molar ratio as an index of zinc bioavailability to rats and humans. *Biological trace element research*, 1989, **19**: 107–117.
36. Reinhold JG et al. Effect of purified phytate and phytate-rich bread upon metabolism of zinc, calcium, phosphorus and nitrogen in man. *Lancet*, 1973, **i**: 283–288.
37. Sandberg AS, Carlsson NG, Svanberg V. *In vitro* studies of inositol tri-, tetra-, penta- and hexaphosphates as potential iron absorption inhibitors. In: Southgate D et al., eds. *Nutrient availability*. London, Royal Society of Chemistry, 1989: 158–160.
38. Cossak ZT, Prasad AA. Effect of protein source on the bioavailability of zinc in human subjects. *Nutrition research*, 1983, **3**: 23–32.
39. Lönnerdal B et al. The effects of individual components of soy-formula and cow's milk on zinc bioavailability. *American journal of clinical nutrition*, 1984, **40**: 1064–1074.
40. Navert B, Sandström B, Cederblad Å. Reduction of the phytate of bran by leavening in bread and its effects on zinc absorption in man. *British journal of nutrition*, 1985, **53**: 47–53.
41. Morris ER, Ellis R. Effect of dietary phytate/zinc molar ratio on growth and bone zinc response of rats fed semi purified diets. *Journal of nutrition*, 1980, **110**: 1037–1045.

42. Sandström B, Kivistö B, Cederblad Å. Absorption of zinc from soy protein meals in humans. *Journal of nutrition*, 1987, **117**: 321–327.
43. Sandström B et al. Effect of protein level and protein source on zinc absorption in humans. *Journal of nutrition*, 1989, **119**: 48–53.
44. Sandström B. Dietary pattern and zinc supply. In: Mills CF, ed. *Zinc in human biology*, London, Springer, 1989: 351–363.
45. Sandström B, Sandberg AS. The effects of penta- and tetra-inositol phosphates on zinc absorption in humans. *FASEB journal*, 1989, **3**: 3090.
46. Lonnerdal B et al. Inhibitory effects of phytic acid and other inositol phosphates on zinc and calcium absorption in suckling rats. *Journal of nutrition*, 1989, **119**: 211–214.
47. Phytase and phytate degradation in humans. *Nutrition reviews*, 1989, **47**: 155–157.
48. Fairweather-Tait SJ et al. Iron and zinc absorption in human subjects from a mixed meal of extruded and non-extruded wheat bran and flour. *American journal of clinical nutrition*, 1989, **49**: 151–155.
49. Kivistö B et al. Extrusion cooking of a high fibre cereal product. II Effects on apparent absorption of zinc, iron, calcium, magnesium and phosphorus in humans. *British journal of nutrition*, 1986, **55**: 255–260.
50. van Dokkum M, Westra A, Schippers FA. Physiological effects of fibre-rich types of bread. *British journal of nutrition*, 1982, **47**: 451–460.
51. Platt SR et al. Protective effect of milk on mineral precipitation by sodium phytate *Journal of food science*, 1987, **52**: 240–241.
52. Forbes RM, Erdman JW. Bioavailability of trace mineral elements. *Annual review of nutrition*, 1983, **3**: 213–231.
53. Hardie-Muncy DA, Rasmussen AL. Inter-relationships between zinc and protein level and source in weanling rats. *Journal of nutrition*, 1979, **109**: 321–329.
54. Erdman JW et al. Zinc and magnesium availability from acid precipitated and neutralised soybean protein products. *Journal of food science*, 1980, **45**: 1193–1199.
55. Rose HE, Quarterman J. The influence of dietary phytic acid and calcium on lead retention in rats. In: Mills CF, Bremner I, Chesters JK, eds. *Trace elements in man and animals—TEMA 5*. Farnham Royal, CAB International, 1985: 524–525.
56. Simpson KM, Morris ER, Cook JD. The inhibitory effect of bran on iron absorption in man. *American journal of clinical nutrition*, 1981, **24**: 1469–1478.
57. Hallberg L, Brune M, Rossander L. Iron absorption in man: ascorbic acid and dose dependent inhibition by phytate. *American journal of clinical nutrition*, 1989, **49**: 140–144.
58. Turnlund JR, Swanson CA, King J. Copper absorption and retention in pregnant women fed diets based on animal and plant proteins. *Journal of nutrition*, 1983, **113**: 2346–2352.
59. Yip R et al. Does iron supplementation compromise zinc nutrition in healthy infants. *American journal of clinical nutrition*, 1985, **42**: 683–687.
60. Hambidge KM et al. Acute effects of iron therapy on zinc status during pregnancy. *Obstetrics and gynaecology*, 1987, **70**: 593–596.
61. Flanagan PR. Trace metal interactions involving the intestinal absorption mech-

anisms of iron and zinc. In: Dintzis FR, Laszlo JA, eds. *Mineral absorption in the monogastric gastrointestinal tract.* New York, Plenum Press, 1989.

62. Solomons NW, Jacob RA. Studies on the bioavailability of zinc in humans: effects of heme and non heme iron on the absorption of zinc. *Journal of clinical nutrition,* 1981, **34**: 475–482.

63. Solomons NW et al. Studies of the bioavailability of zinc to humans: mechanisms of the intestinal interaction of non heme iron and zinc. *Journal of nutrition* 1983, **113**: 337–349.

64. Flanagan PR, Valberg LS. The intestinal interaction of zinc and iron in humans: does it occur with food. In: Prasad AS, ed. *Essential and toxic trace elements in human health and disease.* New York, Alan R. Liss, 1988: 501–507.

65. Sandström B. Effect of inorganic iron on the absorption of zinc from a test solution and a composite meal. In: Mills CF, Bremner I, Chesters JK, eds. *Trace elements in man and animals—TEMA 5.* Farnham Royal, CAB International, 1985: 414–416.

66. Barclay SM et al. Reduced erythrocyte superoxide dismutase activity in low birth weight infants given iron supplements. *Pediatric research,* 1991, **29**: 297–301.

67. Watson WS, Hume R, Moore MR. Oral absorption of lead and iron. *Lancet,* 1980, **ii**: 236–237.

68. Flanagan PR, Chamberlain MJ, Valberg LS. The relationship between iron and lead absorption in humans. *American journal of clinical nutrition,* 1982, **36**: 823–829.

69. Kostial K et al. Effect of iron additive to milk on cadmium, mercury and manganese absorption in rats. *Environmental research,* 1980, **22**: 40–45.

70. Flanagan PR, Haist J, Valberg LS. Comparative effects of iron deficiency induced by bleeding and a low iron diet on the intestinal absorptive interactions of iron, cobalt, manganese, zinc, lead and cadmium. *Journal of nutrition,* 1980, **110**: 1754–1763.

71. Solomons NW. Competitive interaction of iron and zinc in the diet: consequences for human nutrition. *Journal of nutrition,* 1986, **116**: 927–935.

72. Solomons NW. The iron:zinc interaction: does it exist? An affirmative view. In: Prasad AS, ed. *Essential and toxic elements in health and disease.* New York, Alan R. Liss, 1988: 509–518.

73. Yadrick MK, Kenney MA, Wintefeldt EA. Iron, copper and zinc status: response to supplementation with zinc or zinc and iron in adult females. *American journal of clinical nutrition,* 1989, **49**: 145–150.

74. Fischer PWF, Girouse A, L'Abbé MR. Effect of zinc supplementation on copper status in adult man. *American journal of clinical nutrition,* 1984, **40**: 743–746.

75. Al-Rahim AG, Arthur JR, Mills CF. Effects of dietary copper, cadmium, iron, molybdenum and manganese on selenium utilisation by the rat. *Journal of nutrition,* 1986, **116**: 403–411.

76. Haschke F et al. Effect of iron fortification of infant formula on trace mineral absorption. *Journal of pediatric gastroenterology and nutrition,* 1986, **5**: 768–773.

77. Lonnerdal B, Bell JG, Keen CL. Copper absorption from human milk, cow's milk and infant formula using a suckling rat model. *American journal of clinical nutrition,* 1985, **42**: 836–844.

78. Lonnerdal B. Trace element nutrition in infants. *Annual reviews of nutrition*, 1989, 9: 109–125.

79. Blakeborough P, Salter DN. Zinc binding by lactoferrin and human milk. In: Mills CF, Bremner I, Chesters JK, eds. *Trace elements in man and animals—TEMA 5*. Farnham Royal, CAB International, 1985: 420–422.

80. Kiely J et al. Improved zinc bioavailability from colloidal calcium phosphate-free cows' milk. In: Hurley LS et al., eds. *Trace elements in man and animals—TEMA 6*. New York, Plenum Press, 1988: 499–500.

81. Lönnerdal B, Glazier C. Distribution of zinc in human milk and cow's milk after *in vitro* proteolysis. In: Hurley LS eds. *Trace elements in man and animals—TEMA 6*. New York, Plenum Press, 1988: 505–506.

82. Blakeborough P, Gurr MI, Salter DN. Digestion of the zinc in human milk, cows' milk and a commercial babyfood: some implications for human infant nutrition. *British journal of nutrition*, 1986, 55: 209–217.

83. Matovinovic J. Endemic goitre. *Annual review of nutrition*, 1983, 3: 341–412.

84. Arthur JR, Nicol F, Beckett GJ. Hepatic iodothyronine 5-deiodinase: the role of selenium. *Biochemical journal*, 1990, 272: 537–540.

85. Finley EB, Cerklewski FI. Influence of ascorbic acid on copper status in young adult men. *American journal of clinical nutrition*, 1983, 17: 553–556.

86. Milne DB, Klevay LM, Hunt JR. Effects of ascorbic acid supplements and a diet marginal in copper on indices of copper nutrition in women. *Nutrition research*, 1988, 8: 865–873.

87. Snedeker SM, Smith SA, Greger JL. Effect of dietary calcium and phosphorus levels on the utilization of iron, copper, and zinc by adult males. *Journal of nutrition*, 1982, 112: 136–143.

88. Deosthale YG, Gopalan C. The effect of molybdenum levels in sorghum (*Sorghum vulgare* Pers.) on uric acid and copper excretion in man. *British journal of nutrition*, 1974, 31: 351–355.

A

Essential trace elements

4.
Iodine

4.1 Introduction

Iodine is an essential constituent of the thyroid hormones thyroxine [3,5,3'5'-tetraiodothyronine (T_4)] and 3,5,3'-triiodothyronine (T_3). The major role of iodine in nutrition arises from the important part played by the thyroid hormones in the growth and development of humans and animals.

The effects of iodine deficiency on growth and development are now denoted by the term iodine-deficiency disorders (IDD). These effects are seen at all stages of development, and particularly in the fetus, the neonate and the infant, i.e. in periods of rapid growth. Fetal survival and development are both sensitive to iodine deficiency. Brain development in the fetus and neonate is particularly affected, the effects forming a continuum and increasing in proportion to the severity of the iodine deficiency. They result from the influence of a low maternal thyroxine level on the fetus and are associated with levels of intake of iodine less than 25% of normal. Levels less than 50% of normal are associated with goitre. Data indicating that goitrous children have a poorer school performance than non-goitrous children have been reported (see below). All these effects are fully preventable if the iodine deficiency is corrected before pregnancy.

The term "goitre" has been used for many years to describe the effect of iodine deficiency. Goitre is indeed the visually obvious and familiar feature of iodine deficiency, but understanding of the other consequences of iodine deficiency has greatly expanded in the last 25 years so that it is not surprising that the wider designation IDD is now considered more appropriate (Table 4.1) (1).

The clinical effects of a grossly excessive iodine intake (20 mg/day) also include endemic goitre and hypothyroidism. At lower, but still excessive levels (up to 5 mg/day), no ill effects have been observed in the Japanese population (3). The iodine-deficient thyroid in older age groups is particularly sensitive to any increase in iodine intake because of the persistent autonomy of the thyroid. Iodine-induced hyperthyroidism has been described in many countries with a background of iodine deficiency. In contrast, the lack of previous exposure to

Table 4.1. The spectrum of iodine-deficiency disorders[a]

Stage of development	Disorder
Fetus	Abortions
	Stillbirths
	Congenital anomalies
	Increased perinatal mortality
	Increased infant mortality
	Neurological cretinism (mental deficiency, deaf mutism, spastic diplegia, squint)
	Myxoedematous cretinism (dwarfism, mental deficiency)
	Psychomotor defects
Neonate	Neonatal goitre
	Neonatal hypothyroidism
Child and adolescent	Goitre
	Juvenile hypothyroidism
	Impaired mental function
	Retarded physical development
Adult	Goitre with its complications
	Hypothyroidism
	Impaired mental function
	Iodine-induced hyperthyroidism[b]
All ages	Increased susceptibility to nuclear radiation

[a] Adapted, by permission, from Hetzel et al. (*2*).
[b] Regarded as an iodine-deficiency disorder (see page 66).

periods of iodine deficiency accounts for the absence of the condition in Japan and some other countries.

Iodine nutritional status can be assessed by means of goitre surveys, the determination of urinary iodine excretion, and the measurement of levels of thyroid hormones and of the pituitary thyroid-stimulating hormone (TSH).

4.2 Iodine-deficiency disorders

4.2.1 Goitre (see Plate 1, page 51)

Extensive reviews of the global geographical prevalence of goitre have been published (*2, 4, 5*).

Iodine deficiency depletes thyroid iodine stores and reduces daily production of T_4. A fall in the blood level of T_4 triggers the secretion of increased

Plate 1. Goitre due to iodine deficiency, Papua New Guinea

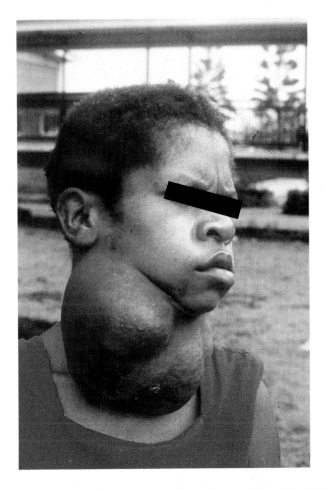

Reproduced by kind permission of CAB International from: Pharoah POD. In: Mills CF, Bremner I, Chesters JK, eds. *Trace elements in man and animals—TEMA 5.* Farnham Royal, CAB International, 1985: 929–932.

amounts of TSH which increases thyroid activity with consequent hyperplasia of the thyroid. The efficiency of the thyroid iodide pump is increased, accompanied by faster turnover of thyroid iodine, as can be demonstrated by an increased thyroidal uptake of the radioactive isotopes iodine-131 and iodine-235. These features were first demonstrated in the field in the classical observations of Stanbury et al. (*6*) in the Andes in Argentina.

51

4.2.2 Fetal iodine deficiency

Iodine deficiency in the fetus is the result of iodine deficiency in the mother. The condition is associated with an increased incidence of stillbirths, abortions and congenital abnormalities, all of which can be avoided by appropriate intervention. The effects are similar to those observed with maternal hypothyroidism, which can be treated by thyroid hormone replacement therapy (7). Controlled trials with iodized oil have shown a significant reduction in recorded fetal and neonatal deaths in treated groups; this is consistent with animal evidence indicating the effect of iodine deficiency on fetal survival (8–10).

Data from Papua New Guinea indicate a relationship between the level of maternal thyroxine and the outcome of current and recent pregnancies, including mortality and the occurrence of cretinism. The rate of perinatal deaths among mothers with very low serum concentrations of total thyroxine, i.e. < 25 µg per ml, was 36.0% as compared with 16.4% in other women with levels > 25 µg per ml; the same was true of free thyroxine (11). These data, which indicate the importance of maternal thyroid function in fetal survival and development, are complemented by extensive animal data (8).

A major effect of fetal iodine deficiency is endemic cretinism (see Plate 2, page 53), which is quite distinct from the sporadic form (9). The former, which occurs with an iodine intake < 25 µg/day in contrast to a normal intake of 80–150 µg/day, is still widely prevalent, affecting for example up to 10% of the populations living in severely iodine-deficient areas in China (12), India (9) and Indonesia (9). In its most common form, it is characterized by mental deficiency, deaf mutism and spastic diplegia; this is referred to as the "nervous" or neurological type in contrast to the less common "myxoedematous" type characterized by hypothyroidism and dwarfism.

Apart from its prevalence in Asia and Oceania (Papua New Guinea), cretinism also occurs in Africa (Zaire) and in South America in the Andean region (Argentina, Bolivia, Ecuador and Peru) (9). In all these areas, with the exception of Zaire, neurological features are predominant (9). In Zaire the myxoedematous form is more common, because of the high intake of cassava (13). However, there is considerable variation in the clinical manifestations of neurological cretinism, including isolated deaf mutism and mental defects of varying degrees. In China, the term "cretinoid" is used to describe the individuals affected.

The apparent spontaneous disappearance of endemic cretinism in southern Europe raised considerable doubts as to the relation of iodine deficiency to the condition. Spontaneous disappearance without iodization was also noted by Costa et al. (14) in northern Italy and by König & Veraguth (15) in Switzerland. A controlled trial in the Western Highlands of Papua New Guinea showed that endemic cretinism could be prevented by correction of iodine deficiency with

Plate 2. Iodine deficiency, Papua New Guinea: endemic cretin showing diplegic adduction

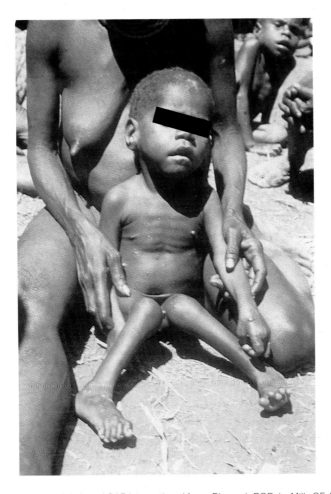

Reproduced by kind permission of CAB International from: Pharoah POD. In: Mills CF, Bremner I, Chesters JK, eds. *Trace elements in man and animals—TEMA 5.* Farnham Royal, CAB International, 1985: 929–932.

iodized oil before pregnancy (*16, 17*). The value of iodized oil injection in the prevention of endemic cretinism has been confirmed in Zaire and in South America (*18*). Mass injection programmes have been carried out in New Guinea in 1971–1972 and in China, Indonesia and Zaire. Recent evaluations of these programmes in China and Indonesia indicate that endemic cretinism has been prevented where iodine deficiency has been corrected (*12, 19*). The apparently spontaneous disappearance of the condition is now attributed to increases in iodine intake as a result of dietary diversification consequent on social and economic development in the more remote rural areas.

4.2.3 Neonatal iodine deficiency

An increased perinatal mortality due to iodine deficiency has been found in Zaire in a trial in which iodized oil injections and control injections were given in the latter half of pregnancy (10). In the treated group, there was a substantial fall in perinatal and infant mortality together with an increase in birth weight. Low birth weight (whatever the cause) is generally associated with a higher rate of congenital anomalies and higher risk throughout childhood.

Apart from its influence on mortality, the importance of the state of thyroid function in the neonate relates to the fact that, at birth, the brain of the human infant has only reached about one-third of its full size and continues to grow rapidly until the end of the second year (20). The thyroid hormone, which depends on an adequate supply of iodine, is essential for normal brain development, as confirmed by animal studies (21, 22).

Data on iodine nutrition and neonatal thyroid function in Europe have recently been published which confirm the continuing presence of severe iodine deficiency affecting neonatal thyroid function and hence constituting a threat to early brain development (23). There is similar evidence from neonatal observations in Zaire, where rates of chemical hypothyroidism of 10% have been found (24). In Zaire, it has been observed that this hypothyroidism persists into infancy and childhood if the deficiency is not corrected, and retardation of physical and mental development results.

These observations indicate a much greater risk of mental defects in severely iodine-deficient populations than is indicated merely by the presence of classical cretinism. The studies of Pharoah et al. (25), which demonstrated depressed cognitive and motor performance in 10–12-year-old children born to women known to have developed iodine deficiency during pregnancy, illustrate both the long-term consequences of a low iodine status during fetal development and the fact that they need not be accompanied by concurrent overt signs of deficiency in the child.

4.2.4 Iodine deficiency in children

Iodine deficiency in children is characteristically associated with goitre. The WHO classification of goitre has been discussed elsewhere (5). The goitre rate increases with age, reaching a maximum at adolescence. Girls have a higher prevalence than boys. Goitre rates in schoolchildren over the age range 6–12 years provide a convenient indicator of the presence of iodine deficiency in a community.

Recent studies on schoolchildren living in iodine-deficient areas in a number of countries indicate impaired school performance and IQs as compared with matched groups from non-iodine-deficient areas (26). These studies are difficult to design because of the problem of establishing appropriate control groups. There are many possible causes both of impaired school performance and impaired performance in IQ tests and these may confound the interpretation of any differences between such areas that might be observed. The iodine-deficient area is likely to be more remote, suffer more social deprivation, and have poorer schools, a lower socioeconomic status and poorer general nutrition. All such factors have to be taken into account, apart from the problem of adapting tests developed in Western countries for use in developing countries. However, several studies indicate that iodine deficiency can impair school performance even when the effect of other factors, such as social deprivation and other nutritional factors, has been taken into account (26).

4.2.5 Iodine deficiency in adults

Iodine administration in the form of iodized salt, bread or oil has been demonstrated to be effective in the prevention of goitre in adults. It may also reduce existing goitre in adults; this is particularly true of iodized oil injections (2). The obvious nature of this effect leads to ready acceptance of the measure by people living in iodine-deficient communities. A rise in circulating T_4 can be readily demonstrated in adults following iodization.

The major determinant of brain and pituitary T_3 is serum T_4 and not, in contrast to liver, kidney and muscle, T_3 (27). Low levels of brain T_3 have been demonstrated in the iodine-deficient rat in association with reduced levels of serum T_4, and these have been restored to normal following correction of iodine deficiency (28). These findings provide an explanation of suboptimal brain function in subjects with endemic goitre and lowered serum T_4 levels, and of its improvement following correction of iodine deficiency. However, it must also be emphasized that relationships between T_4 and T_3 are influenced by the fact that selenium is a component of at least one of the enzymes mediating this conversion. Thus a fall in selenium status (see Chapter 6) reduces T_3 synthesis and may increase the adverse consequences of iodine deficiency (29).

In northern India, a high degree of apathy has been noted in populations living in iodine-deficient areas, which may even affect domestic animals such as dogs. It is apparent that reduced mental function is widely prevalent in iodine-deficient communities, with consequent effects on their capacity for taking the initiative and for decision-making.

Such evidence indicates that iodine deficiency is a major obstacle to the human and social development of communities living in an iodine-deficient environment. Correction of iodine deficiency is thus a major contribution to development.

4.2.6 Iodine deficiency in animals

Epidemiological and experimental studies on animals strongly support the conclusion that reproductive, neurological and other defects are important consequences of iodine deficiency.

Observations on naturally occurring iodine deficiency have been made on farm animals; the consequent reproductive failure and thyroid insufficiency have been fully reported in the older literature (30). In areas of iodine deficiency, the development of the fetus has been retarded or arrested at some stage in gestation, resulting in early death or resorption, abortion and stillbirth, or the birth of weak, hairless offspring, associated with prolonged gestation and parturition and retention of placental membranes. Subnormal thyroid hormone levels in herds of cattle have been accompanied by a high incidence of aborted, stillborn and weak calves (30).

In recent experimental work with animal models (21, 22), severe iodine deficiency has been established before and during pregnancy and the effects on fetal development studied. Iodine deficiency in the sheep (5–8 μg/day for sheep weighing 40 kg) is associated with an increased incidence of abortions and stillbirths. At the end of pregnancy, the body weight of the fetus is reduced, and there is a complete absence of wool growth, deformation of the skull, and retardation of bone development. Brain development is retarded, as indicated both by reduced brain weight and a reduced number of cells (as measured by DNA). Similar effects have been observed in the marmoset (0.3 μg/day for a 340-g animal) (22).

In the light of these data and observations on animal models, it may be concluded that the effects of severe iodine deficiency on fetal development are mediated by a combination of maternal and fetal hypothyroidism, the effect of the former occurring before the onset of fetal thyroid secretion. This would imply an effect on neuroblast multiplication which occurs on days 40–80 of gestation in the sheep and at 11–18 weeks in the human (31). In the rat (whose brain develops postnatally), neuroblast multiplication occurs in the last third of fetal life; an effect of maternal hypothyroidism early in pregnancy is indicated by reduced weight and number of embryos, reduced brain weight and reduced transfer of maternal T_4 (32, 33).

The findings suggest that iodine deficiency has an early effect on neuroblast multiplication that could be important in the pathogenesis of the neurological form of endemic cretinism (*22*).

4.3 Epidemiology and control of iodine-deficiency disorders

Large populations are at risk of IDD because they live in iodine-deficient environments characterized by soil from which iodine has been leached by glaciation, high rainfall or floods. Such leaching occurs most often in mountainous areas, e.g. in the Himalayan region, the Andean region, and the vast mountain ranges of China. However, low-lying areas subject to flooding, as in the Ganges Valley in India and Bangladesh, are also severely iodine-deficient. This means that all the food grown in such soil is low in iodine so that iodine deficiency will persist unless there is dietary diversification, as occurred in Europe late in the 19th century and in the early decades of this century, or some form of iodine supplement is given.

Resolution WHA 43/2, unanimously adopted by the Forty-third World Health Assembly (Geneva, May 1990), to which all Member States are committed, stated that "in view of the progress already achieved, and the promising potential of current and planned national prevention and control programmes, WHO shall aim at eliminating IDD as a major public health problem in all countries by the year 2000." A similar resolution was adopted by the Executive Board of UNICEF in April 1990.

Activities at global, regional and national level since the founding of the International Council for the Control of Iodine Deficiency Disorders (ICCIDD) in 1986 culminated in the preparation of a Global Action Plan by ICCIDD in consultation with WHO and UNICEF. This Plan was formally endorsed by the United Nations Administrative Committee on Coordination/Subcommittee on Nutrition (ACC/SCN) at its sixteenth session in Paris in February 1990; it developed naturally from the close working relationship that has grown up between ICCIDD, WHO and UNICEF.

According to a report to the World Health Assembly in 1994 (*34*), about 1600 million people are at risk of IDD because they live in iodine-deficient environments. Of these, 656 million have goitre (see Table 4.2) and 43 million some degree of mental defect, including 11.2 million overt cretins.

The major concentrations of people suffering from IDD are in Asia, where there has recently been a major increase in IDD control programmes in Bhutan, India, Indonesia, Myanmar and Nepal.

In Latin America, a large measure of control has been achieved in such countries as Argentina, Brazil, Colombia and Guatemala, but there is evidence of a recurrence of the problem in the last two countries associated with political

Table 4.2. Numbers of people at risk of iodine-deficiency disorders and numbers with goitre (in millions) [a]

WHO region	At risk	Goitre
Africa	181	89
Americas	167	63
South-East Asia	486	175
Europe	141	97
Eastern Mediterranean	173	93
Western Pacific	423	139
Total	1571	656

[a] From reference *34.*

and social unrest. Major IDD problems have persisted in Bolivia, Ecuador and Peru, but significant progress has recently been made thanks to a combination of national government initiatives and support from international agencies.

In Africa, the development of IDD control programmes has lagged behind in comparison with the other continents. However, new initiatives have begun following a Joint WHO/UNICEF/ICCIDD Regional Seminar held in Yaoundé, Cameroon, in March 1987. This Seminar set up a joint IDD Task Force and most countries have now begun comprehensive action for the prevention and control of IDD in Africa (*35*).

China has also made rapid progress since the end of the Cultural Revolution in 1976. One-third of the population of China (300 million) is at risk of IDD because of the extensive mountainous areas in that country (*12*).

4.4 Assessment of status

The assessment of the iodine nutritional status of a population or group living in an area or region suspected to be iodine-deficient is important in relation to public health programmes in which iodine supplementation is to be carried out. The recommended methods of assessing status are as follows:

- assessment of the goitre rate, including the rate of palpable or visible goitre classified according to accepted criteria (*36*);
- measurement of urinary iodine excretion;[1]

---

[1] Formerly expressed in relation to creatinine concentration (μg iodine/g). However, the level of creatinine varies with nutritional status and introduces an unnecessary additional variable.

- determination of the level of blood T_4 or TSH in various age groups; particular attention is now focused on the levels in neonates and in pregnant women because of the importance of thyroid function for early brain development.

Goitre severity. A classification of goitre severity has been adopted by WHO (*36*), but there are still minor differences in the techniques used by different observers for determining severity. In general, visible goitre is more readily verified than palpable goitre. Recent observations in the United Republic of Tanzania (*37*) indicate that palpation of the thyroid overestimates the size of the gland as compared with ultrasonography, particularly in children. However, the large-scale assessment of goitre rate, while desirable, is not essential. It is both time-consuming and costly, and limited samples of the population may be sufficient for purposes of determining the rate.

Urinary iodine excretion. The determination of urinary iodine excretion can be carried out on 24-hour samples. However, the difficulties involved in collecting such samples may be insurmountable. For this reason, as originally suggested by Follis (*38*), determinations can be carried out on casual samples from a group of approximately 40 subjects. The iodine levels are expressed as $\mu g/100$ ml and the results plotted as a histogram. This provides a reference point for the level of iodine excretion, which is also a good index of the level of iodine nutrition. The availability of modern automated equipment is making the analysis of large numbers of samples quite feasible, and methods have recently been improved so that reliable results can be obtained (*39, 40*).

Excessive iodine intake can also be most conveniently monitored by the determination of urinary iodine excretion.

Iodine-responsive hormone activity. The determination of the level of serum T_4 or thyroid-stimulating hormone provides an indirect measure of iodine nutritional status. The availability of radioimmunoassay methods with auto mated equipment has greatly assisted this approach. The determination of TSH is now the preferred method because of the greater stability of this hormone under tropical conditions and the easier methodology. Particular attention should be given to levels of TSH in neonates and pregnant women.

Monitoring of neonates. In developed countries, where iodine deficiency in humans does not normally exist, all babies are screened to ensure that their thyroid hormone levels are adequate. In these screening programmes, blood from heel pricks of neonates is spotted onto filter paper, which is then dried and sent to a regional laboratory. Blood levels of either T_4 or TSH or both are measured by immunoassay techniques. The detection rate of neonatal hypo-thyroidism requiring treatment is about 1 per 3500 babies screened. This rate varies little among developed countries (*41*).

Neonatal hypothyroid monitoring has also been started in several iodine-deficient regions in developing countries. Kochupillai et al. in India (42) and, as already noted, Ermans et al. in Zaire (43) have reported severe biochemical hypothyroidism (T_4 concentrations less than 30 μg/l or TSH greater than 50 μIU/ml) in 4% and 10% of neonates, respectively. It is evident from these and other reports (11) that, within an iodine-deficient population, serum T_4 levels are lowest at birth and lower in children than in the adult population. In addition, goitrogens such as those of cassava seem to be much more effective in reducing serum T_4 levels in neonates and children than in adults.

To summarize, the most important information in the determination of the status of iodine nutrition comes from the measurement of the urinary excretion of iodine and from the measurement of blood TSH in neonates or pregnant women. The results of these two determinations indicate the severity of the problem, and can also be used to assess the effectiveness of remedial measures.

The severity of iodine deficiency can be assessed using the criteria shown in Table 4.3, which were considered at a recent WHO/UNICEF/ICCIDD Consultation (44). The Consultation recommended that every effort should be made to ensure the international comparability and reliability of all survey procedures (clinical and biochemical); IDD assessments should be undertaken with the full involvement of the participating communities and both local and national administrations. These assessments should cover a wide range of socio-economic factors as well as the clinical and biochemical ones mentioned above.

Table 4.3. Summary of IDD prevalence indicators and criteria for a significant public health problem[a]

Indicator	Target population	Severity of public health problem (prevalence)		
		Mild	Moderate	Severe
Goitre	SAC	5.0–19.9%	20.0–29.9%	≥ 30.0%
Thyroid volume > 97th centile by ultrasound[b]	SAC	5.0–19.9%	20.0–29.9%	≥ 30.0%
Median urinary iodine level (μg/l)	SAC	50–99	20–49	< 20
TSH > 5 mIU/l whole blood	neonates	3.0–19.9%	20.0–39.9%	≥ 40.0%
Median thyroglobulin (ng/ml serum)[c]	C/A	10.0–19.9	20.0–39.9	≥ 40.0

[a] Adapted from reference 44.
[b] Normative thyroid volume values will be available from WHO and ICCIDD in 1996.
[c] Different assays may have different normal ranges.
SAC, school-age children; C/A, children and adults.

Table 4.4. Average iodine content of foods (in µg iodine/g)

Food	Fresh basis		Dry basis	
	Mean	Range	Mean	Range
Fish (freshwater)	30	17–40	116	68–194
Fish (marine)	832	163–3180	3715	471–4591
Shellfish	798	308–1300	3866	1292–4987
Meat	50	27–97	—	—
Milk	47	35–56	—	—
Eggs	93	—	—	—
Cereal grains	47	22–72	65	34–92
Fruits	18	10–29	154	62–277
Legumes	30	23–36	234	223–245
Vegetables	29	12–201	385	204–1636

[a] Reproduced, by permission, from Koutras (*45*).

4.5 Intake, absorption and bioavailability

The iodine contents of foods (Table 4.4) and of total diets differ appreciably and are influenced by geochemical, soil and cultural conditions which modify the iodine uptake of staple crops and foods of animal origin.

Cooking reduces the iodine content of food below the levels shown in Table 4.4. The data show that frying reduces the iodine content by 20%, grilling by 23% and boiling by as much as 58% (*45*).

Iodine is readily absorbed, and excess intake is controlled by renal excretion. Absorption is usually complete but may be delayed in protein–energy malnutrition. Thyroid hormones in animal foods and other organic iodine compounds are not completely absorbed—there may be a loss of up to 50% (*45*).

The usual recommended level for the population mean intake[1] of iodine is 100–150 µg/day. This level is adequate to maintain the normal thyroid function that is essential for normal growth and development. In the presence of goitrogens in the diet, the intake should be increased to 200–300 µg/day (*4, 5*).

Goitrogens are found in a number of staple foods used in developing countries, including cassava, maize, bamboo shoots, sweet potatoes, lima beans and millets. They are derived from cyanogenic glycosides, which are capable of

---

[1] For most practical purposes, this recommendation will satisfy similar criteria to $I_{Plmin}^{normative}$, the lowest population mean intake of iodine that will meet normative requirements (see Chapter 2).

liberating large quantities of cyanide by hydrolysis. Not only is the cyanide itself toxic, but the metabolite in the body is predominantly thiocyanate, which is a goitrogen. Except in cassava, these glycosides are located in the inedible portions of the plants or, if in the edible portion, are present only in small quantities so that they do not cause a major problem. Cassava, on the other hand, is cultivated extensively in developing countries and represents an essential source of calories for more than 200 million people.

Recent studies indicate that the essential element selenium is a component of the enzyme responsible for converting thyroxine to T_3 (29, 46). It remains to be determined whether the systemic utilization of iodine is impaired in subjects deficient in selenium (see Chapter 6).

In the presence of long-standing iodine deficiency, an increase in intake, even to normal levels, may be associated with hyperthyroidism. This cohort phenomenon, reflecting an autonomous and sustained metabolic response of the thyroid to previous iodine deficiency, does not develop if community prophylaxis with iodine was introduced at an early stage of deficiency.

4.6 Requirements

The recommendations of the Food and Nutrition Board of the National Academy of Sciences in the United States (47) were accepted by the Expert Consultation.[1]

---

[1] Since the time of the Expert Consultation, several WHO/ICCIDD meetings at both regional and global levels have suggested increased iodine requirements, especially for infants and pregnant and lactating women. Pending further information on breast-milk iodine in developing countries, the following table gives recommended mean population iodine intakes.

Recommended intakes of iodine (population requirements)[a]

Age range or state	Intake (μg/day)
0–12 months	50
1–6 years	90
7–12 years	120
12 years to (and through) adulthood	150
Pregnancy	200
Lactation	200

[a] For virtually all practical purposes, these allowances can be regarded as serving the same purpose as estimates of population minimum mean intakes sufficient to meet normative requirements ($I_{Plmin}^{normative}$).

4.7 Correction of iodine deficiency

4.7.1 Iodized salt

Iodized salt was first successfully used in Switzerland in the 1920s (*4*, *5*). Since then, successful programmes have been reported from a number of countries, including some in Central and South America (e.g. Colombia, Guatemala), China and Finland (*4*, *5*).

The difficulties in the production of iodized salt and in maintaining its quality so that it can be supplied to the millions of iodine-deficient people, especially in Asia, have been vividly demonstrated in India, where there has been a breakdown in supply. The difficulties have led to the adoption of the goal of universal salt iodization in India. In Asia, the cost of iodized salt production and distribution at present is of the order of US 3–5 cents per person per year (*2*). This must be considered cheap in relation to the social benefits that have been described earlier in this section.

However, the salt still has to reach the iodine-deficient person. There may be a problem with the distribution or with the preservation of the iodine content—the salt may be left uncovered or exposed to heat. It should be added after cooking to reduce the loss of iodine.

Finally, there are difficulties in relation to the consumption of the salt. While the addition of iodine makes no difference to the taste, the introduction of a new variety of salt in an area where salt is already available and familiar, and much appreciated as a condiment, is likely to be resisted. In the Chinese provinces of Xinjiang and Inner Mongolia, the strong preference of the people for desert salt of very low iodine content led to a mass programme of iodized oil injection in order to prevent cretinism (*12*).

4.7.2 Iodine supplements for animals

The use of iodine supplements for cattle and pigs has been very successful in eastern Germany and deserves to be more extensive. Significant levels are attained in milk and meat, which then act as the vehicle for human dietary intake, resulting in the return of urinary iodine levels to normal values (*48*). In contrast, legislation prohibiting such supplementation in some iodine-deficient countries is probably responsible for the persistence of IDD in a number of them.

4.7.3 Iodized oil by injection

The value of iodized oil injection in the prevention of endemic goitre and endemic cretinism was first established in Papua New Guinea in trials in which injection of saline was used as a control. These trials established the value of the oil in the prevention of both goitre and cretinism (2, 4, 5). Experience in China, South America and Zaire has confirmed the value of this procedure. The quantitative correction of severe iodine deficiency by a single intramuscular injection has been demonstrated (5) for a period of over 4 years (2, 4).

Iodized oil is particularly appropriate for use in the isolated village communities so characteristic of mountainous endemic goitre areas. The striking regression of goitre following iodized oil injection ensures general acceptance of the measure. In a suitable area, the oil (1 ml usually contains 480 mg of iodine) should be administered to all females up to the age of 40 years and all males up to the age of 20 years. A repeat injection may be required in 3–5 years, depending on the dose given and the age of the subject. The need of children for iodine is greater than that of adults, and the recommended dose should be repeated in 3 years if severe iodine deficiency persists (2). Iodized walnut oil and iodized soya bean oil are new preparations developed in China since 1980 (2).

4.7.4 Iodized oil by mouth

Recent studies in China and India show that the effect of oral iodized oil lasts only half as long as that of a similar dose given by injection (2). A recent review indicates the need for more extensive studies to determine the effectiveness of mass intervention (2).

4.7.5 Indications for different methods of iodine supplementation

The most appropriate method of iodine supplementation will depend on the severity of IDD in a population, graded on the basis of urinary iodine excretion and the prevalence of goitre and cretinism (2, 44), as follows:

- *Mild IDD*: goitre prevalence in the range 5.0–19.9% (schoolchildren) and median urinary iodine levels in the range 50–99 µg/l. Mild IDD can be eliminated with iodized salt. It may also disappear with economic development.
- *Moderate IDD*: goitre prevalence of 20.0–29.9% and some hypo-thyroidism, and median urinary iodine levels in the range 20–49 µg/l. Moderate IDD can be controlled with iodized salt (usually 20–40 mg/kg at household level) if this can be effectively produced and distributed. Otherwise, iodized oil, given either orally or by injection, should be administered via the primary health care system.
- *Severe IDD*: a high prevalence of goitre (30.0% or more), endemic cretinism, and median urinary iodine below 20 µg/l. Severe IDD usually requires iodized oil, given either orally or by injection as an interim

measure until an effective iodized salt system is operational, if central nervous system defects are to be completely prevented.

Both iodized salt and iodized oil have been used in major mass supplementation programmes; more than 20 million injections of iodized oil have been given in Asia, and there is evidence that IDD have been successfully prevented.

4.8 Toxicity and hyperthyroidism

4.8.1 Toxicity

Iodine toxicity has been carefully studied in humans, laboratory species, poultry, pigs and cattle. Wolff (49) has defined four degrees of iodide excess in humans, as follows:

1. A relatively modest excess, promoting temporary increases in the absolute uptake of iodine by the thyroid and the formation of organic iodine, but without inhibiting the capacity to release iodine in response to physiological demand.
2. A larger excess, which can inhibit iodine release from the thyrotoxic human thyroid or from thyroids in which iodine release has been accelerated by TSH.
3. A slightly greater intake, which inhibits organic iodine formation and which probably causes iodide goitre (the so-called Wolff–Chaikoff effect).
4. Very high levels of iodide, which saturate the active transport mechanism for this ion. The acute pharmacological effects of iodide can usually be demonstrated before saturation becomes significant.

Wolff (49) has also suggested that human intakes of 2000 μg of iodine/day should be regarded as excessive or potentially harmful. Normal diets composed of natural foods are unlikely to supply as much as this, and most would supply less than 1000 μg of iodine/day. Exceptions occur when diets are exceptionally high in marine fish or seaweed, or where foods are contaminated with iodine from adventitious sources.

Inhabitants of the coastal regions of Hokkaido, the northernmost island of Japan, whose diets contain large amounts of seaweed, have remarkably high iodine intakes, amounting to 50 000–80 000 μg of iodine/day (50). Urinary excretion in five patients exhibiting clinical signs of iodide goitre exceeded 20 mg of iodine/day, or about 100 times the normal amount. Similar findings have been reported from two Chinese villages on the Yellow Sea coast in which large amounts of kelp are consumed (51).

In Japan, it has been shown (3) that:

- Normal subjects can maintain normal thyroid function even when they are consuming several milligrams/day (perhaps 30 mg/day) of dietary iodine.
- The incidences of non-toxic diffuse goitre and toxic nodular goitre are markedly decreased by high dietary iodine.
- The incidences of Graves disease and Hashimoto disease appear not to be affected by high dietary iodine.
- High dietary iodine may, however, induce hypothyroidism in auto-immune thyroid disease and may inhibit the effects of thionamide drugs.

Significant species differences exist in tolerance of high iodine intakes. However, in all species studied, the tolerance is high relative to normal dietary iodine intakes, pointing to a wide margin of safety for this element (52).

4.8.2 Iodine-induced hyperthyroidism

A mild increase in the incidence of hyperthyroidism has been reported following the introduction of programmes for the fortification of salt with iodine in Europe and South America and that of iodized bread in the Netherlands and Tasmania (52, 53). A few cases have been noted following the administration of iodized oil in South America. No cases have yet been described in India, Papua New Guinea or Zaire, probably because of the scattered nature of the population which is distributed among a large number of small villages where opportunities for observation are limited (54). The condition is largely confined to those over 40 years of age—a smaller proportion of the population in developing than in developed countries. Detailed observations have been reported from Tasmania (53, 55).

The condition is readily controlled with antithyroid drugs or radioiodine. Spontaneous remission also occurs. In general, iodization should be avoided in those over the age of 40 because of the risk of hyperthyroidism (56).

However, the correction of iodine deficiency prevents the formation of an autonomous thyroid and thus the development of iodine-induced hyper-thyroidism. For this reason, this condition is also regarded as an "iodine-deficiency disorder".

4.8.3 Safe upper limits of intake

Joseph et al. (57) have reported that iodine intakes of less than 100 μg/day pose no risk for patients with autonomous thyroid tissue caused by previous iodine deficiency; for such subjects the critical intake probably lies between 100 and

200 µg/day. The iodization of bread in Tasmania resulted in thyrotoxicosis for some individuals at levels of iodine intake of about 200 µg/day (*53*). Iodized bread in the Netherlands contributed an additional 120–160 µg of iodine per day and increased the incidence of thyrotoxicosis (*58*). A spring–summer peak of thyrotoxicosis (related to winter milk) in England occurred with average iodine intakes of 236 µg/day for women and 306 µg/day for men (*58*). The absence of previous episodes of iodine deficiency in the population of Japan accounts for the absence of iodine-induced thyrotoxicosis in that country (*3*).

4.9 Recommendations for future research and other activities

- There has been an increase in activity directed towards the establishment of effective national IDD-control programmes throughout the world aimed at the elimination of IDD as a major public health problem by the year 2000; this activity must be maintained.
- There is an urgent need for further investigation of alternative sources of iodine. Currently, iodine is produced mainly as a by-product of natural gas in Japan and from mineral nitrate refining in Chile (*59*).
- There is also a need for research directed towards the acquisition of more detailed data on the effects of iodine deficiency on a total population. This should include, in particular, research on the effects on mental function, on the socioeconomic impact of iodine deficiency, and on the benefits that can be derived from IDD-control programmes.
- The accuracy of the assessment of iodine deficiency is improving as new techniques are developed. Techniques such as ultrasonography for the estimation of thyroid size (*60*) and improved methods of urinary iodine determination and for the determination of TSH in blood spots on filter paper have all been reviewed recently (*45*). The criteria for the interpretation of the data such techniques provide require further verification and international ratification, and further development of these techniques is needed.
- Simpler methods are required for the assessment of central nervous system function that would be suitable for use in epidemiological studies. Such methods could also be used to assess the effects of the correction of iodine deficiency.
- More accurate data on the incidence and prevalence of thyrotoxicosis following iodization programmes are needed.
- Greater attention must be paid to the problem of defining quantitatively the antagonistic effects of organic and inorganic goitrogens on iodine

utilization and requirements. The modifying influence of differences in selenium status on the prevalence and manifestations of IDD must be examined in human subjects living in geographical areas low in both iodine and selenium.

References

1. Hetzel BS. Iodine deficiencey disorders (IDD) and their eradication. *Lancet*, 1983, ii: 1126–1129.
2. Hetzel BS, Dunn JT, Stanbury JB, eds. *The prevention and control of iodine deficiency disorders*. Amsterdam, Elsevier, 1987.
3. Nagataki S. Effects of iodide supplement in thyroid diseases. In: Vichayanrat A et al., eds. *Recent progress in thyroidology*. Bangkok, Crystal House Press, 1987: 31–37.
4. Stanbury JB, Hetzel BS, eds. *Endemic goiter and endemic cretinism: iodine nutrition in health and disease*. New York, Wiley, 1980.
5. Dunn JT et al., eds. *Towards the eradiction of endemic goiter, cretinism, and iodine deficiency*. Washington, DC, Pan American Health Organization, 1986.
6. Stanbury JB et al. *The adaptation of man to iodine deficiency*. Cambridge, MA, Harvard University Press, 1954: 11–209.
7. McMichael AJ, Potter JT, Hetzel BS. Iodine deficiency, thyroid function, and reproductive failure. In: Stanbury JB, Hetzel BS, eds. *Endemic goiter and endemic cretinism*. New York, Wiley, 1980: 445–460.
8. Hetzel BS, Potter BJ, Dulberg EM. The iodine deficiency disorders: nature, pathogenesis and epidemiology. *World review of nutrition and diet*, 1990, **62**: 59–119.
9. Pharoah POD et al. Endemic cretinism. In: Stanbury JB, Hetzel BS, eds. *Endemic goiter and endemic cretinism*. New York, Wiley, 1980: 395–421.
10. Thilly CH. Goitre et crétinisme endémiques: rôle étiologique de la consommation de manioc et stratégie d'éradication. [Endemic goitre and cretinism: etiological role of manioc consumption and eradication strategy.] *Bulletin of the Belgian Academy of Medicine*, 1981, **136**: 389–412.
11. Pharoah POD et al. Maternal thyroid function, iodine deficiency and fetal development. *Clinical endocrinology*, 1976, 5: 159–166.
12. Ma T et al. The present status of endemic goiter and endemic cretinism in China. *Food and nutrition bulletin*, 1982, **4**: 13–19.
13. Delange F, Iteke FB, Ermans AM. *Nutritional factors involved in the goitrogenic action of cassava*. Canada, Ottawa, International Development Research Center, 1982: 1–15.
14. Costa A et al. Endemic cretinism in Piedmont. *Panminerva medical*, 1964, **6**: 250–259.
15. König MP, Veraguth P. Studies of thyroid function in endemic cretins. In: Pitt-Rivers R, ed. *Advances in thyroid research*. London, Pergamon, 1961: 294–298.

16. Pharoah POD, Buttfield IH, Hetzel BS. Neurological damage to the fetus resulting from severe iodine deficiency during pregnancy. *Lancet*, 1971, i: 308–310.

17. Pharoah POD, Connolly KJ. A controlled trial of iodinated oil for the prevention of endemic cretinism: a long term follow up. *International journal of epidemiology*, 1987, 16: 68–73.

18. Pretell EA et al. Prophylaxis of endemic goiter with iodized oil in rural Peru. *Advances in experimental medicine and biology*, 1972, 30: 249–265.

19. Dulberg EM et al. Evaluation of the iodization program in Central Java with reference to the prevention of endemic cretinism and motor coordination defects. In: Ui N et al., eds. *Current problems in thyroid research*. Amsterdam, Excerpta Medica, 1983: 19–22.

20. Dobbing J. The later development of the brain and its vulnerability. In: Davis J, Dobbing J, eds. *Scientific foundations of paediatrics*. London, Heinemann Medical, 1974: 565–577.

21. Hetzel BS, Potter BJ. Iodine deficiency and the role of thyroid hormones in brain development. In: Dreosti I, Smith RM, eds. *Neurobiology of the trace elements*. Totowa, NJ, Humana Press, 1983: 83–133.

22. Hetzel BS, Chavadej J, Potter BJ. The brain in iodine deficiency. *Neuropathology and applied neurobiology*, 1988, 14: 93–104.

23. Delange F et al. Regional variations of iodine nutrition and thyroid function during the neonatal period in Europe. *Biology of the neonate*, 1986, 49: 322–330.

24. Ermans AM et al., eds. *Role of cassava in the aetiology of endemic goiter and cretinism*. Ottawa, International Development Research Center, 1980.

25. Pharoah POD et al. Maternal thyroid hormone levels in pregnancy and the subsequent cognitive and motor performance of the children. *Clinical endocrinology*, 1984, 21: 265–270.

26. Fierro-Benitez R et al. Long-term effect of correction of iodine deficiency on psychomotor and intellectual development. In: Dunn JT et al., eds. *Towards the eradication of endemic goiter, cretinism, and iodine deficiency*. Washington, DC, Pan American Health Organization, 1986: 182–200.

27. Crantz FR, Larsen PR. Rapid thyroxine to 3,5,3'-triiodothyronine conversion binding in rat cerebral cortex and cerebellum. *Journal of clinical investigation*, 1980, 65: 935–938.

28. Obregon MJ et al. Cerebral hypothyroidism in rats with adult-onset iodine deficiency. *Endocrinology*, 1984, 115: 614–624.

29. Arthur JR, Nicol F, Beckett GJ. Hepatic iodothyronine deiodinase: the role of selenium. *Biochemical journal*, 1990, 272: 537–540.

30. Hetzel BS, Maberly GF. Iodine. In: Mertz W, ed. *Trace elements in human and animal nutrition*, 5th ed., Vol. 2. Orlando, Academic Press, 1986: 139–208.

31. Dobbing J, Sands J. Comparative aspects of the brain growth spurt. *Early human development*, 1979, 3: 79–83.

32. Morreale de Escobar G et al. Effects of maternal hypothyroidism on weight and thyroid hormone content of rat embryonic tissues, before and after onset of fetal thyroid function. *Endocrinology*, 1985, 117: 1890–1900.

33. Obregon J et al. L-Thyroxine and 3,5,3'-triiodo-L-thyronine in rat embryos before onset of fetal thyroid function. *Endocrinology*, 1984, **114**: 305–307.

34. *World Health Organization. Forty-seventh World Health Assembly, Geneva, 2–12 May 1994. Resolutions and decisions; annexes.* Geneva, World Health Organization, 1994: 47 (unpublished document WHA47/1994/REC/1).

35. Hetzel BS. Progress in the prevention and control of iodine deficiency disorders. *Lancet*, 1987, **ii**: 266.

36. Thilly CH, Delange F, Stanbury JB. Epidemiologic surveys in endemic goitre and cretinism. In: Stanbury JB, Hetzel BS, eds. *Endemic goitre and endemic cretinism: iodine nutrition in health and disease.* New York, Wiley, 1980: 157–179.

37. Wachter W et al. Use of ultrasonography for goiter assessment in IDD: studies in Tanzania. In: Hetzel BS, Dunn JT, Stanbury JB, eds. *The prevention and control of iodine deficiency disorders.* Amsterdam, Elsevier, 1987: 95–108.

38. Follis Jr RH. A pattern of urinary iodine excretion in goitrous and non-goitrous areas. *American journal of clinical nutrition*, 1963, **14**: 253–268.

39. Belling GB. Further studies on the recovery of iodine as iodine-125 after alkaline ashing prior to assay. *Analyst*, 1983, **108**: 763–765.

40. Garry PJ, Lashley DW, Owen GM. Automated measurement of urinary iodine. *Clinical chemistry*, 1973, **19**: 950–953.

41. Burrow GN, ed. *Neonatal thyroid screening.* New York, Raven Press, 1980.

42. Kochupillai N et al. Neonatal thyroid status in iodine deficient environments of the Sub-Himalayan Region. *Indian journal of medical research*, 1984, **80**: 293–299.

43. Ermans AM et al. Congenital hypothyroidism in developing countries. In: Burrow GN, ed. *Neonatal thyroid screening.* New York, Raven Press, 1980: 61–73.

44. *Indicators for assessing iodine deficiency disorders and their control through salt iodization.* Geneva, World Health Organization, 1994 (unpublished document WHO/NUT/94.6; available on request from Nutrition, World Health Organization, 1211 Geneva 27, Switzerland).

45. Koutras DA. Iodine: distribution, availability, and effects of deficiency on the thyroid. In: Dunn JT et al., eds. *Towards the eradication of endemic goitre, cretinism and iodine deficiency.* Washington, DC, Pan American Health Organization, 1986: 15–27.

46. Arthur JR, Beckett GR. Selenium deficiency and thyroid hormone metabolism. In: Wendel A, ed. *Selenium in biology and medicine.* Berlin, Springer, 1989: 90–95.

47. National Research Council. *Recommended dietary allowances*, 10th ed. Washington, DC, National Academy of Sciences, 1989.

48. Bauch K et al. A five year interdisciplinary control of iodine deficiency in the GDR. *Acta medica austriaca*, 1990, **17**(Suppl. 1): 36–38.

49. Wolff J. Iodide goitre and the pharmacologic effects of excess iodide. *American journal of medicine*, 1969, **47**: 101–124.

50. Suzuki H. Etiology of endemic goiter and iodide excess. In: Stanbury JB, Hetzel BS, eds. *Endemic goiter and endemic cretinism.* New York, Wiley, 1980: 237–253.

51. Zhu XY et al. The present status of endemic goitre and endemic cretinism in China. In: Ui N, ed. *Current problems in thyroid research*. Amsterdam, Excerpta Medica, 1983: 13–15.

52. Connolly RJ, Vidor GI, Stewart JC. Increase in thyrotoxicosis in endemic goitre area after iodation of bread. *Lancet*, 1970, i: 500–502.

53. Stewart JC et al. Epidemic thyrotoxicosis in Northern Tasmania: studies of clinical features and iodine nutrition. *Australian and New Zealand journal of medicine*, 1971, 3: 203–211.

54. Larsen PR et al. Monitoring prophylactic programmes: general consideration. In: Stanbury JB, Hetzel BS, eds. *Endemic goiter and endemic cretinism: iodine nutrition in health and disease*. New York, Wiley, 1980: 551–566.

55. Vidor GI et al. Pathogenesis of iodine-induced thyrotoxicosis: studies in Northern Tasmania. *Journal of clinical endocrinology and metabolism*. 1973, 37: 901–909.

56. Stanbury JB et al. Endemic goitre and cretinism: public health significance and prevention. *WHO chronicle*, 1974, 28: 220.

57. Joseph K et al. Early recognition and evaluation of the risk of hyperthyroidism in thyroid autonomy in an endemic goitre area. *Journal of molecular medicine*, 1980, 4: 21–37.

58. Nelson M, Phillips DIW. Seasonal variations in dietary iodine intake and thyrotoxicosis. *Human nutrition and applied nutrition*, 1985, 39(3): 213–216.

59. Subramanian P, Hetzel BS. Iodine sources for SE Asia—requirement, production and procurement. *IDD Newsletter*, 1989, 5(3): 8–10.

60. Wachter W et al. Use of ultrasonography for goitre assessment in IDD. In: Hetzel BS, Dunn JT, Stanbury JB, eds. *The prevention and control of iodine deficiency disorders*. Amsterdam, Elsevier, 1987: 95–108.

5.
Zinc

5.1 Biochemical function

Most biochemical roles of zinc reflect its involvement in a large number of enzymes or as a stabilizer of the molecular structure of subcellular constituents and membranes. Zinc participates in the synthesis and degradation of carbohydrates, lipids, proteins and nucleic acids. It has recently been shown to play an essential role in polynucleotide transcription and translation and thus in the processes of genetic expression. Its involvement in such fundamental activities probably accounts for the essentiality of zinc for all forms of life.

5.2 Deficiency and toxicity

5.2.1 Deficiency (see Plate 3, page 74)

The principal clinical features of severe zinc deficiency in humans are growth retardation, a delay in sexual and skeletal maturation, the development of orificial and acral dermatitis, diarrhoea, alopecia, a failure of appetite and the appearance of behavioural changes (1). An increased susceptibility to infections reflects the development of defects in the immune system.

The effects of marginal or mild zinc deficiency are less obvious and can readily be overlooked. A reduced growth rate and impaired resistance to infection are frequently the only manifestations of mild deficiency in humans. Several studies have now demonstrated the beneficial effects on growth velocity of supplementing the zinc intake of socially deprived children undergoing nutritional rehabilitation. Responses to zinc occurred even though gross, overt clinical evidence of deficiency was lacking (2–4). Among the many factors influencing the competence of cell-mediated immunity are the structure and biological activity of the hormone thymulin, both of which are largely zinc-dependent, and it has therefore been suggested that a reduced activity of this thymic hormone, which is involved in the differentiation of T-cells, could provide an early indication of mild zinc deficiency (5). Other effects, which it is claimed are the result of a low zinc intake, such as impaired taste and delayed wound healing, are less consistently observed and the conditions under which such effects may appear must be defined more clearly.

Studies on laboratory primates and other experimental animals indicate that zinc deficiency impairs reproductive performance, adversely affects voluntary food consumption, and probably restricts the utilization of dietary vitamin A or its tissue stores. The significance of these and many other observed effects of zinc deficiency, observed experimentally but not yet adequately verified in studies with human subjects, have been reviewed elsewhere (6).[1]

5.2.2 Toxicity

Few instances of acute zinc poisoning have been reported; its manifestations include nausea, vomiting, diarrhoea, fever and lethargy and have been observed, typically, after ingestion of 4–8 g of zinc. Long-term exposure to high zinc intakes substantially in excess of requirements has been shown to result in interference with the metabolism of other trace elements. Copper utilization is especially sensitive to an excess of zinc. This copper/zinc interaction has been responsible for the inadvertent induction of copper deficiency, but has also been deliberately exploited to control copper accumulation in Wilson disease (see references listed in Table 7.1, page 130). A zinc intake of as little as 50 mg/day has been shown to influence copper status, as indicated by a decline in erythrocyte copper–zinc superoxide dismutase activity (7, 8). Low plasma copper and plasma caeruloplasmin levels and anaemia have been observed after higher intakes of zinc (450–660 mg/day) (9, 10). Changes in serum lipid patterns and immune response have also been associated with zinc supplementation (11, 12).

---

[1] *Note added in proof*: The effects, causes and control of zinc deficiency in developing countries have been reviewed recently (Gibson RS. Zinc nutrition in developing countries. *Nutrition research reviews*, 1994, 7: 151–173). Infants, in particular males, in each of eight double-blind studies involving a total of 451 subjects in Bangladesh, Chile, France, and the United States responded significantly to increases in zinc intake by an increased rate of weight gain and/or linear growth. Results of double-blind studies with children aged 2–12 years were less consistent. However, there were positive weight and height responses in 5 of 10 studies, again principally in males. Improvements in dark adaptation, conjunctival integrity and immunocompetence were also noted in some studies of the effects of zinc fortification of diets. Gibson (1994) also reviewed a series of seven studies involving a total of 2734 pregnant women, half of whom received zinc supplements. While supplements had apparently no influence on infant birth weight, fewer preterm deliveries were reported in some studies, parturition had to be induced less frequently and a reduced perinatal death rate was reported from one major study. Effects of supplementation during lactation upon the content of zinc in milk were inconsistent. Gibson (1994) emphasizes the difficulty, in virtually all these studies, of relating the observed physiological effects to the zinc contents of diets when insufficient detail is given of factors that may influence zinc availability (see also p. 292).

Plate 3. Zinc deficiency: child with acute marasmic kwashiorkor and hypozincaemia; the skin lesions responded rapidly once zinc intake was increased

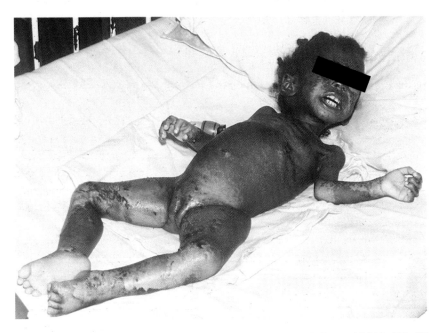

Reproduced by kind permission of CAB International from: Golden BE, Golden MHN. In: Mills CF, Bremner I, Chester JK, eds. *Trace elements in man and animals—TEMA 5*. Farnham Royal, CAB International, 1985.

5.3 Epidemiology of deficiency

The frequency and effects of mild zinc deficiency in "free-living" populations have not yet been adequately investigated; its prevalence is thus unknown. Protein–energy malnutrition is frequently accompanied by a reduced supply of bioavailable zinc and this may well contribute to the widespread stunting in malnourished communities in large areas of the world. Growth-limiting, mild zinc deficiency has been observed in studies on otherwise healthy male American and Canadian infants and preschool children (5, 13, 14) and zinc-responsive growth failure has also been found in adolescents in rural areas of Egypt and the Islamic Republic of Iran (15, 16). The etiology of these conditions, especially in American and Canadian children, is not entirely clear. However, it is becoming evident that male children are particularly susceptible to zinc deficiency and, in the above-mentioned studies, responded significantly to supplementation of their daily intake. It has been suggested that a poor availability of dietary zinc could have contributed to their suboptimal zinc status. The improvement of immunological competence in elderly subjects supplemented with zinc suggests that a marginal zinc status could also develop during old age (R.K. Chandra, personal communication, 1991).

5.4 Assessment of status

Sensitive, pathologically relevant indices of zinc status are at present either lacking or insufficiently validated to permit their use as primary criteria for assessing zinc requirements or as diagnostic criteria in epidemiological surveys. Zinc concentrations, e.g. of plasma, blood cells and hair, and urinary zinc excretion decrease in severe zinc deficiency. However, a number of conditions, unrelated to zinc status, can affect all these indices, particularly plasma zinc. Infection, fever, other stresses and pregnancy tend to reduce it, and it frequently declines following realimentation after brief periods of restricted food intake or protein depletion.

Since the zinc content of organs accessible for sampling and analysis does not reflect the normality of biochemical functions dependent on adequate zinc, a number of functional indices of zinc status have been suggested, e.g. diminished taste acuity and delayed dark adaptation. Changes in these functions are, however, not specific for zinc, and these indices have not so far proved useful in identifying marginal zinc deficiency in humans when used as the sole criteria.

In epidemiological studies, changes in the growth rates of children or in cell-mediated immunocompetence following zinc supplementation could prove to be useful indices of marginal zinc status in a population.

5.5 Metabolism

Zinc is present in all the tissues and fluids of the body. The total body content has been estimated to be approximately 2 g. The zinc concentration of the lean body mass is approximately 30 μg/g. Skeletal muscle accounts for approximately 60% of the total body content, and bone, with a zinc concentration of 100–200 μg/g, for about 30%. Plasma zinc accounts for only about 0.1% of total body content; it has a rapid turnover, and its level appears to be under close homoeostatic control. High concentrations of zinc are found in the choroid of the eye (274 μg zinc/g) and in prostatic fluids (300–500 μg/ml) (1).

There is no "store" of zinc in the conventional sense. Under conditions of bone resorption and tissue catabolism, zinc can be released and, to some extent, reutilized. Human experimental studies with low-zinc diets (2.6–3.6 mg/day) have shown that circulating plasma zinc and the activities of zinc-containing enzymes can be maintained within a normal range over several months (*17, 18*), indicating that some zinc can be made available from tissues.

Zinc is lost from the body via the kidneys, the skin and the intestine. Endogenous intestinal losses can range from 0.5 to 3 mg/day depending on zinc intake. Approximately 0.7 mg of zinc/day is lost in the urine of normal healthy subjects. Starvation and muscle catabolism increase zinc losses in urine and faeces. The loss of zinc in perspiration and desquamated epidermal cells has been estimated to be 0.5 mg/day in adult men, but this also depends on zinc intake (*19*). Strenuous exercise and elevated ambient temperatures could lead to larger losses.

Prostatic fluids have a high concentration of zinc, and a semen ejaculate can contain up to 1 mg (*20*). Zinc losses in menstruation are small (0.01 mg/day) (*21*). Other losses, such as that resulting from the normal daily loss of hair, are probably insignificant.

5.6 Absorption and bioavailability

Zinc absorption is concentration-dependent and takes place throughout the small intestine (*22*). The jejunum appears to be the site of maximum absorption, the colon not playing a significant role (*23*). Intestinal perfusion studies in humans suggest that zinc absorption is a carrier-mediated transport process which is not saturated under normal physiological conditions (*22*). However, recent isotopic studies of zinc absorption from single meals indicate that saturation of absorption is approached if the intake of available forms of zinc by adults exceeds approximately 4 or 5 mg per meal (B. Sandström, personal communication, 1992). Zinc administered in aqueous solution to fasting subjects is absorbed very efficiently (60–70%) and there is no indication of saturation up to doses of 10–15 mg. Absorption of zinc from solid diets is much less efficient and, depending on the content of zinc in meals otherwise identical in composition, can vary widely (see Chapter 3).

Many dietary factors have been identified from experimental studies as potential promoters or antagonists of zinc absorption. Soluble, low molecular weight organic substances, such as many amino and hydroxy acids, act as zinc-binding ligands and facilitate its absorption. In contrast, organic compounds that form stable, poorly soluble complexes with zinc can reduce it. Competitive interactions involving zinc and excessive concentrations of other ions with similar physicochemical properties (e.g. cadmium) can restrict the uptake and intestinal transport of zinc and thus its absorption (see Table 3.1, page 24). The equilibria influencing the net effect of these conflicting processes are not adequately defined and thus their quantitative nutritional significance is often uncertain.

Isotopic studies with human subjects have identified three principal dietary factors influencing zinc absorption and utilization, namely the content of inositol hexaphosphate (phytate), the level and source of protein and the total zinc content of the diet.

An inhibitory effect of phytate on zinc utilization was first identified in animal studies in the early 1960s (24, 25). It is present in bran (25–30 g/kg dry weight), in whole-grain cereals (8–10 g/kg dry weight), in legumes (10–25 g/kg dry weight) and, in smaller amounts, in other vegetables. At the pH values encountered in foods, phytate is strongly negatively charged and thus has a strong potential for binding divalent cations such as zinc. However, during many traditional food-preparation procedures, such as sour dough fermentation of bread and the soaking of grains, the naturally occurring phytase present in grains partially hydrolyses the phytate to penta-, tetra-, or lower phosphorylated analogues of phytic acid. The triphosphorylated or lower analogues have a markedly reduced mineral-binding capacity and probably do not inhibit zinc utilization.

A depressive effect of phytate on zinc absorption has also been demonstrated in human subjects (26–28), and its presence in wholemeal bread and soya-protein-based infant formulae is most probably the reason for the low fractional absorption of zinc ($< 20\%$) from such foods (28–30). In a mixed diet, the effect of phytate on zinc absorption depends, however, on the composition of the total diet. Animal protein improves zinc absorption from a phytate-containing diet (29, 31), while high dietary calcium potentiates its antagonistic effect. However, when milk products are the major source of calcium in the diet, a lower fractional zinc absorption is counterbalanced by the higher zinc content of the meal (31, 32). The zinc-depressing effect of phytate appears to be most pronounced in whole-grain cereal diets. Zinc absorption from diets based on legumes seems comparable to that from animal protein diets with similar zinc and protein contents (31).

When diets are low in zinc-binding substances, their total zinc content, often influenced strongly by zinc derived from the major protein source (see Table 5.1), has important effects both on the fractional efficiency of zinc absorption and on the absolute quantity of zinc absorbed. From low-zinc diets (< 1 mg zinc/MJ), the fractional absorption of zinc can be as high as 40–60%, while absorption from diets higher in zinc is typically 20–30%. However, despite the smaller fraction absorbed, total absorption is usually higher (33).

It is particularly desirable to select diets with a high zinc availability for infants, since requirements during this period of life are high in relation to body weight. Infants probably absorb up to about 80% of the zinc of maternal milk, while adults are only able to absorb about 40% of the zinc from this source, only 30% from cow's milk formulae and about 15% from soya-based formulae

(*30*). Whether absorption from formula milks is reduced in infants to an extent similar to that observed in adults is unknown but seems probable (see p. 93).

5.7 Dietary sources and intake

The zinc content of the total diet is influenced, not only by the range of food items selected, but also by the degree of refinement of any constituent cereals. Fats, from which zinc is virtually absent, tend to dilute zinc from the total diet. The average zinc content of some major food proteins and energy sources is given in Table 5.1. As the primary goal of nutrition in developing countries is to provide sufficient energy, the most appropriate basis for the comparison of foods is the relationship of their zinc content to their energy content. As is evident from Table 5.1, lean, red meat is an outstanding zinc source. Furthermore, its zinc is present in a highly available form. Many staple foods provide amounts of zinc similar to those of foods derived from animal tissues. However, energy sources such as fats, oils, sugar and alcohol have a very low zinc content. Green leafy vegetables and fruits are only modest sources of zinc (as of energy) because of their high water content.

The daily intake of zinc in industrialized countries from diets characteristically high in fat, refined sugar and animal protein has been reported to be

Table 5.1. Zinc contents of food groups on a weight basis and in relation to their protein and energy contents[a]

Food	mg/kg raw wet weight	mg/g protein	mg/MJ
Whole grains, wholemeal bread, unpolished rice	30–50	0.2–0.4	2–4
Pulses, legumes	25–35	0.1–0.2	2–3
Rice (polished) corn	10–12	0.2–0.3	1–2
Wheat, low extraction rate	8–10	< 0.1	< 1
Roots, tubers	3–5	0.1–0.2	< 1
Coconut	5	0.1–0.2	< 0.5
Milk	3–5	0.1	1–2
Cheese	30–40	0.2	2–4
Red meat (lean)	40–50	0.2–0.3	8–10
Red meat (fat)	10–15	0.1	< 0.5
Pork (lean)	20–30	0.1	3–5
Pork (fat)	4–5	< 0.1	< 0.5
Chicken	7–20	< 0.1	1–3
Fish	3–5	< 0.1	≈ 1

[a] B. Sandström, unpublished data.

approximately 10–12 mg or 1.0–1.2 mg zinc/MJ. However, a recent survey of over 2100 adults in the United Kingdom suggested a mean zinc intake of 9.7 ± 3.3 (SD) mg/day (34). A lower zinc intake of 7 mg/day has been reported for a fish-based diet typical of the Amazonas area of Brazil (35). Other low intakes of zinc have been reported for the population of Papua New Guinea, where the principal food sources are roots, tubers and leaves (36). Unrefined cereal- or legume-based diets can, on the other hand, have a higher zinc content. Analyses of Indian vegetarian diets suggest a typical zinc intake of 16 mg (1.4 mg/MJ per day) (37). Other data are considered in Chapter 22.

5.8 Physiological requirements

Requirements for dietary zinc are determined partly by the physiological processes governing tissue demands for zinc and its rate of loss from the body, and partly by the intrinsic characteristics of the diet, which influence the release of potentially absorbable forms of the element during digestion. In this section, the *physiological requirements* for absorbed zinc, both to meet demands for tissue growth and to replace regulated body losses, are considered.

The physiological responses apparently directed towards the maintenance of body zinc status when zinc intake begins to decline also provide the basis for differentiating between "basal" and "normative" requirements. Both are first considered in relation to the needs for *absorbed* zinc (i.e. as variable components of the *physiological requirement*). Section 5.9 deals with those factors which influence the fraction of dietary zinc that becomes available for absorption, and are thus taken into account in translating estimates of the *physiological requirements* for absorbed zinc into the quantities that must be consumed daily to meet the *basal requirements* and *normative requirements* for this element.

5.8.1 Adults

In the absence of adequate epidemiological evidence, the physiological requirement of adults for zinc has been estimated by a factorial technique, i.e. by adding together the requirements for tissue growth, maintenance, metabolism and endogenous losses. The principal problem has been to define the amount of zinc needed to replace obligatory endogenous losses in people adapted to low zinc intakes. Except in young rapidly growing subjects or those in whom zinc losses are enhanced as a consequence of stress or other challenges, it is notable that the activity of zinc-dependent processes can be maintained for several weeks after both the intake and the total absorption of zinc have declined. This is achieved by a means of a substantial reduction in endogenous losses. Extrapolation of data from balance studies carried out on adults introduced to very low zinc intakes (0.2–0.3 mg/day) indicated that initial faecal plus urinary losses of zinc were 0.9 mg/day for women (*19*) and 1.4 mg/day for men (*18*). However, after 4 weeks of negligible zinc intake, average faecal losses declined to 0.3 mg/day for women (*19*) and, after 4–9 weeks, 0.5 mg/day for men (*18*). Urinary zinc output, normally about 0.5 mg/day, decreases at low zinc intakes to less than 0.15 mg/day before a significant decline in serum zinc occurs (*18*). Semen zinc concentration also falls during zinc depletion from an initial value of 0.6 mg per ejaculation to 0.3 mg after prolonged depletion (*18*). A similar reduction has been observed for integumental losses in men. At an intake of 8.3 mg zinc/day, losses of 0.5 mg/day occurred. When zinc intake decreased to 3.4 mg/day, skin losses were approximately 0.3 mg/day after 3 weeks and 0.2 mg after 10 weeks. This decrease occurred even though plasma zinc remained within the normal range (*17*).

The tentative estimates of zinc losses summarized in Table 5.2 suggest that the average *physiological requirement* for absorbed zinc to ensure the maintenance of a metabolically available body-zinc pool in the fully adapted adult is approximately 1 mg/day for men and 0.7 mg/day for women (see Table 5.2).

Table 5.2. Tentative estimates of endogenous losses of zinc from adults adapted or unadapted to low intakes of zinc[a]

A. Before adaptation

Data used for estimates of *normative requirement*	Losses (mg/day)	
	Male	Female
Faecal loss	0.8	0.5
Urinary loss	0.3	0.3
Skin loss	0.3	0.2
Total	1.4	1.0

B. After adaptation

Data used for estimates of *basal requirement*	Male	Female
Faecal loss	0.5	0.3
Urinary loss	0.2	0.2
Skin loss	0.3	0.2
Total	1.0	0.7

[a] Derived principally from the data of references 18, 19 and 38.

The estimate for adult males does not include an allowance for zinc losses in semen.

It should be noted that the continued provision of zinc at a rate only just sufficient to meet these *basal physiological requirements* will fully exploit the potential to exercise homoeostatic control and minimize zinc losses, but will leave no "reserve potential" to adapt to further reductions in zinc intake by increasing the efficiency of zinc retention.

Observations made during the early phase of studies of zinc depletion have also been used to estimate the *normative physiological requirement* of adults for absorbed zinc. As indicated in Table 5.2, total losses of zinc in faeces and urine and from skin during zinc depletion can decrease by approximately 40% if subjects have had a previous opportunity to adapt to the low zinc intake. Data for unadapted clinically normal men receiving diets very low in zinc content indicated that faecal losses after 15 days depletion ranged from 0.55 to 1.1 mg of zinc/day (*38*); corresponding urinary losses were 0.03–1.1 mg/day. It is estimated that epidermal squames could have accounted for an additional 0.3 mg/day. A total of 1.4 mg of zinc must thus be absorbed daily to maintain zinc equilibrium, as compared with the 1.0 mg needed daily to replace losses after adaptation. In women, faecal losses of 0.29–0.59 mg/day and urinary losses of 0.06–0.61 mg/day were reported (*21*) after 11–13 days on a low zinc diet.

Since these differences in zinc loss between adapted and unadapted subjects presumably reflect a protective response to a potentially hazardous reduction of zinc intake, it is reasonable to use them as the basis for estimating normative requirements for zinc. The assumptions involved are justified by the absence of evidence of any alternative store of tissue zinc that can be used to buffer the effects of depletion. *On the basis of such arguments, the normative requirements for zinc has thus been set 40% higher than the basal requirement for all age groups.* For adult males, the estimate of the *normative physiological requirement* for *absorbed* zinc is 1.4 mg/day and for adult females 1.0 mg/day.

Experimental data to support these factorial estimates for adults are scarce. Reduced plasma zinc levels have been observed in a limited number of men on a dietary zinc intake of 4.8 mg/day from a semipurified diet based on soy protein and with a molar ratio of phytate to zinc of approximately 20 (*39*). If the efficiency of absorption from this type of diet is 15% (see Table 5.5 and Fig. 5.2, on pp. 93 and 90, respectively), the diet would yield 0.7 mg of absorbable zinc and thus, according to the above estimates, would be insufficient to cover the basal physiological requirement. In a study of women with an intake of 2.6 mg/day for 6 weeks from a diet low in zinc but containing no identified inhibitors of zinc absorption, circulating zinc levels and urinary zinc excretion were not affected (*18*). From the description of this diet and the criteria outlined in Table 5.5, it appears likely that 35–40% of its zinc would be absorbable, giving at least 0.9 mg of absorbed zinc; it would thus meet the basal physiological requirements for zinc.

5.8.2 Infants, children and adolescents

Endogenous losses at low zinc intakes were measured using stable isotopes in six milk-formula-fed infants ranging in age from 41 days to 244 days (40). This study confirmed the ability of infants to adapt to a lower zinc intake by decreasing faecal endogenous losses of zinc. At an intake of 1 mg/kg per day, endogenous faecal losses were 78 µg/kg per day and decreased to 34 µg/kg per day at an intake of 0.2 mg/kg per day. Urinary zinc losses did not change and were, on average, 25 µg/kg per day during each of the 11-day periods for which these diets were offered.

Data for endogenous losses at the different zinc intakes of other age groups are lacking. To estimate the physiological maintenance requirement for zinc of formula-fed infants, children and adolescents (Table 5.3), differences in basal metabolic rate (41) have been used as the basis for extrapolation from adult data. The derived estimates of endogenous losses of zinc in adults correspond to an average loss of 0.57 µg/basal kcal. In the context of our extrapolations, basal metabolic rate is seen as an indirect measure of lean body mass and body surface, both of which are closely related to zinc losses. The rationale for this approach is as follows:

— body surface can be assumed to be the principal determinant of integumental losses of zinc;
— intestinal length and therefore endogenous intestinal losses in the form of desquamated cells can be assumed to be related to body size;
— energy intake is assumed to influence the volume of intestinal digestive secretions and thus the endogenous losses of zinc in this form.

These assumptions are supported by evidence of sex differences in endogenous losses at very low intakes of zinc and by the substantially higher endogenous losses of zinc per kg of body weight in children with a proportionally higher metabolic rate than adults. The fact that such relationships have been used for the purposes of extrapolation should not be taken as implying the existence of a direct relationship between energy metabolism and zinc requirement.

Attention is also drawn to the possibility that endogenous zinc losses by infants, and thus their zinc requirements for maintenance, may be influenced significantly by the nature of their feed. Previous suggestions that the maintenance requirements of infants fed maternal milk may approximate to 20 µg/kg of body weight (42) rather than about 30 or more µg/kg in formula-fed infants of corresponding age (Table 5.3) appear increasingly plausible in the light of a

Table 5.3. Factorially derived estimates of the average physiological requirements of individuals for absorbed zinc[a]

Age (years)	Sex	Representative weight (kg)	μg/kg of body weight per day			
			Basal			Normative (total)
			Maintenance	Growth	Total	
0–0.25	F	5	40[b]	120	160	(224)[c]
0–0.25	M	5	40[b]	140	180	(252)[c]
0.25–0.5	M + F	7	28.6[b]	42.9	71.5	(100)[c]
0.5–1	F + M	9	33.3[b]	33.3	66.6	93.2
1–3	F + M	12	32.8	16.4	49.2	68.9
3–6	F + M	17	29.1	11.6	40.7	57.0
6–10	F + M	25	24.0	8.0	32.0	44.8
10–12	F	37	18.9	5.4	24.3	34.0
12–15	F	48	16.7	6.3	23.0	32.2
15–18	F	55	14.5	5.5	20.0	28.0
18–60 +	F	55	12.7	—	12.7	17.8
10–12	M	35	22.9	5.7	28.6	40.0
12–15	M	48	18.8	8.3	27.1	37.9
15–18	M	64	17.2	4.7	21.9	30.7
18–60 +	M	65	15.4	—	15.4	21.6

[a] These data take into account neither the absorbability of dietary zinc nor the variability of intake from one individual to another. See Table 5.6 for the dietary equivalents, Zn_R^{basal} or $Zn_R^{normative}$, and Table 5.7 for population minimum mean intakes to meet basal (Zn_{Plmin}^{basal}) or normative ($Zn_{Plmin}^{normative}$) requirements.

[b] The maintenance requirement is assumed to be 20 μg/kg for infants fed exclusively on maternal milk; see text. The total requirements should be amended accordingly.

[c] These specific estimates are probably of very limited applicability. The period 0–0.5 years of infant development is associated with a physiologically normal decline in hepatic zinc stores accumulated during late fetal growth (except in the premature infant). It is questionable whether the normative increments listed would serve any physiologically useful purpose in full-term infants, except where maternal zinc deficiency developed during pregnancy and fetal storage of zinc was thus precluded.

recent study (43). That the lower estimates of endogenous losses for breast-fed infants could be nutritionally significant is suggested by evidence that exclusive breast-feeding will increase the length of the period in which the zinc supply from maternal milk is sufficient to meet the zinc requirements of the infant. A maintenance requirement of 20 μg/kg has been assumed in deriving estimates of mean individual requirements of 0–12-month-old infants for absorbed zinc (Table 5.3) when they are consuming maternal milk (Table 5.6). An endogenous loss of 40 μg/kg has been assumed for other feeds. The maintenance requirements for zinc of infants offered formula feeds or mixed solid/liquid feeds are given in Table 5.3.

There is a marked increase in fetal hepatic zinc in the terminal stages of a normal pregnancy. Although this reserve is apparently used during the first 6 months of normal postnatal life of the infant, the rate at which the reserve declines has yet to be investigated adequately. This makes it particularly difficult to estimate the requirements of 0–0.5-year-old infants. It is questionable, for example, whether an attempt should be made to prevent such a physiologically normal decline in a tissue reserve by supplying additional absorbable zinc. However, the size of this reserve is greatly reduced by premature birth and is probably reduced if maternal zinc intake is inadequate during pregnancy. For all these reasons, indications of the likely magnitude of the "normative" physiological requirements of young infants in these specific situations are given in parentheses in Table 5.3.

5.8.3 Tissue growth

Normal growth

The data required in estimating the physiological requirement for the zinc needed for tissue growth are the net rate of accretion and the zinc content of the newly formed tissues. The estimated zinc increment for infant growth is about 175 μg/kg per day in the first month decreasing to about 30 μg/kg per day at 9–12 months (42). The pubertal growth spurt also increases the zinc requirement substantially; thus the accelerated growth of adolescent males is associated with a zinc increment of 0.5 mg/day. For age groups < 10 years, estimates of the physiological requirement for zinc for growth are based on the assumption that the increment of new tissue contains 30 μg of zinc/g. For adolescent growth, a zinc content of 23 μg per g increase in body weight has been assumed.

"Catch-up" growth

The remit of the Expert Consultation did not include estimates of requirements for recovery from previous periods of nutritional inadequacy. However, it is considered essential to emphasize that rapid catch-up growth during rehabilitation from malnutrition or infection must be expected to increase zinc requirements substantially. Failure to anticipate this has been shown to increase the risks that clinical signs and biochemical evidence of zinc deficiency will develop during rehabilitation from protein–energy malnutrition (44). The magnitude of the effect of accelerated growth on physiological requirements for absorbed zinc is illustrated by the following typical estimate.

Rehabilitation of a 12-month-old previously malnourished male child weighing 8.5 kg (5th weight centile of the WHO reference population (45)) can realistically achieve a weight of 10.4 kg (40th weight centile) in 2 months. The rate of tissue gain, 3.7 g/kg per day, incorporating approximately 30 μg zinc/g tissue would account for a growth increment of 111 μg zinc/kg of initial body weight per day. Adding the maintenance requirement for absorbed zinc of 33 μg/kg (from Table 5.3) gives a total requirement of the rehabilitating child for absorbed zinc of 144 μg/kg per day, which may be compared with 67 μg/kg per day for the normally growing child. The implications of this increment, which is modest compared with estimates recently derived from Caribbean studies of zinc metabolism during rehabilitation (44), are considered in the later discussion of dietary requirements.

5.8.4 Pregnancy

The total amount of zinc retained during pregnancy in the fetus, placental tissue, amniotic fluid, uterine and mammary tissue and maternal blood has been estimated to be 100 mg (46, 47). The physiological requirement for zinc during the three trimesters of pregnancy has been estimated from this value (Table 5.4). Animal studies suggest that the increased physiological demand for zinc during pregnancy is at least partially met by an increase in the efficiency of zinc absorption or a decrease in the endogenous loss of zinc. Whether such adaptive responses can occur in the human female is not known and no allowance has been made for them in estimates of dietary requirements during pregnancy.

5.8.5 Lactation

The zinc concentration in human milk falls during lactation from 2.5 μg/ml in the first month, to 0.9 μg/ml after 3 months, and to 0.7 μg/ml after 4 months (42).

It is estimated from data on maternal milk volume and zinc content (42, 48, 49) during the period 0–3 months postpartum that the daily output of zinc by this route, on average, could amount to 1.4 mg/day. This amount, as compared with the basal requirements of the individual non-pregnant (say, 55-kg) adult woman for 0.7 mg absorbed zinc daily, would substantially increase the requirement for absorbed zinc during early lactation. The corresponding effect of lactation on minimum acceptable mean population intakes of dietary zinc (Zn_{Plmin}^{basal}) would be to increase the value from 4 mg/day to 9 mg/day if dietary zinc is moderately available (Tables 5.7 & 5.8, pages 96 & 97). Any suggestion that such an increase in population mean intakes of zinc in a reasonably available form is essential to reduce the risks of development of zinc deficiency at this time is not supported by direct evidence. Failure to achieve

Table 5.4. Factorially derived estimates of physiological requirements for absorbed zinc (mg/day) during pregnancy and lactation[a]

A. Average individual physiological requirement for pregnancy (mg/day)

Duration of pregnancy	Basal			Normative
	Maintenance	Growth	Total	Total
First trimester	0.7	0.1	0.8	1.1
Second trimester	0.7	0.3	1.0	1.4
Third trimester	0.7	0.7	1.4	2.0

B. Average individual physiological requirement for lactation (mg/day)

Duration of lactation	Basal				Normative			
	For maintenance	For lactation	Amount obtained from endogenous sources	Total	For maintenance	For lactation	Amount obtained from endogenous sources	Total
0–3 months	0.7	1.4[b]	0.5[c]	1.6	1.0	1.4[b]	0.5[c]	1.9
3–6 months	0.7	0.8[b]	—	1.5	1.0	0.8[b]	—	1.8
6–12 months	0.7	0.5[b]	—	1.2	1.0	0.5[b]	—	1.5

[a] These data take into account neither differences in the absorbability of dietary zinc nor the variability of intake from one population to another. See Table 5.8 for lower limits of population mean intakes of dietary zinc to meet Zn_{Pimin}^{basal} and $Zn_{Pimin}^{normative}$ for diets differing in zinc bioavailability.

[b] Increment for lactation estimated from yield and zinc content of breast milk of normal lactating women (42, 48, 49). It is unlikely to change significantly with a modest increase in zinc intake to meet the normative requirement.

[c] Derived from the estimated redistribution of tissue zinc from postnatal skeletal resorption and from involution of uterine tissue during the first 3 months of lactation only (see p. 87)

86

such a marked increase in the voluntary intake of zinc during lactation has not, so far, been associated epidemiologically with an increased frequency of zinc-responsive disorders nor is there consistent evidence that milk zinc content is particularly sensitive to modest changes in dietary zinc content (50).

Studies with laboratory rats indicate that dietary zinc is utilized more efficiently by the lactating female (51). However, no such effect of lactation has been detected in human females nor is there consistent evidence of a significant decline in endogenous losses of zinc during lactation. The apparent paradox of a marked increase in physiological demands for zinc with no consistent evidence of an increased susceptibility to deficiency during early lactation may arise because of a systemic redistribution of tissue zinc during postnatal readaptation to the non-pregnant state. This zinc could originate partly from postnatal involution of the uterus during the first 2 months postpartum and partly from the skeletal mineral matrix, which resorbs during the first 3 months postpartum to meet high lactational requirements for calcium. It is estimated that 970 g of uterine tissue (46) containing typically 25 µg of zinc/g fresh tissue (52) resorbs during this period and could thus liberate up to 0.27 mg of zinc daily. At the same time, skeletal resorption, variously reported to amount to 2% (53), 3% (54) or 4.5% (A Caid, personal communication, 1993) of a skeleton typically containing, overall, 770 mg of zinc (55), could also yield at least 0.23 mg of zinc daily. It is known that zinc liberated from skeletal sources can be utilized physiologically and, since there is no evidence of increased urinary and faecal losses of zinc at this time, it is assumed that the zinc liberated from the involuting uterus in addition to that from the resorbing skeleton might contribute at least 0.5 mg of zinc daily to the demand for lactation during the period 0–3 months postpartum. While this possibility has yet to be verified, it has been taken into account in provisionally estimating demands for zinc at this time (Tables 5.4 and 5.8). Such considerations would not influence requirements for zinc after 3 months postpartum.

In the absence of any evidence that milk zinc output is influenced significantly by typical dietary variations in maternal zinc intake, it has been assumed that diets with zinc contents that just meet the basal or normative requirement will not differ in their influence on the zinc content of maternal milk. Estimates of mean basal and normative requirements of individuals for absorbed zinc during lactation have been given in Table 5.4.

5.9 Dietary requirements

5.9.1 Bioavailability of dietary zinc

Factorially based estimates of average *basal* and *normative physiological requirements* of individuals for *absorbed* zinc have been given in Tables 5.3 and

5.4. The translation of such estimates into requirements for dietary zinc involves the consideration of important variables governing the efficiency with which dietary zinc is absorbed. Firstly, the potential value of the dietary zinc consumed is influenced by the chemical and physical properties of the zinc in foods, its release into the gastrointestinal lumen and the extent of its interactions with other constituents of digesta. All these interacting factors govern the yield of zinc in forms which are soluble and potentially absorbable. Secondly, the evidence derived from a variety of species, including humans, indicates that the efficiency of absorption of these potentially available forms of zinc is inversely related to the dietary intake of zinc and the extent to which this saturates receptors involved in the intestinal transport and tissue uptake of the element.

Such findings imply that the fate of dietary zinc is governed not only by the intrinsic characteristics of the diet but also by physiological variables. Both must therefore be taken into account in deriving corresponding estimates of dietary zinc requirements. Except when the chemical and physical nature of the diet restricts zinc release, it must also be anticipated that the efficiency of zinc utilization at the relatively low intakes of the element needed to meet *basal* and *normative* requirements may often be substantially higher than is typical for many normal populations ingesting substantially greater quantities of zinc.

Much more information is needed to define the independent influence of these two important variables governing the efficiency with which zinc is absorbed. However, their quantitative effects have been tentatively assessed by comparing data describing dose–absorption relationships for zinc in studies monitoring the fate of zinc from a range of isotopically labelled daily intakes from sources that appear likely, from compositional evidence, to differ markedly in their bioavailability. The characterization of diets and foods likely to be associated with a high, intermediate, or low bioavailability of zinc has also drawn on evidence from studies on other, non-human species.

Data pooled from 12 sets of studies indicate that logarithmic relationships exist between the total daily intake of isotopically labelled zinc from highly available dietary sources and the quantity of zinc absorbed therefrom. Data for situations in which diets contained no known inhibitors of zinc absorption are illustrated in Fig. 5.1. These data, replotted as curve A in Fig. 5.2, illustrate the dose- and status-dependent relationship between zinc intake and absorption even for zinc sources of similar characteristics. The use of such information to derive bioavailability "factors" appropriate for the definition of *basal* and *normative* requirements when dietary zinc is derived from sources of high, intermediate and low availability is described in the following example.

It can be calculated from Table 5.3 that the individual average *basal physiological* requirement for *absorbed* zinc of a 65-kg adult man is approxim-

Figure 5.1. Relationships between dietary zinc intake (mg/day) and zinc absorption (mg/day) derived from total-diet studies with stable zinc isotopes and diets not containing any significant inhibitors of zinc absorption (category A, Table 5.5)

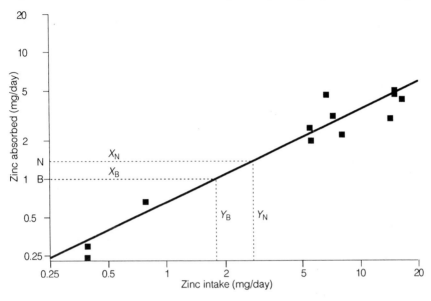

WHO 94658

Note $\log_{10}$ scales of intake and absorption. Intakes and absorptions meeting individual *basal* and *normative* requirements for 65-kg adult males are designated B or N respectively. Availabilities of zinc at intakes meeting *basal* or *normative* requirements are derived from X_B/Y_B or X_N/Y_N respectively.

ately 1 mg/day; the *normative* requirement is approximately 1.4 mg/day. The data of Fig. 5.1 (and thus of Fig. 5.2, curve A) show that, when dietary zinc is highly available, the intake likely to promote absorption of 1 mg of zinc/day must be approximately 1.8 mg/day, corresponding to an efficiency of utilization of 56%. Similar evidence indicates that an intake of 2.8 mg of highly available zinc would just meet the *normative physiological* requirement for 1.4 mg of absorbed zinc, corresponding to an efficiency of utilization of 50%.

Similar arguments were used to define the absorptive efficiencies obtained when diets contained modest dietary concentrations of inhibitors of zinc absorption, such as the phytate of many vegetable protein sources and cereal grains (Table 5.5, category B). However, in these instances, it was necessary to pool data derived from two different types of study, namely the small number of studies in which the total diet was labelled with isotopic zinc and the large number in which an isotopically labelled single meal or individual food was

Figure 5.2. Predicted fractional absorption (%) by 65-kg men of dietary zinc derived from diets in which zinc is highly available (category A), moderately available (category B) or poorly available (category C)

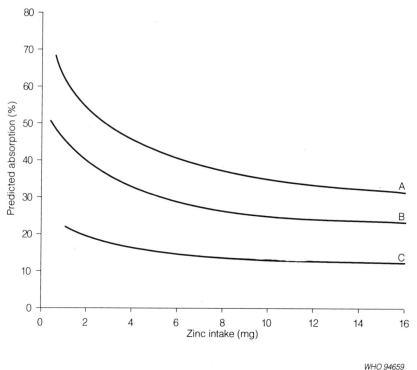

WHO 94659

For information on diets see Table 5.5. Curve A is based on the data of Fig. 5.1. Curves B and C are obtained from adjusted data derived from single-meal isotopic studies of diets of categories B and C.

administered. Once these differences in experimental technique were taken into account, curve B in Fig. 5.2 was drawn for relationships between zinc intake and absorption for diets with zinc in moderately available forms and with phytate/zinc molar ratios ranging between 5 and 15.

Because of a great scarcity of data derived from "total-diet" studies, much less confidence can be attached to the estimates of the bioavailability of zinc from diets very rich in antagonists of zinc absorption, most of which will have phytate/zinc molar ratios above 15 (curve C in Fig. 5.2). For such diets and staple foods, the relationships between log intake and log absorption differ profoundly, are much less influenced by intake, and suggest a much lower efficiency of absorption even when total zinc intake declines. However, the Expert Consultation was confident that the 15% availability suggested for category C foods and diets is not an underestimate. Indeed, several studies of zinc absorption from single meals, either of whole cereal grains or flours rich in phytate or vegetable protein sources with phytate/zinc ratios > 25, indicate the possibility that zinc availability from such foods can decline to 10% or less. Evidence, firstly, that phytate-rich staple foods can increase the phytate/zinc ratios of Moroccan total diets to 33–45 (56), and secondly that a ratio of 27 : 1 can reduce the zinc status of 4–6-year-old infants (57) emphasizes the importance of seeking evidence that the deficits in available zinc supply associated with such dietary regimens may have pathological significance.

The criteria used to discriminate between diets likely to promote high availability of zinc (category A diets), normal availability (category B) or low availability (category C) are summarized in Table 5.5. Preferred estimates of bioavailability at *the intakes adequate to meet the basal and normative requirements for absorbed zinc* (Table 5.3) when the three categories of diet are consumed by the average individual are as follows:

	Bioavailability factor at:	
Diet category	*Basal requirement*	*Normative requirement*
A	55%	50%
B	35%	30%
C	15%	15%

It must be appreciated that the validity of these particular bioavailability estimates is restricted specifically to circumstances that permit absorption of the quantity of zinc just sufficient to meet *basal* or *normative* requirements. Although derived predominantly from experimental data obtained from studies with men and non-pregnant women, the scarcity of appropriate isotopic studies on other categories of subject led the Expert Consultation to suggest that they should be applied to all diets based principally on solid foods until evidence to the contrary is forthcoming. The bioavailability of zinc from maternal milk and other liquid feeds for infants is considered later. With the exception of infants given maternal milk, an approximate indication of bioavailability for categories of subjects other than the adult male may be derived from Fig. 5.2 by modifying the existing scale of units of intake (x_0) as follows:

$$\log x_1 = \log x_0 + \log R_1 - \log R_0$$

i.e. by the ratio of the individual basal or normative physiological requirements of the subject category of interest (R_1) to the corresponding requirements of 65-kg adult males (R_0).

5.9.2 Infants consuming maternal milk or formula feeds

Data on zinc absorption by infants are scarce. Furthermore, in estimating their zinc requirements, it has not been possible to take into account evidence that prenatally accumulated hepatic zinc stores may be redistributed systemically during early infancy and thus confer a brief period of protection against a low intake.

Although the bioavailability of zinc from maternal milk is known to be high, quantitative data are lacking. It has been assumed provisionally that the breast-fed infant absorbs up to 80%. This assumption, coupled with data on the zinc content and daily consumption of maternal milk, results in estimates of the yield of potentially available zinc that are compatible with factorially based estimates of daily basal requirements for the first six months of infant life. For example, Vuori (49) reports median daily intakes of zinc from breast milk at 1, 2 and 3 months postpartum of 440, 250 and 150 μg/kg for male and 250, 190 and 140 μg/kg for female infants which, if 80% is absorbed, would suffice to meet their physiological requirements for absorbable zinc (Table 5.3).

To estimate the lowest acceptable population mean intakes ($Zn_{\text{PImin}}^{\text{basal}}$) for infants up to 6 months of age, it has been assumed that the coefficient of variation (CV) of breast-milk zinc intakes is 12.5% (derived from reference 49); an identical CV has been adopted for liquid formula milks for the same age range, after which a CV of 25% has been assumed (Table 5.7, page 96).

Table 5.5. Provisional criteria for categorizing diets according to the potential availability of their zinc

Nominal category	Principal dietary characteristics
A. High availability	(i) Refined diets low in cereal fibre, low in phytic acid content and with phytate/zinc (molar) ratio < 5; adequate protein content principally from non-vegetable sources, such as meats, fish.
	(ii) Includes semisynthetic formula diets based on animal protein.
B. Moderate availability	(i) Mixed diets containing animal or fish protein.
	(ii) Lacto-ovo, ovovegetarian or vegan diets *not* based primarily on unrefined cereal grains or high-extraction-rate flours.
	(iii) Phytate/zinc molar ratio of total diet within the range 5–15 or not exceeding 10 if more than 50% of the energy intake is accounted for by un-fermented, unrefined cereal grains and flours while the diet is fortified with inorganic calcium salts (> 1 g Ca^{2+}/day).
	(iv) Availability of zinc in category B foods improves when the diet includes animal or protein sources or milks.

Table 5.5 (continued)

Nominal category	Principal dietary characteristics
C. Low availability	(i) Diets high in unrefined, unfermented and un-germinated cereal grain,[a] especially when fortified with inorganic calcium salts and when intake of animal protein is negligible.
	(ii) Phytate/zinc molar ratio of total diet exceeding 15.[b]
	(iii) High-phytate soya-protein products constitute the primary protein source.
	(iv) Diets in which, singly or collectively, approximately 50% of the energy intake is accounted for by the following high-phytate foods: high-extraction-rate (90% +) wheat, rice, maize grains and flours, oatmeal, millet; chapatti flours and "tanok"; sorghum; cowpeas; pigeon peas; grams; kidney beans; blackeye beans; groundnut flours.
	(v) High intakes of inorganic calcium salts (>1 g Ca^{2+}/day), either as supplements or as adventitious contaminants (e.g. from calcareous geophagia), potentiate the inhibitory effects of category C diets; low intakes of animal protein exacerbate these effects.

[a] Germination of many of such grains or fermentation (e.g. leavening) of many flours can reduce antagonistic potency; the diet should then be reallocated to category B.
[b] Vegetable diets with phytate/zinc ratios exceeding 30 are not unknown; for such diets, an assumption of 10% availability of zinc or less may be justified, especially if the protein intake is low and/or that of calcium salts is excessive, e.g. > 1.5 g Ca^{2+} per day.

In contrast to the bioavailability estimate of 80% for the zinc of maternal milk, category B availability, namely 30–35% (Tables 5.3, 5.5 and 5.8), has been assumed for the zinc of infant formulae based on whey-adjusted cow's milk and for the zinc intake of infants not exclusively breast-fed. Category C availability is probably applicable to the zinc of phytate-rich vegetable-protein-based formulae and to weaning foods based on non-fermented whole-grain cereals. As for adults, the fractional absorption of zinc by infants is inversely related to zinc intake. A typical study showed that 16.8% of the zinc was absorbed from a high-zinc formula (1081 µg/kg per day), as compared with 41.1% from a low-zinc formula (237 µg/kg per day) (40). In the light of such evidence, it was considered valid to apply to infants the same bioavailability factors for diet categories B and C that were used to derive the basal and normative requirements of adults.

5.9.3 Estimation of individual requirements

Estimates of *individual* requirements for zinc for subjects consuming diets of categories A, B and C are shown as $\mu g/kg$ of body weight per day of dietary zinc for infants, children and adults in Table 5.6.

5.9.4 Estimation of population requirements

Estimates are given in Tables 5.7 and 5.8 of the lower limits of the *safe ranges of population mean intakes* of zinc for all age ranges and during pregnancy and lactation, respectively, to meet *basal* $(Zn_{\text{PImin}}^{\text{basal}})$ and *normative* $(Zn_{\text{PImin}}^{\text{normative}})$ requirements for zinc under conditions in which populations consume diets of categories A, B or C when the CV of intake is either 25% (for solid diets) or 12.5% (for formula feeds or maternal milk).

5.9.5 Implications and limitations of requirement estimates

The estimates of zinc requirement (Tables 5.6, 5.7 and 5.8) and the proposed criteria for identifying diets differing in their effects on zinc availability must be regarded as provisional until they have been appraised more fully by experimentation or by epidemiological study. Even so, specific features are already of interest or concern.

Recent data (*48, 49*) on the output of zinc in maternal milk indicate that this is fully adequate to meet infant basal requirements for zinc $(Zn_{\text{PImin}}^{\text{basal}})$ up to 6 months of age. However, the estimates of the requirement between 6 and 12 months suggest that the declining daily output of zinc in milk, typically 0.6–0.4 mg/day during this period, will be insufficient to meet infant demands for zinc if maternal milk is the sole source. Unless the increment in the zinc normally incorporated into the tissue of growing infants or their maintenance requirements (Table 5.3) have been seriously overestimated, these estimates indicate a risk that zinc could be one of possibly several nutrients limiting the rate of growth of infants maintained solely on breast milk after 5–6 months of age. The dramatic increases in individual mean and minimum population mean estimates of requirement when infant formulae are based on constituents that reduce the availability of zinc are evident in Tables 5.6 and 5.7. For the reasons indicated on pp. 83–84, estimates of $Zn_{\text{PImin}}^{\text{normative}}$ have not been tabulated for infants less than 6 months of age. Such specific estimates might be appropriate for use only in circumstances where the infant has been born prematurely or exposure to a low maternal intake of zinc during the late stages of intrauterine growth has prevented accumulation of a hepatic reserve of zinc by the fetus. Only for such infants is it suggested, tentatively, that the average individual requirement $(Zn_{\text{R}}^{\text{normative}})$ might decline during the first 6 months from 790 to

Table 5.6. Average individual basal (Zn_R^basal) and normative (Zn_R^normative) requirements for zinc (µg/kg of body weight per day) from diets differing in zinc bioavailability[a]

Age range (years)	Sex	A. High availability		B. Moderate availability		C. Low availability	
		Zn_R^basal[b]	Zn_R^normative[c]	Zn_R^basal[d]	Zn_R^normative[e]	Zn_R^basal[f]	Zn_R^normative[f]
0–0.25	F	175[g]	—	457[h]	—	1067[i]	—
0–0.25	M	200[g]	—	514[h]	—	1200[i]	—
0.25–0.5	M&F	79[g]	—	204[h]	—	477[i]	—
0.5–1	M&F	66[g]	—	—	—	—	—
0.5–1	M&F	121	186	190	311	444	621
1–3	M&F	89	138	141	230	328	459
3–6	M&F	74	114	116	190	271	380
6–10	M&F	58	90	91	149	213	299
10–12	F	44	68	69	113	162	227
12–15	F	42	64	66	107	153	215
15–18	F	36	56	57	93	133	187
18–60 +	F	23	36	36	59	85	119
10–12	M	52	80	82	133	191	267
12–15	M	49	76	77	126	181	253
15–18	M	40	61	63	102	146	205
18–60 +	M	28	43	44	72	103	144

a For information on diets, see Table 5.5.
b Assumed bioavailability of dietary zinc 55%.
c Assumed bioavailability of dietary zinc 50%.
d Assumed bioavailability of dietary zinc 35%.
e Assumed bioavailability of dietary zinc 30%.
f Assumed bioavailability of dietary zinc 15%.
g Applicable exclusively to infants fed maternal milk alone for which the bioavailability of zinc is assumed to be 80% and infant endogenous loss 20 µg/kg.
h Applicable to infants partly breast-fed or fed whey-adjusted cow's milk formula or milk plus low-phytate solids.
i Applicable to infants receiving phytate-rich vegetable-protein-based infant formulae with or without whole-grain cereals.
j See Table 5.3, pages 83–84 and section 5.9.5.

Table 5.7. Lower limits (mg/day) of the safe ranges of population mean intakes of dietary zinc (in mg dietary zinc/day) to meet the requirements for Zn_{Plmin}^{basal} and $Zn_{Plmin}^{normative}$ from diets differing in zinc bioavailability[a]

Age range (years)	Sex	Assumed weight (kg)	A. High availability		B. Moderate availability		C. Low availability	
			Zn_{Plmin}^{basal}	$Zn_{Plmin}^{normative}$	Zn_{Plmin}^{basal}	$Zn_{Plmin}^{normative}$	Zn_{Plmin}^{basal}	$Zn_{Plmin}^{normative}$
0–0.25	F	5	1.2[b]	—	3.1[c]	—[d]	7.1[e]	—[d]
0–0.25	M	5	1.3[b]	—	3.4[c]		8.0[e]	
0.25–0.5	M&F	7	0.7[b]	—	1.9[c]		4.7[e]	
0.5–1	M&F	9	0.8[b]	—	—	—	—	—
0.5–1	M&F	9	2.2[f]	3.3[f]	3.4	5.6	8.0	11.1
1–3	M&F	12	2.1	3.3	3.4	5.5	7.9	11.0
3–6	M&F	17	2.5	3.9	3.9	6.5	9.2	12.9
6–10	M&F	25	2.9	4.5	4.6	7.5	10.7	15.0
10–12	F	37	3.3	5.0	5.1	8.4	12.0	16.8
12–15	F	48	4.0	6.1	6.3	10.3	14.7	20.6
15–18	F	55	4.0	6.2	6.3	10.2	14.6	20.6
18–60+	F	55	2.5	4.0	4.0	6.5	9.4	13.1
10–12	M	35	3.6	5.6	5.7	9.3	13.4	18.7
12–15	M	48	4.7	7.3	7.4	12.1	17.4	24.3
15–18	M	64	5.1	7.8	8.1	13.1	18.7	26.2
18–60+	M	65	3.6	5.6	5.7	9.4	13.4	18.7

a For information on diets, see Table 5.5. Unless otherwise specified, the CV of usual dietary zinc intakes is assumed to be 25%.

b Breast-fed infants receiving maternal milk only; assumed CV of intake 12.5%; assumed availability 80%.

c Formula-fed infants; category B availability for whey-adjusted milk formulae and for infants partly breast-fed or given low-phytate feeds supplemented with other liquid milks; assumed CV 12.5%.

d See text, section 5.9.5.

e Formula-fed infants; category C availability applicable to phytate-rich vegetable-protein-based formulae with or without whole-grain cereals; CV 12.5%.

f Not applicable to infants consuming breast milk only.

Table 5.8. *Lower limits (mg/day) of the safe ranges of population mean intakes of dietary zinc to meet requirements for Zn_{Plmin}^{basal} and $Zn_{Plmin}^{normative}$ during pregnancy and lactation[a]*

Stage	A. High availability		B. Moderate availability		C. Low availability	
	Zn_{Plmin}^{basal}	$Zn_{Plmin}^{normative}$	Zn_{Plmin}^{basal}	$Zn_{Plmin}^{normative}$	Zn_{Plmin}^{basal}	$Zn_{Plmin}^{normative}$
Pregnancy:						
First trimester	2.9	4.4	4.6	7.3	10.7	14.7
Second trimester	3.6	5.6	5.7	9.3	13.3	18.7
Third trimester	5.1	8.0	8.0	13.3	18.7	26.7
Lactation:						
0–3 months	5.8	7.6	9.1	12.7	21.3	25.3
3–6 months	5.3	7.0	8.4	11.7	19.6	23.3
6–12 months	4.2	5.8	6.6	9.6	15.5	19.2

[a] For information on diets, see Table 5.5; the CV of usual dietary zinc intakes is assumed to be 25%.

330 μg/kg per day when the formula offered has category B zinc availability and from 1580 to 660 μg/kg per day for a category C formula.

The proposed lower limits of population mean intakes of zinc to meet *basal* requirements (Zn_{Plmin}^{basal}) when dietary zinc is absorbed with only 15% efficiency (category C) are close to the intakes described for rural areas of Egypt and the Islamic Republic of Iran and where zinc-responsive growth failure in adolescents has been observed (*15, 16, 58, 59*). Diets of this type, relatively rich in zinc-binding ligands, may also increase the physiological requirements for zinc by trapping the zinc of intestinal secretions, preventing its reabsorption and thus increasing its loss in faeces (*33*). No allowance for this possibility has been made in estimating requirements. The proposed Zn_{Plmin}^{basal} for a category C diet is also applicable to many rural African populations. A dietary survey of children in Malawi showed that zinc intake ranged between 6 and 8 mg/day depending on the season. It was calculated that the phytate content of the cereal-based diet in this area was close to 300 mg/MJ and that the phytate/zinc molar ratio was 27, thus justifying the application of category C estimates (*57*). Over half the children were severely stunted and many showed low hair zinc concentrations, suggesting that growth impairment could have been attributable to a low zinc status of dietary origin. In the light of these observations, the proposed minimum population mean intakes appear realistic.

Catch-up growth of infants and children undergoing rehabilitation markedly increases their zinc requirement. It can readily be calculated from the example given on pp. 84–85 and from the data of Table 5.6 that their zinc requirement would increase more than two-fold *even if it is assumed that rehabilitation implies a transition from diets of moderate zinc availability (category B) to therapeutic diets with highly available zinc (category A)*.

The estimates of requirements derived for category B diets are widely applicable. They are frequently appropriate when, for example, data on dietary composition are scarce but there are no reasons to suspect the presence of significant concentrations of inhibitors of zinc absorption. The zinc content of the food sources and the total energy intakes of the individuals or population will determine whether diets of this category meet basal requirements. Zinc-responsive growth failure in Bangladeshi children has been described in subjects receiving diets of this type providing only 3.7 mg of zinc/day while undergoing rehabilitation from malnutrition (*3*).

Data on the zinc intakes of specific groups of individuals from a wide range of countries have now been presented in many reports on dietary surveys. However, only in a few of these studies have sufficient details of dietary composition been given to enable the content of promoters or inhibitors of zinc absorption to be assessed. This frequently precludes the reliable prediction of zinc bioavailability from the diets in question and its influence on zinc requirements. The effect of this situation on the interpretation of data from an international series of dietary surveys is considered in Chapter 22.

5.10 Upper limits of intakes

The proposed upper limits to the safe range of population mean intake of zinc ($Zn_{\text{Plmax}}^{\text{tox}}$) (see Table 5.9) have been defined as those at which the increase in tissue zinc ultimately disturbs the metabolism of other nutrients. The limited human data available indicate that clinically detectable changes or functional impairments can occur at an average zinc intake of 150 mg/day or more. Interactions with other nutrients influencing their absorption and utilization have been detected biochemically at total zinc intakes as low as 60 mg/day when zinc was given in the form of a supplement to a diet that, it is reasonable to assume, already provided 10 mg of zinc/day.

The intakes of those nutrients with which zinc interacts metabolically must also be considered. The risks of pathological consequences from such zinc-related interactions are higher if the intake of essential nutrients with which zinc interacts is low or marginal and the element imbalance is thus accentuated (see Chapter 3). To ensure that very few individuals in a population have an intake of zinc of 60 mg or higher, the Expert Consultation recommended that the adult population mean intake should not exceed 45 mg if a 20% variation in intake is assumed. This figure has been extrapolated to other age and sex groups by using

Table 5.9. Upper limits of the safe ranges of population mean intakes of zinc

Age range (years)	Sex	Weight (kg)	$Zn_{\text{Plmax}}^{\text{tox}}$ (mg/day)
0.5–1	F + M	9	13
1–6	F + M	16	23
6–10	F + M	25	28
10–12	F	37	32
12–15	F	48	36
15–18	F	55	38
18–60 +	F	55	35
10–12	M	35	34
12–15	M	48	40
15–18	M	64	48
18–60 +	M	65	45
Pregnancy and lactation			35

differences in basal metabolic rate. With the possible exception of occasions when the consumption of oysters is excessive, such intakes of zinc are unlikely to be attained with most diets. Adventitious zinc in water from contaminated wells and from newly galvanized cooking utensils could also lead to such high intakes. The manner in which a zinc supplement is given influences the extent to which it is tolerated. Retention of adventitious zinc is usually higher when it is taken in solution, in the fasted state or with liquid food (see Chapter 3). Such circumstances tend to increase the antagonistic effects of high zinc levels on the absorption of other nutrients. In contrast, the retention of high intakes of supplementary zinc consumed simultaneously with food can be markedly influenced by dietary factors known to restrict zinc absorption. There are insufficient data to enable the safe upper levels of zinc intake for different types of diet to be estimated.

5.11 Recommendations for future studies

The estimates of zinc requirements given in this report should be regarded as provisional. If correct, they suggest that a suboptimal supply of available dietary zinc may be much more prevalent than currently appreciated, particularly in rural communities in developing countries. The following recommendations were therefore made:

- Every opportunity should be taken to assess the validity of these estimates and particularly those for children at stages of development at which growth would normally be most rapid.
- There is an urgent need to characterize the early functional effects of zinc deficiency and to define their relationship to clinical and covert pathological changes. This information is needed both for diagnostic purposes and to provide pathologically relevant indicators of changes in zinc status for use during investigations of zinc requirements and bioavailability. The need for a better understanding of the functional roles of zinc is emphasized so as to be able to determine the significance of zinc deficiency in the etiology of stunting and the failure of immunocompetence.
- It is recognized that factors modifying the bioavailability of dietary zinc probably have a major influence on the risk that pathological effects of zinc deficiency may occur. However, many more quantitative data are needed before the influence of dietary composition on the efficiency of zinc utilization can be reliably predicted. Investigations should centre initially on the staple foods and diets of disadvantaged communities in many of the developing countries.

● Metabolic studies of the processes controlling the absorption, retention and endogenous loss of zinc and of variables influencing the ability to adapt to a low zinc intake are needed to determine the extent and physiological costs of such adaptation. Such investigations should cover periods such as early lactation and catch-up growth during rehabilitation, when the partition of zinc between tissues undergoing catabolism and anabolism obviously influences its physiological availability.

References

1. Hambidge KM. Zinc. In: Mertz W, ed. *Trace elements in human and animal nutrition*, 5th ed., Vol. 1. San Diego, FL, Academic Press, 1987: 1–137.
2. Simmer K et al. Nutritional rehabilitation in Bangladesh—the importance of zinc. *American journal of clinical nutrition*, 1988, **47**: 1036–1040.
3. Walravens PA, Hambidge KM, Koepfer DM. Zinc supplementation in infants with a nutritional pattern of failure to thrive: a double-blind, controlled study. *Pediatrics*, 1989, **83**: 532–538.
4. Walravens PA, Krebs NF, Hambidge KM. Linear growth of low income preschool children receiving a zinc supplement. *American journal of clinical nutrition*, 1983, **38**: 195–201.
5. Prasad AS et al. Serum thymulin in human zinc deficiency. *Journal of clinical investigation*, 1988, **82**: 1202–1210.
6. Mills CF, ed. *Zinc in human biology*, Berlin, Springer-Verlag, 1989 (ILSI Human Nutrition Reviews).
7. Fischer PWF, Giroux A, L'Abbé MR. Effect of zinc supplementation on copper status in adult man. *American journal of clinical nutrition*, 1984, **40**: 743–746.
8. Yadrick MK, Kenney MA, Winterfeldt EA. Iron, copper, and zinc status: response to supplementation with zinc or zinc and iron in adult females. *American journal of clinical nutrition*, 1989, **49**: 145–150.
9. Patterson WP, Winkelmann M, Perry MC. Zinc-induced copper deficiency: megamineral sideroblastic anemia. *Annals of internal medicine*, 1985, **103**: 385–386.
10. Porter KG et al. Anaemia and low serum-copper during zinc therapy. *Lancet*, 1977, **ii**: 774.
11. Hooper PL. Zinc lowers high-density lipoprotein-cholesterol levels. *Journal of the American Medical Association*, 1980, **244**: 1960–1962.
12. Chandra RK. Excessive intake of zinc impairs immune responses. *Journal of the American Medical Association*, 1984, **252**: 1443–1446.
13. Hambidge KM, Krebs NF, Walravens PA. Growth velocity of young children receiving a dietary zinc supplement. *Nutrition research*, 1985, **1**: 306–316.
14. Gibson RS et al. A growth-limiting, mild zinc-deficiency syndrome in some Southern Ontario boys with low height percentiles. *American journal of clinical nutrition*, 1989, **49**: 1266–1273.
15. Sandstead HH et al. Human zinc deficiency, endocrine manifestations, and response to treatment. *American journal of clinical nutrition*, 1967, **20**: 422–442.

16. Halsted JA et al. Zinc deficiency in man: the Shiraz experiment. *American journal of medicine*, 1972, **53**: 277–284.

17. Lukaski HC et al. Changes in plasma zinc content after exercise in men fed a low-zinc diet. *American journal of physiology*, 1984, **247**: E88–93.

18. Milne DB et al. Ethanol metabolism in postmenopausal women fed a diet marginal in zinc. *American journal of clinical nutrition*, 1987, **46**: 688–693.

19. Milne DB et al. Effect of dietary zinc on whole body surface loss of zinc: impact on estimation of zinc retention by balance method. *American journal of clinical nutrition*, 1983, **38**: 181–186.

20. Baer MJ, King JC. Tissue zinc levels and zinc excretion during experimental zinc depletion in young men. *American journal of clinical nutrition*, 1984, **39**: 556–570.

21. Hess FM, King JC, Margen S. Zinc excretion in young women on low zinc intakes and oral contraceptive agents. *Journal of nutrition*, 1977, **107**: 1610–1620.

22. Lee HH et al. Zinc absorption in human small intestine. *American journal of physiology*, 1989, **256**: G87–G91.

23. Sandström B et al. Retention of zinc and calcium from the human colon. *American journal of clinical nutrition*, 1986, **44**: 501–504.

24. O'Dell BL, Savage JE. Effect of phytate on zinc availability. *Proceedings of the Society of Experimental Biology and Medicine*, 1960, **103**: 304–309.

25. Oberleas D, Muhrer ME, O'Dell BL. Some effects of phytic acid on zinc availability and parakeratosis in swine. *Journal of animal science*, 1962, **21**: 57–61.

26. Turnlund JR et al. A stable isotope study of zinc absorption in young men: effects of phytate and α-cellulose. *American journal of clinical nutrition*, 1984, **40**: 1071–1077.

27. Lönnerdal B et al. The effect of individual components of soy formula and cow's milk formula on zinc bioavailability. *American journal of clinical nutrition*, 1984, **40**: 1064–1070.

28. Nävert B, Sandström B, Cederblad Å. Reduction of the phytate content of bran by leavening in bread and its effect on absorption of zinc in man. *British journal of nutrition*, 1985, **53**: 47–53.

29. Sandström B et al. Zinc absorption from composite meals. I. The significance of wheat extraction rate, zinc, calcium and protein content in meals based on bread. *American journal of clinical nutrition*, 1980, **33**: 739–745.

30. Sandström B, Cederblad Å, Lönnerdal B. Zinc absorption from human milk, cow's milk and infant formulas. *American journal of diseases of children*, 1983, **137**: 726–729.

31. Sandström B et al. Effect of protein level and protein source on zinc absorption in humans. *Journal of nutrition*, 1989, **119**: 48–53.

32. Sandström B, Kivistö B, Cederblad Å. Absorption of zinc from soy protein meals in humans. *Journal of nutrition*, 1987, **117**: 321–327.

33. King JC, Turnlund JR. Human zinc requirement In: Mills CF, ed. *Zinc in human biology*. Berlin, Springer-Verlag, 1989: 335–350.

34. Gregory J et al. *The dietary and nutritional survey of British adults*. London, HMSO, 1990.

35. Shrimpton R. Food consumption and dietary adequacy according to income in 1,200 families, Manaus, Amazonas, Brazil. *Archivos latinoamericanos de nutrición*, 1984, **34**: 615–629.

36. Ross J, Gibson RS, Sabry JH. A study of seasonal trace element intakes and hair trace element concentrations in selected households from the Wosera, Papua New Guinea. *Tropical and geographical medicine*, 1986, **38**: 246–254.

37. Soman SD et al. Daily intake of some major and trace elements. *Health physics*, 1969, **17**: 35–40.

38. Taylor CM et al. The homeostatic regulation of zinc absorption and endogenous losses in zinc deprived man. *American journal of clinical nutrition*, 1991, **53**: 755–763.

39. Rabbani PI et al. Dietary model for production of experimental zinc deficiency in man. *American journal of clinical nutrition*, 1987, **45**: 1514–1525.

40. Ziegler EE et al. Effect of low zinc intake on absorption and excretion of zinc by infants studied with ^{70}Zn as extrinsic tag. *Journal of nutrition*, 1989, **119**: 1647–1653.

41. *Energy and protein requirements. Report of a Joint FAO/WHO/UNU Expert Consultation.* Geneva, World Health Organization, 1985 (WHO Technical Report Series, No. 724).

42. Krebs NF, Hambidge KM. Zinc requirements and zinc intakes of breast-fed infants. *American journal of clinical nutrition*, 1986, **43**: 288–292.

43. Krebs NF et al. Zinc absorption and fecal excretion of endogenous zinc in the breastfed infant. In: Anke M, ed. *Trace elements in man and animals—TEMA 8.* Dresden, Media Verlag Touristik, 1993: 1110–1113.

44. Golden BM. *Zinc metabolism during recovery from malnutrition* [MD Thesis]. Belfast, University of Belfast, 1989.

45. *Measuring change in nutritional status.* Geneva, World Health Organization, 1983.

46. Body composition during pregnancy. In: *Geigy scientific tables*, Vol. 3. Basel, CIBA-Geigy, 1984: 291.

47. Swanson CA, King JC. Zinc and pregnancy outcome. *American journal of clinical nutrition*, 1987, **46**: 763–771.

48. Casey CE, Neville MC, Hambidge KM. Studies in human lactation: secretion of zinc, copper and manganese in human milk. *American journal of clinical nutrition*, 1989, **49**: 773–785.

49. Vuori E. Intake of copper, iron, manganese and zinc by healthy, exclusively breast-fed infants during the first 3 months of life. *British journal of nutrition*, 1979, **42**: 407–411.

50. Krebs NF et al. The effect of zinc supplements during lactation on maternal Zn status and milk Zn concentration. *FASEB journal*, 1991, **5**: A1289.

51. Davies NT, Williams RB. The effect of pregnancy and lactation on the absorption of zinc and lysine by the rat duodenum in situ. *British journal of nutrition*, 1977, **38**: 417–423.

52. Tipton JH, Cook MJ. Trace elements in human tissue. II. Adult subjects from the United States. *Health physics*, 1963, **9**: 103–145.

53. Hayslip CC et al. The effects of lactation on bone mineral content in healthy post partum women. *Obstetrics and gynecology*, 1989, **73**: 588–592.
54. Krebs NF et al. Longitudinal measurement of bone metabolism and bone density during lactation. *FASEB journal*, 1992, **6**: A1083.
55. Jackson MJ. Physiology of zinc: general aspects. In: Mills CF ed. *Zinc in human biology*. London, Springer, 1989: 1–14.
56. Essetera MB, Faddouli M, Aloui L. Phytate, Ca, P, Zn and Cu levels in the major food items and diets in Morocco. In: Mills CF, Bremner I, Chester JK, eds. *Trace elements in man and animals — TEMA 5*. Farnham Royal, CAB International, 1985: 622–625.
57. Ferguson EL et al. Dietary calcium, phytate, and zinc intakes and the calcium, phytate, and zinc molar ratios of the diets of a selected group of East African children. *American journal of clinical nutrition*, 1989, **50**: 1450–1456.
58. Maleki M. Food consumption and nutritional status of 13 year old village and city schoolboys in Fars province, Iran. *Ecology, food and nutrition*, 1973, **2**: 39–42.
59. Reinhold JG et al. Decreased absorption of calcium, magnesium, zinc and phosphorus by humans due to increased fiber and phosphorus consumption as wheat bread. *Journal of nutrition*, 1976, **106**: 493–503.

6.
Selenium

6.1 Biochemical function

Until recently, the only known metabolic role for selenium in mammals was as a component of the enzyme glutathione peroxidase which, together with vitamin E, catalase and superoxide dismutase, is a component of one of the antioxidant defence systems of the body (1). Recently, Burk and his colleagues have made great strides in the purification and characterization of their "selenoprotein-P", but so far they have been unable to clarify its function in people or in animals (2). Several different selenium-containing enzymes have been described in microorganisms (1), and it is likely that selenoproteins other than glutathione peroxidase remain to be discovered in higher animals. There is, for example, growing evidence that an additional selenoenzyme protein is involved in the synthesis of the hormone triiodothyronine from thyroxine (3–5).

6.2 Deficiency and toxicity

6.2.1 Deficiency

Keshan disease is a selenium-responsive endemic cardiomyopathy that mainly affects children and women of child-bearing age in certain areas of China (6). This disease was considered a "water and soil" disease because residents of these areas felt that some component of the local water or soil caused it. The fact that domestic animals raised in these areas suffered from white muscle disease (a concurrent deficiency of selenium and vitamin E in livestock) suggested that selenium could be lacking in the environment, and indeed soil samples from Keshan disease areas were found to be low in selenium (6). This endemic disease therefore has a biogeochemical basis in that a deficit of selenium in the soil reduces the flow of this essential trace element into the food chain.

An increased incidence of Keshan disease has now been associated with low selenium levels in staple cereals and in samples of human blood, hair and tissue (6). Moreover, several field trials of selenium supplementation involving thousands of children provide strong evidence for the prophylactic effect of selenium against Keshan disease. None the less, certain epidemiological aspects of the disease (e.g. its seasonal variation) are difficult to explain solely on the basis of selenium deficiency and suggest that an infectious component, such as a virus, is also involved. Other dietary factors, such as low intakes of vitamin E, protein, methionine, and other trace elements and excesses of erucic acid, toxins, etc., have also been considered as possibly relevant to the etiology of Keshan disease (see references 6 and 7 and Chapter 8 on molybdenum).

Keshan disease can be categorized clinically into four types depending on its severity, namely acute, subacute, chronic and insidious (6). Once the disease is established, selenium is of little or no therapeutic value. Treatment generally follows the standard procedures employed in cases of congestive heart failure. The major histopathological feature of the disease is a multifocal myocardial necrosis. The coronary arteries are essentially unaffected. Ultrastructural studies show that membranous organelles, such as mitochondria or sarcolemma, are affected earliest. The precise biochemical connection between the metabolic function of selenium in glutathione peroxidase and the significance of a decline in the activity of this selenoenzyme in the pathogenesis of Keshan disease is not yet clear.

Kashin–Beck disease is an endemic osteoarthropathy that has also been linked with low selenium status (6). This disease primarily affects children between the ages of 5 and 13 years living in certain regions of China and the former Soviet Union. Advanced cases of the disease are characterized by enlargement and deformity of the joints. The principal pathological change is multiple degeneration and necrosis of hyaline cartilage tissue. Epidemiologically, Kashin–Beck disease has characteristics similar to those of Keshan disease but its distribution is less stable. Some studies have suggested that selenium may prevent Kashin–Beck disease, but this work needs further confirmation (6).

Although studies of the etiology of Keshan and Kashin–Beck diseases in human subjects have indicated that a deficit of soil selenium may be the primary cause, it is important to recognize that many instances of selenium-responsive disease in animals reflect the distribution of soils in which, rather than being deficient, soil selenium is fixed in an unavailable form. It is reasonable to expect that the geochemical variables involved also influence the selenium status of humans.

The pathological effects of "pure" selenium deficiency (i.e. independent of vitamin E deficiency) have only recently been recognized in animals. Many of the conditions associated with selenium deficiency (liver necrosis in rats, exudative diathesis in chicks, and white muscle disease in cattle and sheep) are actually combined deficiencies of both selenium and vitamin E and respond favourably to either of these nutrients (1). For several years, nutritional pancreatic atrophy in the chick was considered the best model of pure selenium deficiency but even this condition has now been shown to be prevented by vitamin E (8). However, in addition to its adverse effects on growth (9), other manifestations of "pure" (i.e. vitamin E-independent) selenium deficiency are now recognized in several non-human species. Neutrophil microbicidal activity declines, and recent studies (3) show that selenium deficiency markedly reduces the activity of the 5'-deiodinase enzymes responsible for the production of triiodothyronine (T_3) from thyroxine (T_4). This fundamentally important selenium/iodine interaction is likely to influence the human response to iodine deficiency in areas (e.g. Zaire) where subjects are concurrently deficient in both selenium and iodine (10). It may well be involved in the etiology of cases of iodine-responsive disorders whose prevalence is difficult to explain solely on the basis of environmental deficiencies of iodine.[1]

---

[1] *Note added in proof:* The role of selenium in thyroid hormone metabolism as a constituent of iodothyronine 5'-deiodinase continues to receive attention, with the suggestion that combined deficiencies of iodine and selenium may have adverse effects on neonatal growth, development and survival (Arthur JR, Beckett GJ. New metabolic roles for selenium. *Proceedings of the Nutrition Society*, 1994, 53: 616–624). The nationwide selenium supplementation programme in Finland has now been in place for about a decade but no drastic changes in the incidence of, or mortality from, cancer or cardiovascular diseases have been seen since the start of the programme (Varo P et al. Nationwide selenium supplementation in Finland. In: Burk RF, ed. *Selenium in biology and human health*. New York, Springer, 1994: 199–218). The incidence of Keshan disease in China has declined to such low levels that it is no longer considered to be a major public health problem (Xia Y et al. Keshan disease and selenium status of populations in China. In: Burk RF, ed. *Selenium in biology and human health*. New York, Springer, 1994: 183–196). This appears to be a consequence of selenium supplementation in the endemic areas and an overall improvement in the diet of the rural population because of better economic conditions. Although selenium deficiency is considered the fundamental underlying condition that predisposes to Keshan disease, marginal vitamin E deficiency may also be involved, and a role for infection-induced oxidant stress has also been suggested (Xia et al., 1994). Building on earlier Chinese work, Beck and colleagues have shown that either vitamin E or selenium deficiency can increase the cardiotoxicity to mice of an enterovirus similar to the coxsackievirus B_3 isolated from people with Keshan disease (Beck MA et al. Vitamin E deficiency intensifies the myocardial injury of coxsackievirus B3 infection of mice. *Journal of nutrition*, 1994, 124: 345–358; Beck MA et al. Increased virulence of a human enterovirus (coxsackievirus B3) in selenium-deficient mice. *Journal of infectious disease*, 1994, 170: 351–357). Moreover, selenium deficiency in the host mice allows a normally benign strain of the coxsackievirus B_3 to convert to a virulent form, apparently as a result of some genetic change in the parental strain (Beck MA et al. Benign human enterovirus becomes virulent in selenium-deficient mice. *Journal of medical virology*, 1994, 43: 166–170). These results showing the selenium or vitamin E deficiency can have a major impact on the outcome of viral infection, presumably by altering viral genetics, could have great public health significance concerning the relationship between nutrition and resistance to infection, especially if the results are generalizable to other RNA viruses such as those responsible for influenza, hepatitis, polio or AIDS. In response to these recent findings, attempts are being made to devise selenium-enriched food products suitable as delivery vehicles for increasing dietary selenium intake by the general population should that prove to be desirable on a large scale even in selenium-adequate areas.

6.2.2 Toxicity

Chronic selenium poisoning in people is characterized primarily by loss of hair and changes in fingernail morphology (11). In some cases, skin lesions (redness, blistering) and nervous system abnormalities (paresthesia, paralysis, hemiplegia) are also observed. In animals, particularly rats, liver damage is a common feature of chronic selenosis (12) but evidence suggestive of hepatic functional defects is less convincing in humans (13).

The biochemical mechanisms of selenium toxicity have not been clearly established. Some features of its deleterious effects reflect the chemical form of the particular selenium compound to which exposure has been excessive (14). For example, selenite is a potent catalyst for the oxidation of sulfhydryl groups, and this may be the basis of its inhibitory effect on protein biosynthesis. On the other hand, selenomethionine can be incorporated as such into proteins by mimicking methionine and can thereby increase the susceptibility of certain proteins to denaturation by heat or treatment with urea (15).

6.3 Epidemiology of deficiency and toxicity

Intake criteria for human selenium deficiency and toxicity have been established and are discussed in detail later. However, attempts have also been made to associate anomalous intakes of selenium with the risks of certain degenerative diseases such as cancer, cardiovascular disease and cerebral thrombosis.

The possibility that increased intakes of selenium might protect against the development of cancer in humans has generated great interest (16). However, a number of epidemiological studies have now been reported which show no relationship between selenium status and cancer risk (17). Moreover, a recent analysis of the relationship between selenium and cancer suggests that "the question of whether selenium protects against cancer is still wide open" (18). Furthermore, an increased intake of selenium appears to stimulate tumorigenesis in some animal models of pancreatic and skin cancer (19). The protective effect of higher physiological exposures to selenium observed in several studies on experimental animals, together with small but statistically significant differences in selenium blood plasma levels detected in some retrospective–prospective studies of subgroups of people developing cancer, explains the continuing interest in the anticarcinogenic potential of selenium. However, it should be noted that the levels of exposure in several experiments were higher than the typical upper limits of physiological exposures to selenium. The results of prospective–retrospective studies had no individual predictive value and could, even on a group basis, have reflected non-specific influences. The association between low selenium intake and high cancer risk, while clearly of some interest, is in need of further investigation before a definite conclusion can be reached.

Although a plausible biochemical mechanism can be postulated whereby selenium could protect against heart disease by influencing platelet aggregability through an effect on the prostacyclin–thromboxane ratio, the epidemiological evidence linking selenium status and risk of cardiovascular disease is still equivocal (17).

It has been suggested that excessive selenium exposure plays a role in a variety of conditions (dental caries, reproductive problems, amyotrophic lateral sclerosis), but the evidence is not convincing (12).

6.4 Assessment of status

Several different human tissues, including blood, plasma, hair and toenails, have been analysed for their selenium content as a way of assessing nutritional selenium status (20). In general, these tissues can provide a reasonable estimate of selenium status if dietary selenium intake is relatively uniform. However, blood and plasma selenium levels can be affected by variables other than dietary selenium intake (21), and animal experiments show that the selenium content of hair and nails is a function of several factors including the form and level of dietary selenium, the age of the animal and intake of sulfur-containing amino acids (22). Glutathione peroxidase activity has been used as an index of selenium status in humans over the nutritional range of selenium intake, but is useless for this purpose once the activity of the enzyme is saturated (12). Thus, in countries such as the USA, where diets are relatively rich in selenium, glutathione peroxidase activity is maximal in most people and the enzyme loses its value as a index of selenium status.

A significant handicap in research on selenium toxicity is the lack of a selective and sensitive indicator of selenium overexposure in humans (12). Hair loss and nail changes seem to be the most convenient indicators of human selenosis in the field (13), but the selenium intake needed to produce these effects goes beyond acceptable exposure levels. A shift in the ratio of selenium in plasma to that in red blood cells has been suggested as a more sensitive criterion of overexposure (13), but the physiological significance of this phenomenon is unknown. More research is needed to develop better methods of monitoring elevated selenium exposure.

6.5 Absorption and bioavailability

Selenium compounds are generally very efficiently absorbed by humans, and selenium absorption does not appear to be under homoeostatic control (12). For example, absorption of selenite selenium is greater than 80%, while that of selenium as selenomethionine or as selenate is greater than 90% (12, 23). Thus, the rate-limiting step in determining the overall bioavailability of dietary selenium is not likely to be its absorption but rather its conversion within tissues to its metabolically active forms (e.g. its incorporation into glutathione peroxidase or 5′-deiodinase).

A number of depletion–repletion experiments have now been carried out on animals to estimate the bioavailability of selenium in foods consumed by humans (24). The availability values thus obtained can be a complex function of the response criterion selected, the dietary level of selenium and possibly other unknown dietary factors. Based on the restoration of glutathione peroxidase activity in depleted rats, the bioavailability of the selenium in wheat is quite good, usually 80% or better. The selenium in Brazil nuts and beef kidney also appears readily available (90% or more by most criteria). The selenium in tuna seems of lesser availability (perhaps only 20–60% of that from selenite), whereas the availability of selenium from certain other seafoods (shrimp, crab and Baltic herring) is high. The selenium in a variety of mushrooms appears to be of uniformly low availability to rats.

Data on the nutritional bioavailability of selenium to humans are sparse. A supplementation study carried out in Finnish men of relatively low selenium status showed that selenate selenium was as effective as the selenium in seleniferous wheat in increasing platelet glutathione peroxidase activity (25). The wheat selenium, however, increased plasma selenium levels more than selenate selenium and, once the supplements were withdrawn, platelet gluta-thione peroxidase activity declined less in the group given wheat. This study showed the importance of estimating not only short-term availability but also long-term retention and the convertibility of tissue selenium stores into the biologically active form.

6.6 Dietary intake

Typical values of the selenium content of various foods have been reported as follows (mg/kg wet weight): liver, kidney and seafood, 0.4–1.5; muscle meats, 0.1–0.4; cereals and cereal products, < 0.1– > 0.8; dairy products, < 0.1–0.3; and fruits and vegetables, < 0.1 (12). Apart from these natural differences in the selenium content of foods, the amount of selenium ingested in the diet is a function of the food habits of the individual (i.e. consumption patterns) and particularly of the geographical origin of the food (i.e. whether it comes from regions with selenium-rich or selenium-poor soils). For example, predominantly vegetarian populations living in areas with soils of low selenium content or availability would be particularly at risk of developing a low selenium status. Not only would important selenium sources, such as organ meats and fish and muscle meats, be missing from their diets but the plant foods consumed would also be of low selenium content if produced locally.

Thus the contribution of various food groups to the overall dietary intake of selenium can differ markedly from one country to another. Cereals furnish about 75% of the total 149 μg/day dietary intake of selenium in Canada, whereas these foods provided less than 10% of the total 30 μg/day selenium intake in Finland before 1985 (26, 27). The general dietary patterns in these two countries are probably rather similar, but the differences in dietary selenium intake and in the role of cereals in determining that intake are striking. It should be noted that, since the summer of 1985, fertilizers used for grain crops in Finland have been fortified with selenium. In consequence, the selenium content of the Finnish food supply has gradually increased to levels similar to those in North America (28).

Food consumption patterns would also affect the proportion of dietary selenium that is bioavailable. If most of the dietary selenium is derived from cereals, its bioavailability will be higher than if it is derived from certain fish, such as tuna (see the previous discussion of selenium bioavailability).

There is a high degree of day-to-day variation in the usual dietary selenium intake among individuals of the same sex and the same or similar age group. Welsh et al. (29) analysed 132 composites of self-selected daily diets of 11 male and 11 female subjects ranging from 14 to 64 years of age. The mean selenium intake furnished by these individual daily diets was 81 ± 41 (± SD) μg/day. The distribution of intakes was skewed upwards by a few relatively high selenium levels (median = 74 μg/day). Levander et al. (30) analysed 423 individual 1-day diet composites collected from 23 lactating and 13 non-lactating women at 37 weeks of gestation to 6 months postpartum. The overall dietary selenium intake of these women was 80 ± 37 μg/day (mean of daily diets ± SD). The range of intakes represented by these daily composites was 0.6–221 μg/day. Consolidation of the data into 3-day dietary collections reduced this range considerably to 14–154 μg/day. Mutanen et al. (31) also found a wide dispersion of individual selenium intakes, since the mean values (± SD) based on daily diet composites of 40 Finnish men were 53 ± 32 and 50 ± 20 μg/day in September and December 1981, respectively; the distribution of selenium contents also showed a slight upwards skew. Mutanen calculated that single-day dietary observations gave an error of nearly 90% when used to estimate the "real" long-term selenium intake for an individual (32). She also estimated that 7-day observations would come within 35% of the subject's "true" long-term intake with 95% confidence. Nearly 3 weeks of dietary observations would be needed in order to derive an estimate within 20% of the usual mean selenium intake.

As part of a year-long mineral balance study of North Americans, Levander & Morris (33) analysed four 7-day food composites collected during the various seasons of the year from 12 men and 15 women ranging in age from 19 to 50 years. The mean dietary selenium intake (± SD) calculated on the basis of an average of the four weekly composites was 90 ± 14 and 74 ± 12 μg/day for the men and women, respectively (SD recalculated from Levander & Morris (33)). These results suggest that, for the population investigated (young to middle-aged adults consuming a moderately high-selenium mixed Western diet), the CV of the interindividual variability of usual dietary selenium intakes is about 16%.

6.7 Requirements and safe range of population mean intakes

Because of the scarcity of human data, the first dietary standard for selenium was based on the extrapolation of the results of studies on animals (34). It was noted that a diet with a selenium content of 0.1 μg/g was sufficient for maximal growth and reproductive performance in all mammalian species examined. If it is assumed that adult humans consume 500 g of a mixed diet daily (dry basis), such a selenium content would result in a selenium intake of 50 μg/day. This figure was adopted as the lower limit of the Estimated Safe and Adequate Daily Dietary Intake proposed in 1980 by the United States National Research Council (34). To allow for the possible influence of other dietary factors on selenium metabolism and in order to take into account the effect of individual variation on requirement, a range of 50–200 μg/day was suggested as safe and adequate for adults, with correspondingly lower levels for infants and children. No recommendation was made for pregnant or lactating women.

In an attempt to pinpoint more closely the human requirement for selenium, several balance studies were carried out in various countries (17). When the results were compared internationally, however, it soon became apparent that balance techniques for the determination of mineral requirements were particularly inappropriate for selenium because of the marked ability of individuals to adapt and maintain balance at many levels of selenium intake by modifying the faecal and urinary excretion of the element in line with changes in selenium status.

6.7.1 Requirements of adults, adolescents and infants

With the discovery of Keshan disease, the selenium-responsive juvenile cardiomyopathy endemic in certain areas of China (6), it became possible to use epidemiological data to establish a population basal requirement for selenium.

By conducting dietary surveys in areas of China that are endemic and non-endemic for Keshan disease, the Chinese investigators were able to show that Keshan disease did not appear in regions where the population mean intake of selenium by 60-kg adult men was 19.1 μg or more per day (6). Since the Expert Consultation used a standard reference body weight of 65-kg for men and the selenium requirement may be a function of body weight (33), the following correction is necessary: $19.1 \times 65/60 = 21$ μg/day. Since this mean selenium intake is the lowest associated with freedom from pathological defects in a population otherwise at risk of selenium deficiency, it is reasonable to regard it as indicating the *population minimum mean intake* of selenium likely to meet basal requirements ($Se_{Pl\,min}^{basal}$) (see Table 6.2, page 116).

The Chinese dietary survey was carried out in rural areas, and the peasant diet consisted largely of grain and vegetables with little milk, meat or fish. About 70% of the dietary selenium intake came from cereal products (35). If it is assumed that the bioavailability of selenium from other grains is similar to that from wheat (about 80%, judging from repletion experiments with rats; see page 110) the estimates of requirement in Table 6.2, which are derived essentially from these Chinese data, must be regarded as applicable to diets containing selenium of relatively good bioavailability. Populations receiving most of their dietary selenium from other sources would have to make appropriate adjustments.

The data used to derive *normative requirements* for selenium are taken from a Chinese experimental study by Yang et al. (35) of the relationship between plasma glutathione peroxidase activity and selenium intake in adult men. This study was carried out on subjects who were residents of a Keshan disease area and hence had naturally low selenium reserves. Five groups of eight or nine healthy male adults 18–42 years of age were given graded doses of selenium orally in the form of DL-selenomethionine, namely 0, 10, 30, 60 and 90 μg/day. Plasma glutathione peroxidase activity responded similarly to the three highest levels of selenium supplementation after 5–8 months. These results show that a dietary selenium intake of 41 μg/day (30 μg from supplement plus 11 μg from the usual diet) was sufficient to saturate plasma glutathione peroxidase activity fully in 60-kg men.

Although attainment of the maximum activity of glutathione peroxidase has been regarded as a desirable nutritional goal by others (36), the method used by the Expert Consultation to calculate the *normative requirements* for selenium was to estimate the dietary intake needed to achieve two-thirds of the maximum attainable activity of glutathione peroxidase. This level, as opposed to the maximum enzyme activity, is arbitrary but is based on the observation that abnormalities in the ability of blood cells to metabolize hydrogen peroxide become apparent only when the glutathione peroxidase activity in these cells

113

declines to one-quarter or less of normal (H. J. Cohen, personal communication, 1990).

Recalculation of the data of Yang et al. based on plasma glutathione peroxidase activities after 8 months of selenium supplementation, yields the following equation (correlation coefficient, $r = 0.97$):

$$Y = 2.19X + 13.8$$

where Y is the plasma glutathione peroxidase activity expressed as a percentage of the maximum attainable value and X is the daily intake of selenium in μg. Solution of this equation for $Y = 67\%$ yields a value of 24.3 μg/day of selenium. Thus, for the standard 65-kg reference man, the average *normative requirement* of individuals for selenium ($Se_R^{normative}$) is estimated to be 26 μg/day (24.3 $\times$ 65/60). From the average *normative requirement*, it is possible to calculate that the lower limit of the safe range of population mean intakes of selenium that will meet the normative requirement ($Se_{PImin}^{normative}$) of most adult males is approximately 40 μg/day (20/0.68) if an interindividual variability of dietary selenium intake of 16% is assumed. It is also assumed that a diet of relatively high selenium bioavailability is being consumed. Since selenomethionine, the form of selenium used in the study by Yang et al. (35), is very efficiently absorbed and utilized by humans, the estimates given here are correspondingly applicable only to diets containing selenium of relatively high bioavailability.

From these estimates of $Se_{PImin}^{normative}$ for 65-kg men it is possible to derive requirements for other age and sex groups by extrapolation. Although the best factor to use in extrapolating such values is debatable, the basal metabolic rate may provide a reasonable basis for the calculations. Calculated figures for the individual requirements of the various age and sex groups derived by extrapolation from the adult male values based on the basal metabolic rate are shown in Table 6.1, corresponding estimates of the lower limits of the safe range of population mean intake are given in Table 6.2.

6.7.2 Pregnancy and lactation

Lactation and pregnancy are special physiological states, so that increased selenium requirement during these periods cannot be estimated by extrapolation from data obtained with adult men, as was done above for non-lactating or non-pregnant women, children or infants.

The increased need for selenium during pregnancy was estimated by a factorial method and from the total maternal and fetal selenium demand. The selenium content of skeletal muscle was found to be about 0.3 and 1.2 μg/g of protein in samples obtained in New Zealand and the United States, respectively (37, 38), on the assumption that human skeletal muscle contains about 20%

Table 6.1. Average individual basal (Se_R^{basal}) and normative ($Se_R^{normative}$) requirements (in μg selenium/kg of body weight) for dietary selenium[a]

Age range (years)	Sex	Se_R^{basal}	$Se_R^{normative}$
0–0.25	M & F	0.41	0.82
0.25–0.5	M & F	0.49	0.87
0.5–1.0	M & F	0.45	0.91
1–3	M & F	0.57	1.13
3–6	M & F	0.48	0.96
6–10	M & F	0.38	0.68
10–12	F	0.29	0.55
12–15	F	0.23	0.43
15–18	F	0.20	0.37
18–60[b] +	F	0.20	0.39
10–12	M	0.31	0.58
12–15	M	0.27	0.51
15–18	M	0.22	0.43
18–60 +	M	0.22	0.42

[a] It is assumed that 80% of dietary selenium is bioavailable.
[b] For pregnancy and lactation, see text and Table 6.3.

protein (10). If it is assumed that about 925 g of protein are deposited during pregnancy (36) and that it is desirable that the selenium content of such protein should be similar to that of skeletal muscle, the increment of selenium associated with pregnancy is 278 and 1110 μg in selenium-poor and selenium-rich countries, respectively. Despite evidence from blood analyses of a generally low selenium status, pathological effects of selenium deficiency have not been documented in the general population of New Zealand, so that it seems reasonable to assume that the increased maternal and fetal retention of 278 μg during pregnancy in New Zealand women could be used to calculate the Se_R^{basal} for pregnancy. This corresponds to an increment of 1 μg of absorbed selenium daily or, for 80% bioavailability of dietary selenium, to an increased dietary intake of 1.25 μg/day. Added to the individual mean basal requirement of the 55-kg non-pregnant woman (11 μg/day, Table 6.1) the Se_R^{basal} for pregnancy becomes approximately 12 μg/day and, with a population CV of 16%, $Se_{Pl\,min}^{basal}$ becomes 18 μg/day. If it is assumed that the estimates of increased retention during pregnancy in the United States (1110 μg, or on a daily basis, 4 μg of absorbed selenium) can be taken to reflect the normative accumulation of

Table 6.2. Lower limits of the safe ranges of population mean intakes of dietary selenium (in µg/day)[a]

Age range (years) or duration of pregnancy or lactation	Sex	Weight (kg)	Se_{PImin}^{basal}	$Se_{PImin}^{normative}$
0–0.25	M & F	5	3	6
0.25–0.5	M & F	7	5	9
0.5–1.0	M & F	9	6	12
1–3	M & F	12	10	20
3–6	M & F	17	12	24
6–10	M & F	25	14	25
10–12	F	37	16	30
12–15	F	48	16	30
15–18	F	55	16	30
18– > 60	F	55	16	30
10–12	M	35	16	30
12–15	M	48	19	36
15–18	M	64	21	40
18– > 60	M	65	21	40
Pregnancy[b]				
First trimester			18	39
Second trimester			18	39
Third trimester			18	39
Lactation[c]				
0–3 months			21	42
3–6 months			25	46
6–12 months			26	52

[a] It is assumed that 80% of dietary selenium is bioavailable and that the CV of dietary intake of selenium is 16%.

[b] For derivation, see text and Table 6.3.

[c] To meet requirements of milk-fed infants on the assumption that 80% of milk selenium is bioavailable and that the CV of milk selenium intake is 12.5%. See text and Table 6.3.

selenium, the corresponding estimated values of $Se_{R}^{normative}$ and $Se_{PImin}^{normative}$ are 27 µg/day and 39 µg/day respectively.

The increased selenium requirements during lactation were estimated by determining the amounts of selenium that must be provided in the breast milk of lactating women if their infants are to receive sufficient to meet their Se_{PImin}^{basal} or $Se_{PImin}^{normative}$ requirements. These increments were adjusted to allow for an assumed bioavailability of 80% for the selenium of both maternal milk and the maternal diet before they were added to the corresponding average individual dietary selenium requirements of non-pregnant women. For example, for the first and second 3-month postpartum periods, infants whose selenium intake was just sufficient to meet their Se_R^{basal} would have to consume 2.7 or 4.5 μg of selenium per day from maternal milk, respectively. If dietary bioavailability was 80% and a CV of 12.5% is assumed for milk selenium output, the lactating women would have to consume an additional 3.4 or 5.7 μg of selenium daily to replace these lacteal losses. These amounts, added to the 11.0 μg/day Se_R^{basal} of non-lactating women (Table 6.3), give a total of 14.4 or 16.7 μg/day needed daily to meet the Se_R^{basal} during the first and second 3-month periods of lactation. The corresponding estimates of $Se_R^{normative}$ for lactating women would amount to 29 and 32 μg/day (Table 6.3).

6.8 Tolerance of high dietary intakes

From data derived from endemic outbreaks of human selenosis in China (11), it is possible to derive tentative estimates of the chronic toxicity of dietary selenium. The results obtained in a recent field study carried out in the endemic selenosis zone suggest that persistent clinical signs (morphological changes in the fingernails) could develop with dietary selenium intakes of about 900 μg/day (12). This figure, estimated from a regression equation relating blood selenium to the dietary intake of this element, is based on the lowest blood selenium level observed in one of five patients with long-persisting distinct signs of selenosis (fingernail changes) in a study population of 349 residents living in the high-selenium area.

A serious handicap to further progress in selenium toxicology research is the lack of a specific and/or sensitive biochemical marker of selenium over-exposure. This contrasts with the monitoring of nutritional intakes of the element, for which glutathione peroxidase activity has served as an extremely useful indicator for assessing selenium status. Lack of such an index has hindered toxicologists in their efforts to define the dietary exposure at which selenium begins to have a harmful, as opposed to a beneficial, effect. In the Chinese studies (13), a remarkable reduction in the ratio of selenium in plasma to that in erythrocytes was seen at dietary intakes of about 750 μg/day. This is the first biochemical change to be observed at intakes that do not lead to clinical signs of malfunction and, as such, offers a promising new approach to investigating biochemical changes in selenosis before clinical changes appear. In the future, more sensitive indices of selenium overexposure may be discovered so that the normative dietary selenium toxicity may have to be re-evaluated.

Based on their extensive field experience with selenosis, Yang and his colleagues suggested a marginal level of daily safe dietary selenium intake of

Table 6.3. Average individual basal and normative requirements (in μg dietary selenium/day) for dietary selenium, Se_R^{basal} and $Se_R^{normative}$, for pregnancy and lactation[a]

Pregnancy

Stage	Basal			Normative		
	Accretion by fetus and adnexa[b]	Non-pregnant basal requirement	Total (Se_R^{basal})	Accretion by fetus and adnexa[b]	Non-pregnant normative requirement	Total ($Se_R^{normative}$)
All stages	1.2	11.0	12	5.0	21.5	27

Lactation

Stage	Basal			Normative		
	Increment for maternal milk selenium for infant basal requirement[b,c]	Non-pregnant basal requirement	Total (Se_R^{basal})	Increment for milk selenium for infant normative requirement[b,c]	Non-pregnant normative requirement	Total ($Se_R^{normative}$)
0–3 months	3.4	11.0	14	7.1	21.5	29
3–6 months	5.7	11.0	17	10.2	21.5	32
6–12 months	6.8	11.0	18	13.7	21.5	35

[a] It is assumed that 80% of dietary selenium is bioavailable. The data are insufficient to enable changes in requirements at different stages of pregnancy to be determined.
[b] Includes an allowance for the 80% bioavailability of dietary selenium.
[c] Includes allowances for the 80% bioavailability of maternal milk selenium and for a CV of 12.5% for milk selenium output.

Table 6.4. Upper limits of the safe ranges of adult population mean intakes of selenium (in $\mu g/day$) (Se_{Plmax}^{tox})[a]

Age (years)	Sex	Se_{Plmax}^{tox}
15–60 +	F	400
15–60 +	M	400

[a] The data are insufficient to enable Se_{Plmax}^{tox} to be determined for other age groups or for lactating or pregnant women.

750–850 μg (*13*). This was defined as "the level of Se intake at which few individuals have functional signs of excessive intake and above which the tendency to exhibit functional signs is apparent and symptoms may first appear among ... susceptible individuals [whose] Se intake [is] further increased". Because of the uncertainty surrounding the harmful dose of selenium for humans, a maximal daily safe dietary selenium intake of 400 μg was suggested for adults. This figure was derived arbitrarily by dividing the mean marginal level of daily safe dietary selenium intake defined above (800 μg) by two. The value of 400 μg daily as Se_{Plmax}^{tox} for adult males and females was accepted by the Expert Consultation (Table 6.4). There are insufficient data from which to estimate the safe upper limit to population mean intakes of selenium for most other age groups or for pregnant or lactating women, so that the estimates of the safe range of population intakes of selenium ($Se_{SRI}^{normative}$) are restricted to adults.

6.9 Recommendations for future studies

- The merits and limitations of erythrocyte glutathione peroxidase as a marker of selenium status should be investigated more thoroughly. The diagnostic potential of measurement of tissue 5'-deiodinase for detecting cases in which a low selenium status may be retarding growth should also be explored. In particular, more comparative data are required for populations whose selenium status is apparently lower than normal, as in areas of China where low selenium is associated with selenium-responsive disease and in New Zealand where a low selenium status apparently has no pathological consequences.

- More adequate consideration should be given to the possibility, clearly indicated in animal studies, that the expression of the effects of selenium deficiency may be modified by differences in tissue or dietary antioxidant status in humans.

● Biochemical techniques for the early detection of pathological effects arising from overexposure to dietary selenium should be developed. Data are needed from which acceptable upper limits for selenium intake can be defined for infants, children, adolescents and pregnant or lactating women.

References

1. Combs GF Jr, Combs SB. *The role of selenium in nutrition.* Orlando, FL, Academic Press, 1986.
2. Yang JG, Hill KE, Burk RF. Dietary selenium intake controls rat plasma seleno-protein P concentration. *Journal of nutrition,* 1989, **119**: 1010–1012.
3. Arthur JR, Beckett GR. Selenium deficiency and thyroid hormone metabolism. In Wendell A, ed. *Selenium in biology and medicine.* Springer-Verlag, Berlin, 1989: 90–95.
4. Contempré B et al. Effect of selenium supplementation in hypothyroid subjects of an iodine and selenium deficient area. *Journal of clinical endocrinology and metabolism,* 1991, **74**: 213–215.
5. Arthur JR, Nicol F, Beckett GJ. Hepatic iodothyronine deiodinase: the role of selenium. *Biochemical journal,* 1990, **272**: 537–540.
6. Yang G et al. Selenium-related endemic diseases and the daily selenium requirement of humans. *World review of nutrition and diet,* 1988, **55**: 98–152.
7. Laryea MD et al. Low selenium state and increased erucic acid in children from Keshan endemic areas—a pilot study. In: Wendel A, ed. *Selenium in biology and medicine.* Berlin, Springer-Verlag, 1989: 277–280.
8. Whitacre ME et al. Influence of dietary vitamin E on nutritional pancreatic atrophy in selenium-deficient chicks. *Journal of nutrition,* 1987, **117**: 460–467.
9. McCoy KEM, Weswig PH. Some selenium responses in the rat not related to vitamin E. *Journal of nutrition,* 1969, **98**: 383–389.
10. Forbes GB. *Human body composition,* New York, Springer, 1987.
11. Yang GQ et al. Endemic selenium intoxication of humans in China. *American journal of clinical nutrition,* 1983, **37**: 872–881.
12. *Selenium.* Geneva, World Health Organization, 1987 (Environmental Health Criteria, 58).
13. Yang G et al. Studies of safe maximal daily dietary Se-intake in a seleniferous area in China. Part II: Relation between Se-intake and the manifestation of clinical signs and certain biochemical alterations in blood and urine. *Journal of trace elements and electrolytes in health and disease,* 1989, **3**: 123–130
14. Levander OA. Selenium: biochemical actions, interactions and some human health implications. In: Prasad AS, ed. *Clinical, biochemical and nutritional aspects of trace elements.* New York, Alan R Liss, 1982: 345–368.
15. Huber RE, Criddle RS. The isolation and properties of β-galactosidase from *Escherichia coli* grown on sodium selenate. *Biochimica et biophysica acta,* 1967, **141**: 587–599.

16. Combs GF, Clark LC. Can dietary selenium modify cancer risk? *Nutrition reviews*, 1985, **43**: 325–331.

17. Levander OA. A global view of human selenium nutrition. *Annual review of nutrition*, 1987, **7**: 227–250.

18. Willett WC, Stampfer MJ. Selenium and cancer. *British medical journal*, 1988, **297**: 573–574.

19. Birt DF, Pour PM, Pelling JC. The influence of dietary selenium on colon, pancreas, and skin tumorigenesis. In: Wendel A, ed. *Selenium in biology and medicine*. Berlin, Springer-Verlag, 1989: 297–304.

20. Levander OA. The need for measures of selenium status. *Journal of the American College of Toxicology*, 1986, **5**: 37–44.

21. Burk RF. Selenium and cancer: meaning of serum selenium levels. *Journal of nutrition*, 1986, **116**: 1584–1586.

22. Salbe AD, Levander OA. Effect of various dietary factors on the deposition of selenium in the hair and nails of rats. *Journal of nutrition*, 1990, **120**: 200–206.

23. Patterson BK et al. Human selenite metabolism: a kinetic model. *American journal of physiology*, 1989, **257**: R556–R567.

24. Mutanen M. Bioavailability of selenium. *Annals of clinical research*, 1986, **18**: 48–54.

25. Levander OA et al. Bioavailability of selenium to Finnish men as assessed by platelet glutathione peroxidase activity and other blood parameters. *American journal of clinical nutrition*, 1983, **37**: 887–897.

26. Varo P, Koivistoinen P. Mineral element composition of Finnish foods. XII. General discussion and nutritional evaluation. *Acta agriculturae scandinavica*, 1980, **22** (Suppl.): 165–171.

27. Thompson JN, Erdody P, Smith DC. Selenium content of food consumed by Canadians. *Journal of nutrition*, 1975, **195**: 274–277.

28. Varo P et al. Selenium intake and serum selenium in Finland: effects of soil fertilization with selenium. *American journal of clinical nutrition*, 1988, **48**: 324–329.

29. Welsh SO et al. Selenium intake of Maryland residents consuming self-selected diets. *Journal of the American Dietetic Association*, 1981, **79**: 277–285.

30. Levander OA, Moser PB, Morris VC. Dietary selenium intake and selenium concentrations of plasma, erythrocytes, and breast milk in pregnant and postpartum lactating and nonlactating women. *American journal of clinical nutrition*, 1987, **46**: 694–698.

31. Mutanen M et al. Comparison of chemical analysis and calculation method in estimating selenium content of Finnish diets. *Nutrition research*, 1985, **5**: 693–697.

32. Mutanen M. Dietary intake and sources of selenium in young Finnish women. *Human nutrition: applied nutrition*, 1984, **38A**: 265–269.

33. Levander OA, Morris VC. Dietary selenium levels needed to maintain balance in North American adults consuming self-selected diets. *American journal of clinical nutrition*, 1984, **39**: 809–815.

34. National Research Council. *Recommended dietary allowances*, 9th ed. Washington, DC, National Academy of Sciences, 1980.

35. Yang GQ et al. Human selenium requirements in China. In: Combs GF et al., eds. *Selenium in biology and medicine*. New York, Van Nostrand Reinhold/AVI, 1987: 589–607.

36. National Research Council. *Recommended dietary allowances,* 10th ed. Washington, DC, National Academy of Sciences, 1989.

37. Casey CE et al. Selenium in human tissues from New Zealand. *Archives of environmental health,* 1982, **37**: 133–135.

38. Schroeder HA, Frost DV, Balassa JJ. Essential trace metals in man: selenium. *Journal of chronic diseases,* 1970, **23**: 227–243.

7.

Copper

7.1 Tissue distribution

Copper is widely distributed in biological tissues, where it occurs largely in the form of organic complexes, many of which are metalloproteins and function as enzymes. Copper enzymes are involved in a variety of metabolic reactions, such as the utilization of oxygen during cell respiration and energy utilization. They are also involved in the synthesis of essential compounds, such as the complex proteins of connective tissues of the skeleton and blood vessels, and in a range of neuroactive compounds concerned in nervous tissue function. It has been estimated that the adult human body contains 80 mg of copper, with a range of 50–120 mg. Tissue copper levels range from < 1 μg/g (dry weight) in many organs to > 10 μg/g (dry weight) in the liver and brain (1, 2). Copper levels in the fetus and young infant differ from those in the adult. Concentrations of copper may be 6–10-fold greater in the liver of infants where, during the first 2 months of postnatal life, it presumably serves as a store of copper to tide the infant over the period when intake from breast milk is relatively small (3).

Copper in human blood is principally distributed between the erythrocytes and the plasma. In erythrocytes, most copper (60%) occurs as the copper–zinc metalloenzyme superoxide dismutase, the remaining 40% being loosely bound to other proteins and amino acids. Total erythrocyte copper in normal humans is around 0.9–1.0 μg/ml of packed red cells (1, 2).

In plasma, about 93% of copper is firmly bound to the enzyme caeruloplasmin, believed to be involved in iron mobilization by maintaining the supply of oxidized iron transported after its incorporation into transferrin. The remaining plasma copper (7%) is bound less firmly to albumin and amino acids, and constitutes transport copper capable of reacting with receptor proteins or of diffusing, probably in the form of charged complexes, across cell membranes (1). Plasma or serum copper in normal humans is in the range 0.8–1.2 μg/ml and is not significantly influenced by cyclical rhythms or by feeding. The mean value for females is about 10% higher than that for males and is elevated by a factor of up to 3 in late pregnancy and in women taking estrogen-based oral contraceptives.

Hypocupraemia is defined as a serum copper level of 0.8 μg/ml or less, and since about 93% of serum copper is normally bound to caeruloplasmin, is usually accompanied by hypocaeruloplasminaemia (2). Hypercupraemia occurs naturally during pregnancy and is associated with the so-called "acute phase" reactions of a number of diseased states. It is almost always accompanied by hypercaeruloplasminaemia (2).

7.2 Biochemical function

Many of the well established physiological functions of copper in the body arise directly from its role in a number of copper-containing metalloenzymes (e.g. cytochrome oxidase, lysyl oxidase, caeruloplasmin, superoxide dismutase, monophenol monooxygenase (tyrosinase), dopamine β-monooxygenase) (4), and possibly also indirectly from the effect that a change in copper status may have on other enzyme systems which do not contain copper (4).

7.3 Symptoms of deficiency and toxicity

7.3.1 Deficiency (see Plate 4, pages 125 & 126)

A variety of symptoms have been associated with copper deficiency in animals, many of which are seen also in humans; they include hypochromic anaemia, neutropenia, hypopigmentation of hair and skin, abnormal bone formation with skeletal fragility and osteoporosis, vascular abnormalities and uncrimped or steely hair (1, 2, 5, 6). There is no single specific indicator of copper deficiency. Measurements which, despite major limitations, are currently considered to be of value in establishing a range for normal copper status include serum copper (normal range 0.64–1.56 μg/ml), caeruloplasmin (0.18–0.40 mg/ml), urinary copper (32–64 μg/24 h) and hair copper (10–20 μg/g), all of which are depressed in frankly copper-deficient subjects but are less sensitive to a marginal copper status (5). The possibility that a decline in erythrocyte copper–zinc superoxide dismutase, normally 0.47 ± 0.07 (SEM) mg/g of haemoglobin, may provide a more suitable and early indication of deficiency is being investigated.

Neutropenia is nowadays regarded as a sufficiently constant feature of copper deficiency in humans to be of diagnostic value (7), while evidence of a rapid decline in plasma enkephalins (8) warrants further investigation.[1]

---

[1] *Note added in proof*: Immunocompetence is probably prejudiced if the copper intake of adults is below 0.4 mg/day (Kelley DS et al. Effects of low-copper diets on human immune response. *American journal of clinical nutrition*, 1995, 62: 412–416).

7.3.2 Toxicity

In humans, acute copper poisoning is rare and usually results from contamination of foodstuffs or beverages by copper containers or from the accidental or deliberate ingestion of gram quantities of copper salts (9). Symptoms of acute copper poisoning include salivation, epigastric pain, nausea, vomiting and

Plate 4. Skeletal manifestations of copper deficiency in infant (5 months of age)

(A) Femur: thin bone with generalized osteopenia, metaphyseal cupping and "spur" formation (arrow)

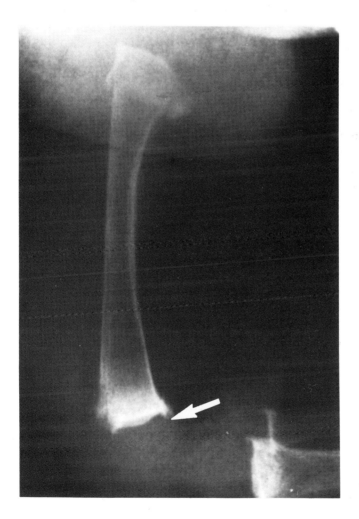

Plate 4 *(continued)*

(B) Radius, ulna and hand: osteopenia with retarded bone age, metaphyseal irregularities with cupping and "spur" formation (arrow)

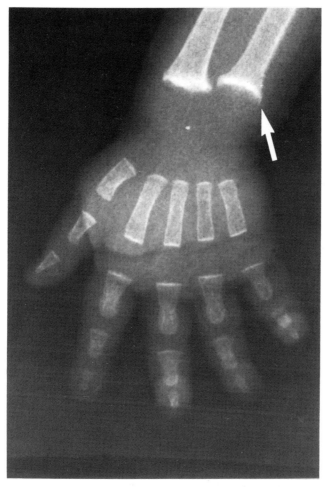

Reproduced with the kind permission of Dr B. Pontz, Kinderklinik und Poliklinik der Technischen Universität München, Germany.

diarrhoea, all of which are probably due to the irritant effect of copper on the gastrointestinal mucosa (1, 9). In addition, copper poisoning may be accompanied by severe intravascular haemolysis and jaundice, hepatic necrosis and failure, haemoglobinuria, proteinuria, hypotension, tachycardia, acute renal tubular failure, vascular collapse and death (9).

The clinical symptoms of chronic copper toxicity are less obvious and only appear when the capacity for protective hepatic sequestration of copper is exceeded, leading to hepatitis, liver cirrhosis, jaundice and, infrequently, a haemolytic crisis similar to that accompanying acute copper toxicity (10). The consumption by early weaned infants of milk-based formulae heavily contaminated with copper after storage in brass vessels is usually a significant feature of Indian childhood cirrhosis, which is frequently fatal. Liver failure is associated in this instance with a massive accumulation of liver copper (10).

7.4 Epidemiology of deficiency

Although the existence of uncomplicated nutritional copper deficiency has not been unequivocally demonstrated in humans, several abnormal situations can provoke a clinically significant copper deficiency (1, 2, 10, 11). Such situations are known to develop in infants with "cow's milk anaemia" and during rehabilitation from malnutrition using inadequately fortified formulae, in adults during protein–energy malnutrition, in various enteropathies, and during total parenteral nutrition with inadequately supplemented preparations. Until recently, it was widely believed that most ostensibly healthy individuals consumed diets which provided more than 2 mg of copper/day. Recent studies have indicated, however, that many diets provide significantly less copper than this, which suggests the possibility either that marginal deficiency may occur more widely than hitherto appreciated or that previous estimates of the lower safe intake (e.g. 2.0 mg/day (12)) have been too high (13). Until more is known of the nutritional requirement of humans for copper and tolerable minimum intakes have been more precisely defined, it would seem unwise to dismiss too readily speculation on the possible extent to which a suboptimal copper status exists in populations in which overt signs of deficiency are absent. These uncertainties are increased by the shortcomings of currently used indices of copper status, which lack the sensitivity to detect marginal copper deficits (5). In consequence, decisions as to the diagnostic value of biochemically evident responses to a low copper status (4) must await more extensive appraisal of the pathological relevance of the changes observed. Thus, although deficiency influences the metabolism of cholesterol (14), the "maturation" of connective tissue proteins, and the metabolism of neuroamines, neuropeptides and catecholamines, and changes in all of these potential indices are detectable by plasma analysis (8), the pathological significance of such changes at early stages of copper depletion has yet to be defined for humans, if not for other species.

7.5 Dietary intake and bioavailability

Copper is widely distributed in plants and animals. The copper content of vegetable crops is not greatly influenced by that of the soils on which they have grown but can increase markedly if leaf surfaces are contaminated by pollutants high in copper. Substantial species differences exist in the copper content of animal tissues used as food. Thus, ruminant liver and kidney can be high in copper. Good dietary sources of copper (> 2 μg/g) include seafood, organ meats, legumes and nuts. Refined cereals, sugar, milk and many other dairy products are low (< 2 μg/g) in the metal (15–17).

In 1980, when setting the Safe and Adequate Daily Dietary Intake of adults for copper at 2–3 mg/day, the United States Food and Nutrition Board was guided to some extent by the evidence then current that the dietary intake of copper in the USA was of that order (12). However, more recent studies based on the analysis of duplicate diets suggest that the actual intakes of adults may be much lower and in the range 1–1.5 mg/day (18–22). In the light of the advantages conferred by improvements in methodology, it is probable that the data from these recent studies more accurately reflect typical adult intake of copper.

Often overlooked, but nevertheless of potential significance, is the contribution copper pipes can make to copper intake from drinking-water. This can vary from less than 0.1 mg/day in hard water areas to 10 times that level with some extremely acid soft waters (2).

Soluble forms of copper are absorbed from the intestine with an efficiency usually in the range 40–60% and involving at least two mechanisms with both saturable and non-saturable components (23, 24).

Several constituents occurring naturally in food have been found to affect the absorption of copper from the intestine and to increase or decrease its bioavailability. Apart from a low intake of dietary copper, which appears to increase the efficiency of copper absorption (5, 25), the other main dietary factor which enhances the bioavailability of copper appears to be a high level of protein intake (100–150 g/day) (13).

Factors inhibiting the absorption of copper from the intestinal lumen and reducing its general bioavailability tend either to reduce its intraluminal solubility or to provoke competitive interactions with processes concerned with the transport of copper through the mucosa (26). In the first instance, the chemical form in which copper occurs in the gut lumen markedly affects its absorption. Highly soluble species of the metal such as the sulfate or nitrate are readily absorbed, while others such as copper carbonate are absorbed only after dissolving in the acid secretions of the stomach. Less soluble forms, e.g. copper oxide, are utilized less readily, while insoluble copper compounds, such as copper sulfide, or insoluble copper complexes such as copper porphyrin, are not utilized at all. Other factors modifying copper bioavailability are presented in Table 7.1 and Chapter 3. Current evidence suggests that the levels of antagonists likely to be encountered in normal diets are unlikely to have significant effects on copper utilization. However, their quantitative effects have not been adequately defined and the possibility exists that some may influence copper absorption from unusual diets.

Few of the dietary factors affecting copper availability appear to have as significant an influence on susceptibility to copper deficiency as does a low intake of the element. However, the enhanced absorption of copper at low intakes confers a limited protection against the development of deficiency. In

Table 7.1. Substances that, when present in excess, reduce the bioavailability of copper

Substance	Effect	Reference
Ascorbic acid	High intakes (> 1500 mg/day) may restrict copper absorption, but this is controversial	27, 28
Calcium/phosphorus	Excessive intakes (> 2 g/day) increase faecal losses of copper	2, 29
Cadmium[a]	Typical ranges of dietary cadmium probably have little influence on copper utilization by humans, but the osteoporosis of itai-itai disease may be related to impaired copper and calcium absorption (see Chapter 16)	13
Drugs and medications	Penicillamine and thiomolybdates used to restrict copper accumulation in Wilson disease; excessive use of "antacids" inhibits copper absorption	5
Fibre/phytate/lignin[a]	Effects variable and, though clearly established for experimental animals, probably not of importance to humans	1, 2, 6, 13, 25, 29, 30, 31
Iron	May restrict copper utilization by infants if intake exceeds 10 mg/day; also depends on dietary levels of zinc and calcium	2, 32, 33
Lead[a]	Probably of little relevance to humans as the effect of lead on copper absorption occurs only at dietary intakes > 250 μg/g	34
Maillard reaction-products and phytate/amino acid complexes	Antagonistic influence on utilization of calcium, iron and zinc clearly established; speculative whether utilization of copper is also impaired	13

Table 7.1 (continued)

Substance	Effect	Reference
Sucrose/fructose[a]	Exacerbatory effects on pathological consequences of copper deficiency in experimental animals are inconsistent and, when present, appear only with very high sugar intakes	35, 36
Zinc	The extent of the zinc:copper imbalance needed to depress copper absorption is inadequately defined; exploited therapeutically for control of Wilson disease	1, 2, 6, 13, 37–39

[a] Evidence derived from studies on experimental animals; human relevance has not been adequately established.

contrast, the bioavailability of copper has been found to decrease at the levels of zinc supplementation (> 100 mg of zinc/day) frequently recommended in quasi-scientific nutritional or medical reports. The enhanced absorption of copper associated with high levels of dietary protein appears to occur only at intakes above 100 g/day, which reduces its practical relevance. The nutritional relevance of the supposed effects of plant fibre and phytic acid, simple sugars and ascorbic acid is also questionable as their deleterious effects only seem to occur at very elevated levels of intake (i.e. fibre > 50 g/day; sugars > 35% of energy; ascorbic acid > 1500 mg/day). There is, however, a need to evaluate the importance of the phytate–fibre–copper interaction in countries where the consumption of plant products may be sufficiently high to restrict copper utilization as a consequence of this antagonism. It is also suspected that diets promoting sulfide generation through bacterial action on sulfates of sulfur-containing amino acids in the lower digestive tract may, if dietary molybdenum is also high, reduce the utilization of copper. The thiomolybdates that are likely to form and be absorbed under such conditions are potent systemic copper antagonists; advantage has been taken of this in their therapeutic use to restrict excessive copper uptake and storage in cases of Wilson disease.

7.6 Requirements and safe ranges of population mean intakes

7.6.1 Adult basal requirement

From the copper-responsive clinical and biochemical changes that occur when copper intake is low, it appears likely that the average adult *basal* requirement for copper (Cu_R^{basal}) is probably about 0.6 mg/day for women and 0.7 mg/day for men, i.e.approximately 11 μg/kg of body weight for either sex. The effects of copper deficiency in adults include decreased plasma copper levels, decreased caeruloplasmin and erythrocyte copper–zinc superoxide dismutase activities, increased low-density lipoprotein cholesterol, decreased high-density lipoprotein cholesterol, cardiac arrhythmia, electrocardiographic abnormalities and elevated blood pressure. Such evidence suggests that physiologically relevant signs of copper deficiency can appear in individuals after the experimental consumption of diets providing 0.7–1.0 mg of copper/day for at least 4 weeks, but not if the copper intake is higher (*14, 27, 40–43*). However, inconsistent responses within this range of intakes and the fact that in some cases (*14, 42, 43*) these experimentally initiated low intakes of copper were accompanied by other

Table 7.2. Average individual basal (Cu_R^{basal}) and normative ($Cu_R^{normative}$) requirement for dietary copper (μg/kg of body weight per day)

Age range (years)	Sex	Representative weight (kg)	Cu_R^{basal}	$Cu_R^{normative}$
0–0.25[a]	M&F	5	—	50–80[a]
0.25–0.5[a]	M&F	7	—	40–70[a]
0.5–1	M&F	9	—	40[b]
1–3	M&F	12	25	28[c]
3–6	M&F	17	18[c]	20[c]
6–10	M&F	25	16[c]	18[c]
10–12	F	37		
12–15	F	48	11	12.5
15–18	F	55		
18–60 +	F[d]	55		
10–12	M	35		
12–15	M	48	11	12.5
15–18	M	64		
18–60 +	M	65		

[a] Refers to formula-fed infants and a copper bioavailability of 30–50% (see page 135); copper intake from maternal milk during early infancy (*46*) can decline to 25 μg/kg of infant body weight per day without clinical or other evidence of deficiency but intrinsic stores of copper laid down during growth *in utero* may be drawn on; it is thus difficult to determine the absolute requirement for copper during infancy.

[b] Derived by interpolation from infant (0–0.5 years) and adult data.

[c] Derived by extrapolation from adult data; values on a body-weight basis for young children are proportionately higher.

[d] For pregnancy and lactation, see text.

significant dietary factors (e.g. high dietary fructose, ascorbic acid or zinc, very low energy content, collagen as the sole protein source), suggest that unidentified variables may have affected either the utilization or absorbability of dietary copper or the validity of the clinical or biochemical criteria used as indices of copper status.

In one experiment involving an otherwise uncomplicated dietary situation, only hypercholesterolaemia and decreased high-density lipoprotein cholesterol in men (40, 41) were linked to low copper intakes (< 0.8 mg/day). Women consuming fairly conventional diets providing 0.67 mg of copper/day for up to 84 days showed no changes in plasma cholesterol, although the activity of the copper-dependent respiratory enzyme cytochrome oxidase was significantly depressed in blood platelets, neutrophils and leukocytes, and there was an increase in stress-induced systolic blood pressure (27). The recent study by Turnlund et al. (44) is also relevant to the estimation of copper requirement, as these workers found no effect on cholesterol levels or heart function in 11 young men receiving only 0.78 mg of copper/day for 42 days.

Some further indication of the requirement of adults for copper can be gained from studies on copper balance in patients receiving total parenteral nutrition. Recent studies (45) suggest that *infusion* of 0.3 mg/day is sufficient to maintain copper balance in a stable 70-kg adult. If it is assumed that the efficiency of absorption of dietary copper is approximately 40% (see later), this would correspond to a dietary intake of 0.75 mg. Together, these clinical and biochemical data suggest that 0.6 and 0.7 mg of copper/day approach the average Cu_R^{basal} of individual women and men, respectively. These conclusions are based on evidence of the maintenance of enzyme function and prevention of clinical symptoms and include an allowance for the marked capacity of the body to increase its efficiency of copper utilization as copper intake declines (44).

7.6.2 Adult normative requirement

The copper intake deemed adequate to meet the *normative* requirement ($Cu_R^{normative}$) of adults for copper under practically all dietary conditions is set at 0.7 and 0.8 mg/day, respectively, for women and men. This represents an increment of 15% above the average basal requirement, firstly, to ensure that copper absorption and retention do not have to operate at maximum capacity and, secondly, to allow for some degree of copper storage. These normative estimates accord reasonably with the assessment by Turnlund et al. (44) that, for men, 0.8 mg of copper/day is probably in excess of requirement.

Table 7.2 presents estimates of average individual copper requirements of humans of all ages; the data are expressed in terms of μg of copper required/kg of body weight per day.

7.6.3 Minimum population mean intakes

To estimate the safe minimum mean copper intake of populations ($Cu_{\text{Plmin}}^{\text{normative}}$), it is necessary to assess the variation of "usual intakes" among active individuals. Such information is scarce. Two large studies of 7-day intakes of copper in the United Kingdom (22) and Australia (47) showed appreciable skewing in the distribution of intake data. The variability of intake to be taken into account in estimating population minimum mean intakes of copper was thus estimated by the procedure for the analysis of skewed survey data outlined in Annex 2. From the difference between the 2.5th centile and the *median* of adult intakes of copper, derived from United Kingdom and Australian survey data (0.6–0.7 mg copper/day), it appeared reasonable to assume that the CV of intake below the mean would be approximately 20%. Surveys of copper intake with smaller numbers of preschool children and adolescents in the United Kingdom (48), with a group of Canadian women (49) and with Canadian preschool children (50) suggested that the CV for interindividual intake could vary from 6% to 25%. Except for infants (see later), a CV of intake of 20% was assumed in the present report, from which:

$$Cu_{\text{Plmin}}^{\text{normative}} = 1.67\, Cu_{\text{R}}^{\text{normative}}$$

where $Cu_{\text{Plmin}}^{\text{normative}}$ is the lower limit of the safe range of population mean intakes of copper.

Estimates of $Cu_{\text{Plmin}}^{\text{normative}}$ obtained in this way are presented in Table 7.3. From pooled data for adults of both sexes, the estimated value was 1.25 mg of copper/day. Allowing for differences in body weight, this is equivalent to about 1.2 mg/day for women and 1.3 mg/day for men, or approximately 20 μg/kg per day. Table 7.3 also gives estimates of the lower acceptable limits of mean population intakes of copper to meet basal requirements ($Cu_{\text{Plmin}}^{\text{basal}}$).

The very tentative nature of these estimates must again be emphasized. They are based on estimates of basal and normative requirement derived using criteria of copper deficiency and adequacy that need further verification and inadequately defined individual differences in requirement. The variability of population intakes of copper needs to be investigated more widely, especially in different ethnic groups.

7.6.4 Requirements of infants

Human breast milk usually contains 200–400 μg of copper/l (51) and, typically, initially provides 50 μg/kg of infant body weight per day, declining to approximately 13 μg/kg after 6 months of lactation (46). Other estimates occasionally suggest even lower intakes. Copper equilibrium has been reported in infants receiving 27 μg/kg per day from breast milk (52). Furthermore, no

Table 7.3. Lower limits (mg/day) of the safe ranges of population mean intakes of dietary copper (in mg copper/day) to meet basal (Cu_{Plmin}^{basal}) and normative ($Cu_{Plmin}^{normative}$) dietary requirements[a]

Age range (years) or state	Sex	Representative weight (kg)	Cu_{Plmin}^{basal}	$Cu_{Plmin}^{normative}$
0–0.25	M&F	5	—	0.33–0.55[b]
0.25–0.5	M&F	7	—	0.37–0.62[b]
0.5–1	M&F	9	—	0.60
1–3	M&F	12	0.50	0.56
3–6	M&F	17	0.51	0.57
6–10	M&F	25	0.67	0.75
10–12	F	37	0.68	0.77
12–15	F	48	0.88	1.00
15–18	F	55	1.01	1.15
18–60 +	F	55	1.01	1.15
10–12	M	35	0.64	0.73
12–15	M	48	0.88	1.00
15–18	M	64	1.17	1.33
18–60 +	M	65	1.19	1.35
Pregnancy			1.01[c]	1.15[c]
Lactation			1.11	1.25

[a] Unless otherwise specified, the CV of usual dietary copper intakes is assumed to be 20% (see page 133).

[b] For formula-fed infants only; CV of intake assumed to be 12.5% (see page 135); the bioavailability of copper is in the range 30–50% (see page 135).

[c] From evidence from other species, it is assumed that the small increase in demand during pregnancy (see page 136) is met by an increased efficiency of copper absorption.

clinical problems associated with copper deficiency have been reported in infants receiving breast milk alone at intakes of copper in the range 15–30 μg/kg per day (53; C.F. Mills, personal communication 1992).

By contrast, clinical copper deficiency, as shown by growth retardation, respiratory tract infection, osteoporosis, neutropenia, leukopenia, anaemia and biochemical changes indicative of a low copper status, has been reported by several workers for infants receiving up to 50 μg of copper/kg per day from formula diets (54–61). These ostensibly conflicting findings possibly reflect a less efficient absorption of copper from these foods than from breast milk. Such differences in the efficiency of copper absorption have been found in experimental model studies in which weanling rats absorbed 25% of human-breast-milk copper but only 10% of copper from a soya-based formula. Preterm infants absorbed 50% of breast milk copper, and virtually none from soya-based formulae (62), whereas, in normal infants, the corresponding figures were 44–57% and 32–33% respectively (C.F. Mills, personal communication 1992). However, no clinical problems associated with copper deficiency have been reported from any infant diet providing more than 50 μg/kg per day. Furthermore, positive copper balances have been reported regularly in infants receiving this or higher intakes of copper (52, 56, 58, 59, 61, 63, 64; C.F. Mills, personal communication 1992).

Accordingly, it can tentatively be assumed that all infants (0–6 months of age) not given breast milk should receive cow's-milk-based or other formula diets providing at least 50 μg/kg per day. This intake may have to be increased in formulae where the bioavailability of copper is likely to be reduced (e.g. soya-based diets), although it appears unlikely that even in these situations $Cu_R^{normative}$ will exceed 100 μg/kg per day.

Estimates of the average individual requirements of infants for copper are presented in Table 7.2; corresponding estimates of minimum population mean intakes of copper from formula diets are given in Table 7.3. It is assumed in both tables that the CV of copper intake from formula diets is 12.5%.

The estimates given above are in reasonably good agreement with the factorial calculation of the total copper requirement of 123 μg/day needed to meet the growth requirement (28 μg/day) and to replace the endogenous losses (95 μg/day) of a 3-month-old infant (estimated from references 65 and 66). These data translate into a physiological requirement for *absorbed* copper of 20 μg/kg per day, probably equivalent to the ingestion of about 40 μg/kg for the infant given breast milk and 60 μg/kg when soya-based formulae are given.

7.6.5 Basal and normative requirements of children and adolescents

Clinical and biochemical studies during the development of copper deficiency in children and while their copper intakes are monitored are very rare. Higuchi et al. (67) describe young patients receiving a low-copper enteral diet providing approximately 0.15 mg of copper/day (4.5–8.5 μg/kg per day) who displayed symptoms of neutropenia, leukopenia, hypocupraemia, hypocaeruloplasminaemia, anaemia and loss of bone density, none of which signs were seen in subjects receiving 0.48–0.80 mg of copper/day (23–46 μg/kg per day). From an examination of the relationships between plasma copper, caeruloplasmin activity, clinical condition and copper intake of these subjects, it was concluded (67) that the adolescent $Cu_R^{normative}$ is probably less than 20 μg/kg per day; this is compatible with that proposed here for adults. Data on copper intakes required to establish equilibrium between input and output differ widely, ranging from 35 to 2000 μg/kg per day (1, 68). Although most suggest that balance can be established at intakes in the range 50–100 μg/kg per day (1, 69, 70), most sets of data also reflect the difficulty of interpreting copper balance studies when the copper status of experimental subjects has not been previously defined.

7.6.6 Requirements for pregnancy and lactation

Limited balance data indicate positive copper balances in pregnant women receiving 2.8 mg/day and 1.4–2.5 mg/day (71). Most significantly, pregnancy was found to improve copper retention by about 4% or 0.08 mg/day, which would be sufficient to accumulate the 21 mg of copper needed for the fetus and its adnexa without any additional copper intake from the diet (71). Pregnancy is therefore not considered to increase the dietary requirement for copper. During lactation, the loss of copper in milk amounts initially to around 0.2 mg/day but declines to approximately 0.1 mg/day after 6 months (46). From studies on other species, it is reasonable to assume that half of this is provided by enhanced maternal absorption of copper during lactation and therefore does not represent an increased dietary requirement. The remainder, 0.1–0.05 mg/day, must be provided from the diet and is often met from the increased (25%) energy intake, and thus of food intake, associated with the period of milk production.

7.6.7 Safe upper limits of population mean intakes

In humans, acute copper poisoning occurs infrequently and results mainly from the accidental ingestion of gram quantities of copper in contaminated foodstuffs and beverages, or occasionally as a consequence of deliberate, suicidal consumption. Intakes of this order cause serious systemic effects of copper toxicity, including haemolysis and jaundice, liver damage, convulsions, hypotension, coma and death (2, 72). Because of the irritant effect of copper ions on mucosal membranes, even milligram quantities can cause vomiting and diarrhoea. Daily intakes of copper ranging from 2 to 32 mg in drinking-water have been reported to cause symptoms of general gastric irritation (73). While this evidence is compatible with the United States drinking-water "action level" of 1.3 mg/l (74), the Expert Consultation considered that additional evidence was needed to show that intakes as low as 2 mg/day from water (about 1 mg/l) could produce an adverse reaction. The Consultation recommended that, until such evidence was available, the WHO provisional guideline value of 2 mg/l of drinking-water should be used as the criterion for looking into the need to limit access to adventitious sources of copper (75).

In the assessment of a safe level of intake for copper, it is important to distinguish ionic copper ingested in water or as a supplement from dietary copper in foods, which is largely present in the form of organic compounds. While there is little doubt that the uncontrolled ingestion of soluble inorganic copper salts in milligram quantities should be regarded with caution, levels of copper in food up to around 10 mg/day seem to have no detrimental effect on human health. The upper limit to the safe range of population mean intakes, Cu^{tox}_{Plmax}, for adults has accordingly been set at 12 mg/day for men and 10 mg/day for women (Table 7.4). This will take account of the quantity likely to be consumed from the usual diet (< 10 mg/day) and will limit both the amount of copper that can be introduced by dietary fortification and the quantity of contaminating copper that can be regarded as tolerable.

While copper intoxication of breast-fed infants is very rare, newborn and young children are more sensitive to excess copper than normal adults. Such susceptibility is apparent in Indian childhood cirrhosis, which is frequently fatal; in this disease hepatic necrosis and inflammation are associated with the weaning of infants onto cow or buffalo milk stored, and sometimes boiled before use, in brass vessels, and thus being contaminated with copper. Milk so treated has been shown to contain 2.66 ± 0.60 (SD) mg of copper/l rather than, typically, 0.086 ± 0.001 (SD) mg/l (12, 72).

Taking into account the adult recommendation, the Expert Consultation set the Cu^{tox}_{Plmax} for infants at 150 μg/kg. Lower population maximum mean intakes have been suggested for young children (1–10 years) because of their potentially higher exposure to non-dietary sources of copper and because of suspicions that

Table 7.4. Upper limits of the safe range of population mean intakes of copper (in mg/day)

Age range (years) or state	Sex	Assumed weight (kg)	Cu^{tox}_{Plmax}
0–1.0	M&F	—	150[a]
1–6	M&F	16	1.5
6–10	M&F	25	3.0
10–12	F	37	6.0
12–15	F	48	8.0
15–60 +	F	55	10.0
10–12	M	35	6.0
12–15	M	48	8.0
15–60 +	M	65	12.0
Pregnancy			10.0
Lactation			10.0

[a] In μg/kg.

some contaminants of food or drinking-water may promote hepatic copper accumulation in this age group.

7.6.8 Comparison of reference values with dietary intakes

A comparison of the proposed values for $Cu_{Plmin}^{normative}$ (men 1.3 mg/day; women 1.2 mg/day) with the data on copper intake from dietary surveys summarized in Chapter 22 shows that dietary copper supply is marginal or possibly inadequate in a number of countries. Comparison with the lower limits of population mean intakes of copper indicates that, in the 136 dietary surveys examined, 30 mean values were below $Cu_{Plmin}^{normative}$ and 17 below Cu_{Plmin}^{basal}. In only one of 10 recent highly controlled IAEA studies were intakes below the basal minimum mean population copper intake. In contrast, a recent survey in the United Kingdom (22) suggests that the copper intake of at least 2.5% of the 2220 individuals investigated aged 16–65 years was less than the estimate of individual mean copper requirements, $Cu_R^{normative}$, given here for both men and women. The significance of this finding has yet to be investigated.

7.7 Recommendations for future studies

In Chapter 22, a small but significant number of dietary surveys are considered which suggest that mean population intakes of copper are frequently lower than the estimates given here of the minimum likely to meet the normative requirement for this element. A smaller number are lower than the estimates of minimum basal population mean intakes. Cases of severe, chronic copper deficiency are likely to remain confined to infants and children subject to incorrect dietary planning during rehabilitation from malnutrition induced by famine or social deprivation. However, there is a significant degree of uncertainty as to the pathological consequences for humans of the less severe degrees of deficiency already known to influence adversely the health of other species when copper intake per unit weight is close to the estimates of basal requirements.

- It is recommended that closer attention be given initially to the definition and later to the monitoring of the many physiological processes that are directly or indirectly responsive to changes in copper status. The involvement of copper in a variety of key oxidative and synthetic processes may well imply that mild deficiency has generalized rather than diagnostically specific effects.
- As a prelude to further epidemiological or experimental studies with human subjects, it is also recommended that sensitivity to cardiovascular structural and functional defects and to neurological metabolic lesions be

more widely investigated in animal models mildly depleted of copper. Such studies should include the monitoring of copper-responsive bio-chemical changes that may suggest appropriate indices for the early detection of pathologically relevant changes in subsequent studies with human subjects.

- Better diagnostic indices are needed for the detection of chronic intoxication with copper to resolve doubts as to the significance of a high copper burden in Indian childhood cirrhosis and controversies relating to the pathological significance of high levels of copper in some highly contaminated water supplies.

References

1. Mason KE. A conspectus of research on copper metabolism and requirements of man. *Journal of nutrition*, 1979, **109**: 1979–2006.
2. Underwood EJ. *Trace elements in human and animal nutrition*, 4th ed. New York, Academic Press, 1977: 56–108.
3. Walravens PA. Nutritional importance of copper and zinc in neonates and infants. *Clinical chemistry*, 1980, **26**: 185–189.
4. Prohaska JR. Biochemical functions of copper in animals. In: Prasad AS ed. *Essential and toxic trace elements in human health and disease*. New York, Alan R. Liss, 1988: 105–124.
5. Turnlund JR. Copper nutriture, bioavailability and the influence of dietary factors. *Journal of the American Dietetic Association*, 1988, **88**: 303–308.
6. O'Dell BL. Biochemical basis of the clinical effects of copper deficiency. In: Prasad AS, ed. *Clinical, biochemical and nutritional aspects of trace elements*. New York, Alan R. Liss, 1982, 301–313.
7. Mills CF. Biological roles of trace elements. In: Harper AE, Davis GK, eds. *Nutrition in health and disease*. New York, Alan R. Liss, 1981: 179–188.
8. Bhathena SJ et al. Decreased plasma enkephalins in copper deficiency in man. *American journal of clinical nutrition*, 1986, **43**: 42–46.
9. Williams DM. Clinical significance of copper deficiency and toxicity in the world population. In: Prasad AS, ed. *Clinical, biochemical and nutritional aspects of trace elements*. New York, Alan R. Liss, 1982: 277–299.
10. Tanner MS. Indian childhood cirrhosis. *Recent advances in paediatrics*, 1986, **8**: 103–120.
11. *Trace elements in human nutrition. Report of a WHO Expert Committee*. Geneva, World Health Organization, 1973 (WHO Technical Report Series, No. 532).
12. National Research Council. *Recommended dietary allowances*, 9th ed., Washington, DC, National Academy of Sciences, 1980.
13. Sandstead HH. Copper bioavailability and requirements. *American journal of clinical nutrition*, 1982, **32**: 908–914.
14. Reiser S et al. Indices of copper status in humans consuming a typical American diet

containing either fructose or starch. *American journal of clinical nutrition*, 1985, **42**: 242–251.

15. Pennington JT, Calloway DH. Copper content of foods. *Journal of the American Dietetic Association*, 1974, **63**: 143–153.

16. Paul AA, Southgate DH. *McCance and Widdowson's the composition of foods*, 4th ed. London, HMSO, 1978: 235–251.

17. Mertz W. Mineral elements: new perspectives. *Journal of the American Dietetic Association*, 1980, **77**: 258–263.

18. Klevay LM et al. The human requirement for copper. 1. Healthy men fed conventional American diets. *American journal of clinical nutrition*, 1980, **33**: 34–50.

19. Patterson KY et al. Zinc, copper and manganese intake and balance for adults consuming self-selected diets. *American journal of clinical nutrition*, 1984, **40**: 1397–1403.

20. Pennington JAT et al. Mineral content of foods and total diets: the selected minerals in foods survey. *Journal of the American Dietetic Association*, 1986, **86**: 876–891.

21. Schwarts R, Apgar BJ, Wien EM. Apparent absorption and retention of Ca, Cu, Mg, Mn and Zn from a diet containing bran. *American journal of clinical nutrition*, 1986, **43**: 444–455.

22. Gregory J et al. *The diet and health of adults in the United Kingdom*. London, HMSO, 1990.

23. King JC, Reynolds WL, Margen S. Absorption of stable isotopes of iron, copper and zinc during oral contraceptive use. *American journal of clinical nutrition*, 1978, **31**: 1198–1203.

24. Hoadley JE, Cousins RJ. Regulatory mechanisms for intestinal transport of zinc and copper. In: Prasad AS, ed. *Essential and toxic trace elements in human health and disease*. New York, Alan R. Liss, 1988: 141–155.

25. Turnlund JR et al. A stable isotope study of copper absorption in young men: effect of phytate and α-cellulose. *American journal of clinical nutrition*, 1985, **42**: 18–23.

26. Mills CF. Dietary interactions involving the trace elements. *Annual review of nutrition*, 1985, **5**: 173–193.

27. Milne DB, Klevay LM, Hunt JR. Effects of ascorbic acid supplements and a diet marginal in copper on indices of copper nutriture in women. *Nutrition research* 1988, **8**: 865–873.

28. Jacob RA et al. Effect of varying ascorbic acid intakes on copper absorption and ceruloplasmin levels in young men. *Journal of nutrition*, 1987, **117**: 2109–2115.

29. Snedeker SM, Smith SA, Greger JL. Effect of dietary calcium and phosphorus levels on the utilization of iron, copper and zinc by adult males. *Journal of nutrition*, 1982, **112**: 136–143.

30. Kelsay JL et al. Mineral balances of men fed a diet containing fiber in fruits and vegetables and oxalic acid in spinach for six weeks. *Journal of nutrition*, 1988, **118**: 1197–1204.

31. Hallfrisch J et al. Mineral balances of men and women consuming high fiber diets with complex or simple carbohydrate. *Journal of nutrition*, 1987, **117**: 48–55.

32. Aggett PJ. Physiology and metabolism of essential trace elements: an outline. *Clinics in endocrinology and metabolism*, 1985, **14**: 513–543.

33. Haschke F et al. Effect of iron fortification in infant formula on trace mineral absorption. *Journal of pediatric gastroenterology and nutrition*, 1986, **5**: 708–733.

34. Mylroie AA, Boseman A, Kyle A. Metabolic interactions between lead and copper in rats ingesting lead acetate. *Biological trace element research*, 1986, **9**: 221–231.

35. Redman RS et al. Dietary fructose exacerbates the cardiac abnormalities of copper deficiency in rats. *Atherosclerosis*, 1988, **74**: 203–214.

36. Holbrook J, Smith JC, Reiser S. Dietary fructose or starch: effects on copper, zinc, iron, manganese, calcium and magnesium balances in humans. *American journal of clinical nutrition*, 1986, **49**: 1295–1301.

37. Oestreicher P, Cousins RJ. Copper and zinc absorption in the rat: mechanisms of mutual antagonism. *Journal of nutrition*, 1985, **115**: 159–166.

38. Festa MD et al. Effect of zinc intake on copper excretion and retention in man. *American journal of clinical nutrition*, 1985, **41**: 285–292.

39. Turnlund HR et al. Copper absorption in young men fed adequate and low zinc diets. *Biological trace element research*, 1988, **17**: 31–41.

40. Reiser S et al. Effect of copper intake on blood cholesterol and its lipoprotein distribution in men. *Nutrition reports international*, 1987, **36**: 641–649.

41. Klevay LM et al. Increased cholesterol in plasma in a young man during experimental copper depletion. *Metabolism*, 1980, **33**: 1112–1117.

42. Lukaski HC et al. Effects of dietary copper on human autonomic cardiovascular function. *European journal of applied physiology*, 1988, **58**: 74–80.

43. Lowy SL et al. Zinc and copper nutriture in obese men receiving very low calorie diets of soy or collagen protein. *American journal of clinical nutrition*, 1986, **43**: 272–287.

44. Turnlund JR et al. Copper absorption and retention in young men at three levels of dietary copper by use of the stable isotope ^{65}Cu. *American journal of clinical nutrition*, 1989, **49**: 870–878.

45. Shike M et al. Copper metabolism and requirements in total parenteral nutrition. *Gastroenterology*, 1981, **81**: 290–297.

46. Casey CE, Neville MC, Hambidge KM. Studies in human lactation; secretion of zinc, copper and manganese in human milk. *American journal of clinical nutrition*, 1989, **49**: 773–785.

47. Baghurst K et al. *The Victorian Nutrition Survey, Part 2*, Adelaide, CSIRO Division of Human Nutrition, 1987: 66–67.

48. Nelson M et al. Between and within subject variation in nutrient intake from infancy to old age: estimating the number of days required to rank dietary intakes with desired precision. *American journal of clinical nutrition*, 1989, **50**: 155–167.

49. Gibson RS, Gibson IL, Kitching J. A study of inter- and intra-subject variability in seven day weighed dietary intakes with particular emphasis on trace elements. *Biological trace element research*, 1986, **8**: 79–91.

50. Vanderkooy PDS, Gibson RS. Food consumption patterns of Canadian pre-school children in relation to zinc and growth status. *American journal of clinical nutrition*, 1987, **45**: 609–616.

51. *Minor and trace elements in breast milk. Report of a joint WHO/IAEA collaborative study.* Geneva, World Health Organization, 1989.

52. Aggett PJ et al. Evaluation of the trace metal supplements for a synthetic low lactose diet. *Archives of disease in childhood*, 1983, **58**: 433–437.

53. Salmenpera L et al. Cu nutrition in infants during prolonged exclusive breast-feeding: low intake but rising serum concentrations of Cu and ceruloplasmin. *American journal of clinical nutrition*, 1986, **43**: 251–257.

54. Sturgeon P, Brubaker C. Copper deficiency in infants. *AMA journal of diseases of children*, 1956, **92**: 254–265.

55. Castillo-Duran C et al. Controlled trial of copper supplementation during recovery from marasmus. *American journal of clinical nutrition*, 1983, **37**: 898–903.

56. Castillo-Duran C, Torres RP, Guzman EC. Plasma copper response in humans with restricted diet: effect of zinc supplementation. *Nutrition research*, 1988, **8**: 163–167.

57. Levy Y et al. Copper deficiency in infants fed cows milk. *Journal of pediatrics*, 1985, **106**: 786–788.

58. Cordano A, Placko RP, Graham GG. Hypocupremia and neutropenia in copper deficiency. *Blood*, 1966, **28**: 280–283.

59. Graham GG, Cordano A. Copper depletion and deficiency in the malnourished infant. *Johns Hopkins medical journal*, 1969, **124**: 139–150.

60. Tanaka Y et al. Nutritional copper deficiency in a Japanese infant on formula. *Journal of pediatrics*, 1980, **96**: 255–256.

61. Sutton AM et al. Copper deficiency in the pre-term infant of very low birth weight. *Archives of disease in childhood*, 1985, **60**: 644–651.

62. Mendelson RA, Bryan MH, Anderson GH. Trace mineral balances in preterm infants fed their own mother's milk. *Journal of pediatric gastroenterology and nutrition*, 1983, **2**: 256–261.

63. Friel JK et al. A comparison of the zinc, copper and manganese status of very low birth weight preterm and full term infants during the first 12 months. *Acta pediatrica scandinavica*, 1984, **73**: 596–601.

64. Thorn JM. Mineral and trace element supplement for use with synthetic diets based on comminuted chicken. *Archives of disease in childhood*, 1978, **53**: 931–938.

65. Widdowson EM, Dickerson JWT. Chemical composition of the body. In: Comar CL, Bronner F, eds. *Mineral metabolism, 2.* New York, Academic Press, 1961.

66. Zlotkin SH, Buchanan BE. Meeting copper intake requirement in the parenterally fed pre-term and full-term infant. *Journal of pediatrics*, 1983, **103**: 441–446.

67. Higuchi S et al. Nutritional copper deficiency in severely handicapped patients on a low copper enteral diet for a prolonged period. *Journal of pediatric gastroenterology and nutrition*, 1988, **7**: 583–587.

68. Alexander FW, Clayton B, Delves HT. Mineral and trace-metal balances in children receiving normal and synthetic diets. *Quarterly journal of medicine*, 1974, **113**: 2346–2352.

69. Daniels AL, Wright OE. Iron and copper retentions in young children. *Journal of nutrition*, 1934, **8**: 125–138.

70. Scoular FI. A quantitative study by spectrographic analysis of copper in nutrition. *Journal of nutrition*, 1938, **16**: 437–450.

71. Turnlund JR, Swanson CA, King JC. Copper absorption and retention in pregnant women fed diets based on animal and plant proteins. *Journal of nutrition*, 1983, **113**: 2346–2352.

72. Moffit AE. Effects of nutrient toxicities in animals and man: copper. In: Rechcigl Jr M, ed. *Nutritional disorders*, Vol 1. Palm Beach, FL, CRC Press, 1978: 195–202 (CRC Handbook Series in Nutrition and Food, Section E).

73. *Summary review of the health effects associated with copper.* Cincinnati, US Environmental Protection Agency, 1987.

74. *Copper.* Washington, DC, National Academy of Sciences, 1977: 117.

75. *Guidelines for drinking-water quality*, 2nd ed. *Volume 1. Recommendations.* Geneva, World Health Organization, 1993.

8.
Molybdenum

8.1 Biochemical function

Aspects of the biochemistry and biological significance of molybdenum have been reviewed elsewhere (1–4). In plants and lower organisms, molybdenum-dependent enzymes are involved in nitrogen fixation, in the conversion of nitrate to ammonia and in a series of other oxidation–reduction reactions. The three principal molybdenum-containing enzymes of human and animal tissues, namely xanthine dehydrogenase/oxidase, aldehyde oxidase and sulfite oxidase share a common cofactor, molybdopterin, a substituted pterin to which molybdenum is bound by two sulfur atoms (2).

Discovery of molybdenum in the enzyme xanthine dehydrogenase/oxidase involved in the conversion of tissue purines to uric acid provided the first evidence of the essentiality of this element. Normally the enzyme acts as a dehydrogenase but, when reacting with oxygen, it initiates the production of a series of highly reactive oxygen-rich free radicals believed to be responsible for some features of tissue damage induced by physical injury and a wide variety of toxins, including excess molybdenum.

A reduced tissue activity of this enzyme has been associated with xanthin-uria, a genetic defect characterized by a low output of uric acid and high concentrations of xanthine and hypoxanthine in blood and urine. Clinical manifestations become apparent only after renal calculi have formed or after deposition of xanthine and hypoxanthine in muscles has resulted in a mild myopathy.

Low molybdenum intakes also reduce tissue xanthine dehydrogenase activity, but there is no convincing evidence that changes in molybdenum intake from conventional diets sufficiently influence enzyme activity to cause clinical changes in mammals. Furthermore, while a low xanthine dehydrogenase activity in tissues or changes in its substrate/product relationships (e.g. of the xanthine + hypoxanthine/uric acid ratio in plasma) may reflect a low molybdenum status, such responses are insufficiently specific to be of diagnostic value. Thus xanthine dehydrogenase activity also decreases if protein intake is low and in cases of hepatoma. Conversely, activity increases if protein intake is high, if vitamin E status is low, or if interferon or agents stimulating its release are

144

given. Claims that high intakes of molybdenum stimulate tissue xanthine dehydrogenase activity await verification (see page 147). The molybdenoenzyme aldehyde oxidase is structurally and chemically similar to xanthine oxidase, exhibits a similar distribution between tissues and shares some substrates. However, other biochemical properties differ and its principal metabolic roles are not known (5).

An additional molybdenoenzyme, sulfite oxidase, responsible for the conversion of sulfite derived from cysteine, methionine and related compounds into inorganic sulfate, has been isolated from the liver of humans and other species. Instances of genetic "deficiency" of sulfite oxidase have been detected in early human infancy and have a lethal outcome at the age of 2–3 years. The lesion results in severe neurological abnormalities, mental retardation and ectopy of the lens. Urinary outputs of sulfite, thiosulfate and S-sulfo-L-cysteine all increase and urinary sulfate decreases (6). These pathological changes may result either from the accumulation of toxic concentrations of sulfite in some critical organs or from inadequate production of the sulfate required for synthesis of sulfolipids, proteins and sulfate-conjugates. Other inborn metabolic disorders are associated with genetically related deficiencies of aldehyde oxidase, xanthine oxidase and sulfite oxidase caused by failure to synthesize their molybdopterin cofactor (2, 7).

8.2 Deficiency and toxicity

8.2.1 Deficiency

A nutritional deficiency of molybdenum giving rise to clinical symptoms suggestive of a deficiency of sulfite oxidase has been reported by Abumrad et al. (6) in a human patient subjected to prolonged total parenteral nutrition. The clinical symptoms included irritability leading to coma, tachycardia, tachypnoea and night blindness. A reduced intake of protein and sulfur-containing amino acids alleviated the symptoms, whereas they were exacerbated by infusion of sulfite. Tissue sulfite oxidase activity was low, thiosulfate excretion increased 25-fold, sulfate output declined by 70% and plasma methionine increased markedly. The clinical symptoms of molybdenum deficiency were totally eliminated by supplementation with 300 µg of ammonium molybdate (147 µg of molybdenum) daily. Further evidence of the essentiality of molybdenum came from a study of two young adults with Crohn disease maintained on total parenteral nutrition after ileal resection. Both had extensive losses of trace minerals including molybdenum (350–530 µg of molybdenum/day) from the intestinal tract. Parenteral infusion of 500 µg of ammonium molybdate (225 µg of molybdenum) increased uric acid levels in the plasma and urine of these patients (8).

Although proving the essentiality of molybdenum to humans, these studies do not provide sufficient data from which requirements for the element can be estimated. Thus, extensive intestinal losses in the above patients could well have disturbed molybdenum homoeostasis and, furthermore, the molybdenum content of the infusates given when molybdenum-responsive disorders were developing is not stated in either of the reports considered above.

Evidence as to the other possible consequences of molybdenum depletion must be drawn from studies on animals or from tissue culture data. Thus, in goats, a molybdenum-deficient diet (24 μg of molybdenum/kg of dietary dry matter) caused a decline in conception rate, an increase in abortion rate and a significant rise in the mortality of molybdenum-deficient dams and their offspring (9). Chinese studies suggest that both molybdenum and selenium are essential for the survival, growth and normal electrophysiological function of rodent cardiomyocytes.

8.2.2 Toxicity (molybdenosis)

Molybdenum intoxication is accompanied by a wide range of symptoms, some possibly attributable to the induction of a secondary deficiency of copper. Typical features of acute, uncomplicated molybdenosis include defects in osteogenesis possibly caused by deranged phosphorus metabolism and leading to skeletal and joint deformities, spontaneous subepiphyseal fractures, and mandibular exostoses (10). Alkaline phosphatase activity and the proteoglycan content of cartilage both decrease.

Development of a "conditioned" copper deficiency as a consequence of high intakes of molybdenum occurs principally in ruminants. However, some aspects of the response of other species to high molybdenum intakes suggest that, even in non-ruminants, including humans, the utilization of copper may be impaired (3, 11). Typical manifestations are the induction of anaemia, cardiac hypertrophy, and achromotrichia arising from the development of defects in melanin synthesis in hair.

The basis for the antagonistic effect of molybdenum on copper utilization is, firstly, the reaction of molybdate with sulfide generated by bacterial reduction of sulfate within the gastrointestinal tract and, secondly, the reaction with copper of the thiomolybdates thus produced to yield derivatives in which the copper cannot be utilized. Large amounts of sulfide can be generated within the human colon if sulfate intake is more than 0.7 g/day (12). Extrapolation of data from other species suggest that the high human intakes of molybdenum in epidemiological studies reported by Yang et al. (13) and Kovalsky et al. (14) would be sufficient to promote thiomolybdate formation and thus induce systemic antagonistic effects on copper utilization. Other consequences of molybdenum intoxication *per se* in non-human species include inhibition of the synthesis of "active" sulfate (phosphoadenosine phosphosulfate), inhibition of estrus, and interstitial testicular degeneration possibly mediated through effects on estrogen- or androgen-receptor activities. Their relevance to humans has not been studied.

8.3 Epidemiology of deficiency and toxicity

The intake of molybdenum by humans, like that of farm animals, is high both when soil molybdenum levels are high and when its uptake into foods and forages is promoted by neutral or alkaline conditions, particularly where soils are poorly drained. Thus, the human intake of molybdenum in parts of Armenia where such conditions prevail can amount to 10–15 mg of molybdenum/day. Workers employed in molybdenum-roasting plants are exposed to similar intakes from the inhalation of molybdenum dust. In both situations, elevated serum molybdenum values and abnormally high activities of xanthine dehydrogenase activity have been associated with increases in uric acid concentrations in blood and urine. Claims that these changes are relevant to the abnormally high incidence of gout in the high-molybdenum provinces of the Ankavan and Kajaran regions of Armenia (*14*) require closer investigation.

8.3.1 Cancer

It has been claimed that molybdenum status influences susceptibility to certain forms of cancer and that the high incidence of oesophageal cancer among the Bantu in Transkei (South Africa) is associated with a deficiency of this element in locally available food (*15*). Studies in Henan province, China, suggest that a high incidence of oesophageal cancer is associated with lower than normal contents of molybdenum in drinking-water and food as well as in serum, hair and urine. Oesophageal cancer tissue also had a lower molybdenum content than normal. It may well be relevant that inclusion of 2 or 20 µg of molybdenum/g in the diet of rats has been found to inhibit oesophageal and stomach cancer following the administration of N-nitrososarcosine ethyl ester (*16*). Molybdenum in the drinking-water of rats at a concentration of 10 mg/l inhibited mammary carcinogenesis induced by N-nitroso-N-methylurea.

8.3.2 Dental caries

Epidemiological studies claiming that molybdenum exerts an anticariogenic effect in humans have been critically reviewed by Hadjimarkos (*17*), who found the evidence contradictory and inconclusive. Nevertheless, teeth accumulate molybdenum and dental enamel is relatively rich in this element (18). The implications of these findings merit further investigation.

8.3.3 Keshan disease

While there is clear evidence that a deficiency of selenium is a predisposing factor in the pathogenesis of myocardial defects in Keshan disease (see Chapter 6), other factors, as yet unidentified, are also involved. Some data indicate that the molybdenum content of cereal grains and drinking-water is particularly low in areas where Keshan disease is endemic (19). It is claimed that the incidence of Keshan disease has been reduced in such areas by fertilization of staple food crops with molybdenum salts (20). Such data and the evidence referred to earlier that cardiomyocyte viability and function are improved by fortification of cell culture media with molybdenum have led to the suggestion that molybdenum deficiency coexisting with selenium deficiency may be obligatory for the development of Keshan disease (19). In contrast, other reports (13) provide striking evidence of abnormally high molybdenum contents of rice, wheat and soya in areas where Keshan disease is endemic, together with data illustrating remarkably high tissue and hair molybdenum in subjects from Keshan disease areas. In the face of such conflicting evidence, the outcome of investigations designed to determine the significance or otherwise of anomalies in the molybdenum status of Keshan disease subjects is awaited with interest.

8.4 Absorption and bioavailability

Our understanding of the factors influencing the absorption and bioavailability of molybdenum is based almost entirely on evidence from studies with ruminants or laboratory animals. Hexavalent molybdenum compounds are readily absorbed from the digestive tract. This applies to water-soluble molybdates, the molybdenum of herbage and thus, presumably, to the molybdenum of green vegetables. Although the molybdenum of insoluble molybdenum(IV) sulfide is not absorbed, water-soluble thiomolybdates and oxythiomolybdates are readily absorbed both by ruminants and by rats.

Intestinal absorption of molybdate is inhibited by high intraluminal concentrations of the sulfate anion, presumably because of the competition between the latter and the molybdate ion for a common carrier. Sulfate also reduces the utilization of molybdenum by various tissues and increases the urinary excretion of the element (3). Such effects of the sulfate anion on molybdenum metabolism are highly specific. Sulfate generated from protein breakdown and the oxidation of methionine, cysteine or thiosulfate is as active as dietary sulfate as a molybdenum antagonist. Mutually antagonistic interactions between soluble dietary molybdates and silicates have been found to restrict the tissue uptake of both elements (21).

Molybdate is rapidly absorbed from the gastrointestinal tract. Approximately 40% of the dose appears in major organs after oral administration, as compared with almost 80% when molybdate is administered intravenously (22). According to the International Commission for Radiation Protection, "reference" man can be expected to absorb only 5% of an orally administered dose of molybdenum(IV) sulfide, whereas most other molybdenum compounds may be absorbed with an efficiency of approximately 80%. According to other studies (23), soluble molybdates are absorbed from the digestive tract with an efficiency of approximately 50% and typically exhibit a gut residence time of 14 days.

8.5 Dietary intake

Estimates of the daily intake of molybdenum differ widely. This may be attributable partly to the technical difficulties of estimating dietary molybdenum accurately. However, extreme regional variations occur both in the soil availability of molybdenum and in the extent to which this is reflected by its content in food crops. Representative ranges of mean estimates of molybdenum intake are summarized in Table 22.2 (page 273), which also includes data from an international survey of dietary trace-element intakes conducted with rigorous analytical control under the supervision of the IAEA.

8.5.1 Infants and children

Data from several countries suggest that the molybdenum intakes of breast-fed infants 0–3 months of age vary, typically, from 0.1 to 0.5 μg/kg of body weight per day (24,25). Many such intakes are substantially less than those previously recommended by WHO (2 μg of molybdenum/kg of body weight per day) (26) and the United States National Academy of Sciences (30–60 μg of molybdenum/ day) (27). High contents of molybdenum in some samples of breast milk have been reported from India and the Philippines; whether these reflect a higher maternal intake of molybdenum is not known. With these exceptions, it appears likely that infant intakes of molybdenum substantially lower than previous estimates of minimum requirements may prove adequate for normal health and development, so that a reappraisal of these estimates is probably required.

Molybdenum intakes between weaning and 3 years of age appear to be higher (5–7 μg/kg of body weight per day) but decline thereafter to, typically, 1.5–3 μg/kg of body weight per day. Higher intakes reported from Asian countries may be partly due to the predominantly vegetarian diet in these countries, but the data await verification since the sampling and analytical techniques used were unsatisfactory.

8.5.2 Adolescents and adults

Typical intakes of molybdenum are probably in the range 1.5–2.5 μg/kg of body weight per day. Values below this range have been reported from New Zealand and Switzerland, while it is suggested that the substantially higher values found in the Indian subcontinent may be associated with high intakes of sorghum and other cereals having a relatively high molybdenum content. Representative total diets from 11 countries analysed in an IAEA programme (28) revealed an average dietary molybdenum concentration of 0.23 ± 0.02 (SEM) mg/kg of dry matter. This corresponds to a daily dietary intake of approximately 100 μg of molybdenum/day for adults.

Animal products, with the exception of liver, are generally poor sources of molybdenum, whereas vegetables, especially those grown on neutral or alkaline soils, are rich in the element. In contrast, vegetables grown on leached acid soils may be molybdenum-deficient. Vegetation grown on soils derived from shales, mineralized granites and some peats tend to have an elevated molybdenum content, which may give rise to molybdenum toxicity in farm livestock and possibly to threshold molybdenum toxicity in humans. Industrial pollution has resulted in high molybdenum contents of crops in the environment of molyb-denum-processing plants (4).

8.5.3 Tissue status

There are insufficient data from which to derive reliable estimates of the tissue molybdenum status of normal individuals. Estimates of blood serum molyb-denum range over four orders of magnitude (for review, see reference 29). Estimates of the molybdenum concentration in human liver are in the range 1.3–2.9 mg/kg of dry matter (30). The mean molybdenum contents of other organs have been reported as: kidney 1.6, lung 0.15, brain 0.14 and muscle 0.14 mg/kg of dry matter. The reported mean molybdenum concentration of human hair ranges from 0.07 to 0.16 mg/kg (31, 32). Defects in liver function, whether induced by infection, tumours or drugs, are frequently accompanied by increases in serum molybdenum content. Elevated blood molybdenum has also been reported in uraemia, rheumatic disorders and cardiovascular diseases.

8.6 Requirements

In 1973, a WHO Expert Committee suggested (26) that 2 μg of molybdenum per kg of body weight per day would be adequate to maintain normal health. This tentative estimate was derived by extrapolation from a small series of balance studies with subjects ranging in age from 2 years to adulthood. The estimates of the Food and Nutrition Board of the United States National Research Council (27) of the lower limit of the range of "safe and adequate" dietary intakes of molybdenum, are lower than that suggested by the WHO Expert Committee, for example between 1.2 and 1.5 μg/kg of body weight per day for adults and children. Despite the scarcity of reliable analytical data from which to estimate human intakes of molybdenum, it is nevertheless apparent that normal health and development can be maintained on substantially lower intakes of molybdenum than the above.

The clearest evidence of the clinical consequences of a suboptimal molybdenum intake is provided by the report (6) describing the effects of deficiency in a subject maintained on total parenteral nutrition. Unfortunately, as already mentioned, the molybdenum content of the "deficient" infusate that produced clinical lesions rectified by molybdenum fortification was not recorded; parenteral infusion of 147 μg of molybdenum/day as inorganic molybdate rapidly corrected the deficiency. A more recent investigation (33) suggests that biochemical changes indicative of a functional deficiency of molybdenum can develop if the diet of adults provides approximately 25 μg of molybdenum/day. Subjects exposed to such a low molybdenum intake for 102 days doubled their excretion of xanthine and decreased uric acid excretion after purine loading by 20%, suggesting that this dietary regimen depressed the tissue activity of the molybdenoenzyme xanthine oxidase. Other evidence of anomalies of nicotinamide metabolism indicative of a failure of aldehyde oxidase also suggested that such a low molybdenum intake was insufficient to maintain normal biochemical functions. Although no clinical signs of deficiency developed in these experimental subjects, the metabolic anomalies were eliminated when the diet provided 475 μg of molybdenum/day.

The above data suggesting that the daily requirement of the human adult may be lower than previously believed (26) are reasonably consistent with the results of a study on the effects of a low molybdenum intake in rats. Thus Wang et al. (34) reported that female rats offered diets containing only 25 μg of molybdenum/kg exhibited abnormally low xanthine dehydrogenase/oxidase activities in liver and intestinal mucosa and sulfite oxidase activity in liver. These molybdoenzymes regained full activity when the diet provided $\geqslant$ 50 μg of molybdenum/kg. Extrapolation from one species to another solely on the basis of differences in daily dry matter intake suggests that the adult human basal requirement for molybdenum could be approximately 25 μg of molybdenum/day. Until further studies have been undertaken, it is suggested tentatively that such an intake, corresponding to approximately 0.4 μg of molybdenum/kg of body weight, should be regarded as the average basal requirement (Mo_R^{basal}) for this element. There are insufficient data from which to derive even tentative estimates of the requirements for infants or for pregnant or lactating women.

8.7 Safe population mean intake

Chappel (35) has concluded from an extensive review of studies of molybdenum toxicity in a range of species that the lowest level at which adverse effects from high molybdenum levels are likely to be encountered in humans lies between 0.14 and 0.20 mg of molybdenum/kg of body weight if the ingested element is in the form of soluble molybdate. This conclusion accords with data from studies conducted in areas of Armenia where molybdenum is present at high levels in staple food crops and it has been suggested that a high incidence of gout associated with defects in purine metabolism may be caused by the consumption of natural diets providing up to 10–15 mg of molybdenum/day (14). Evidence from further studies is needed before a maximum tolerable population mean intake of molybdenum can be derived with confidence.

Despite this uncertainty, it should be noted that the molybdenum intakes in the various studies (> 150 µg/kg of body weight per day) are substantially higher, by a factor of approximately 3, than those known to result in conversion of molybdate to thiomolybdate in experimental animals if dietary intakes of sulfate permit the generation of free sulfide (S^-) in the lower digestive tract (12). Thiomolybdate intoxication causing diarrhoea, skeletal lesions and ultimately anaemia has developed under such circumstances when diets of experimental animals provided only 5 mg of molybdenum/kg (3). Human dietary intakes of sulfate and amino-acid sulfur that are sufficient to induce sulfide generation in the colon may not be tolerable in areas where molybdenum intake is high (12).

References

1. Coughlan MP. The role of molybdenum in human biology. *Journal of inherited metabolic disease*, 1983, **6** (Suppl. 1): 70–77.
2. Rajagopalan KV. Molybdenum. In: Frieden E, ed. *Biochemistry of the essential ultratrace elements*. New York, Plenum Press, 1984: 147–174.
3. Mills CF, Davis GK. Molybdenum. In: Mertz W, ed. *Trace elements in human and animal nutrition*, 5th ed., Vol. 1. San Diego, Academic Press, 1987: 429–463.
4. Anke M, Groppel B. Toxic action of essential trace elements (Mo, Cu, Zn, Fe, Mn). In: Brätter P, Schramel P, eds. *Trace element analytical chemistry in medicine and biology*. Berlin, de Gruyter, 1987: 203–208.
5. Coughlan MP. Aldehydeoxidase, xanthine oxidase and xanthine dehydrogenase. In: Coughlan MP, ed. *Molybdenum and molybdenum-containing enzymes*. Oxford, Pergamon, 1980: 119–185.

6. Abumrad NN et al. Amino acid intolerance during prolonged total parenteral nutrition reversed by molybdate therapy. *American journal of clinical nutrition*, 1981, 34: 2551–2559.

7. Rajagopalan KV. Molybdenum—an essential trace element. *Nutrition reviews*, 1987, 45: 321–328.

8. Rajagopalan KV. Molybdenum: an essential trace mineral in human nutrition. *Annual reviews of nutrition*, 1988, 8: 401–427.

9. Anke M et al. Molybdenum supply and status in animals and human beings. *Nutrition research*, 1985, Suppl. 1: 180–186.

10. Ostrom CA, Van Reen R, Miller CW. Changes in the connective tissue of rats fed toxic diets containing molybdenum salts. *Journal of dental research*, 1961, 40: 520–527.

11. Halverson AW, Phifer JH, Monty KJ. A mechanism for the copper–molybdenum inter-relationship. *Journal of nutrition*, 1960, 71: 95–100.

12. Christl SU et al. Role of dietary sulphate in the regulation of methanogenesis in the human large intestine. *Gastroenterology*, 1992, 33: 1234–1238.

13. Yang G-Q et al. Human selenium requirements in China. In: Combs GF et al., eds. *Selenium in biology and medicine*, part B. New York, van Nostrand, 1978: 589–607.

14. Kovalsky VV, Jarovaja GA, Samavonjan DM. [Changes in purine metabolism in man and animals in various molybdenum rich biogeochemical provinces.] *Zhurnal obshchei biologii (Moskva)*, 1961, 22: 179–192.

15. Burrell RJ, Roach WA, Shadwell A. Esophageal cancer in the Bantu of Transkei associated with mineral deficiency in garden plants. *Journal of the National Cancer Institute* 1966, N36: 201–209.

16. Wei H-J. Effects of molybdenum and tungsten on mammary carcinogenesis in SD-rats. *Journal of the National Cancer Institute*, 1989, 74: 469.

17. Hadjimarkos DM. Trace elements in dental health. *Trace substances in environmental health*, 1973, 8: 23–30.

18. Losee F, Cutress TW, Brown R. Trace elements in human dental enamel. *Trace substances in environmental health*, 1973, 8: 19–24.

19. Zhang X. The relationship between endemic diseases and trace elements in the natural environment of Jilin province of China. *Trace substances in environmental health*, 1986, 20: 381–391.

20. Wang F et al. Pathogenic factors of Keshan Disease in the grains cultivated in endemic areas. In: Combs JR et al., eds. *Selenium in biology and medicine*, part B. New York, van Nostrand, 1987: 896–901.

21. Carlisle EM. A silicon-molybdenum interrelationship *in vivo*. *Federation proceedings*, 1979, 38: 553.

22. Moskalev JuI. [*Mineral metabolism.*] Moscow, Medicina, 1985: 190–193.

23. Cumbrovsky J, Wiesener W. Spurenelementgehalt menschlicher Organe in Abhängigkeit von Umweltfaktoren. [Trace element content of human organs in relation to environmental factors.] In: Fiedler HJ, Rösler HJ, eds. *Spurenelemente in der Umwelt.* [*Trace elements in the environment.*] Jena, Gustav Fischer, 1987: 205–215.

24. Casey CE, Neville MC. Studies in human lactation. 3. Molybdenum and nickel in human milk during the first month of lactation. *American journal of clinical nutrition*, 1987, **N45**: 921–926.

25. Iyengar GV. *Elemental composition of human and animal milk*. Vienna, International Atomic Energy Agency, 1982 (IAEA TECDOC 269).

26. *Trace elements in human nutrition. Report of a WHO Expert Committee*. Geneva, World Health Organization, 1973 (WHO Technical Report Series, No. 532).

27. National Research Council. *Recommended dietary allowances*, 10th ed. Washington, DC, National Academy of Sciences, 1989.

28. Parr RM. An international collaborative research program on minor and trace elements in total diets. In: Brätter P, Schramel P, eds. *Trace element analytical chemistry in medicine and biology*. Berlin, de Gruyter, 1987, 157–164.

29. Versieck J. Molybdän. [Molybdenum.] In: Zumkley H, ed. *Spurenelemente*. [*Trace elements.*] Stuttgart, Thieme, 1983, 152–165.

30. Iyengar GV. Normal values for the elemental composition of human tissues and body fluids: new look at an old problem. *Trace substances in environmental health*, 1985, **29**: 227–295.

31. Ward NJ, Minski MJ. Comparison of trace elements in whole blood and scalp hair of multiple sclerosis patients and normal individuals. *Trace substances in environmental health*, 1982, **26**: 252–260.

32. Anke M, Risch MA. *Haaranalyse und Spurenelementstatus*. [*Hair analysis and trace element status*.] Jena, Gustav Fischer, 1979: 176–193.

33. Chiang G, Swenseid ME, Turnlund J. Studies of biochemical markers indicating molybdenum status in humans. *FASEB Journal*, 1989, **Abstracts 3**: A4922.

34. Wang X, Yang MT, Yang SP. Molybdenum requirement of female rats. *FASEB journal*, 1989, **Abstracts 3**: A4923.

35. Chappel WR. Use of surface area for the extrapolation of non-carcinogenic risks from animals to humans. *Trace substances in environmental health*, 1985, **19**: 326–327.

9.
Chromium

Studies of the nutritional significance of chromium have been reviewed in several recent publications (1–6).

9.1 Biochemical function

Chromium is an essential nutrient that potentiates insulin action and thus influences carbohydrate, lipid and protein metabolism. However, the nature of the relationship between chromium and insulin function has not been defined.

Mertz et al. (4) suggested that the biologically active form of chromium (glucose tolerance factor) is a complex of chromium, nicotinic acid and possibly the amino acids glycine, cysteine and glutamic acid. Many attempts have been made to isolate or synthesize the glucose tolerance factor; none has been successful. Thus, the precise structure of the glucose tolerance factor, and whether it is the biologically active form of chromium, remain uncertain.

Chromium may have a biochemical function that affects the ability of the insulin receptor to interact with insulin. For example, it has been found that *in vitro* RNA synthesis directed by free DNA is enhanced by the binding of chromium to the template (7); this suggests that chromium may act similarly to zinc in regulating gene expression, so that it may be regulating the synthesis of a molecule that potentiates insulin action. This suggestion is supported by the finding that there is a 4-hour lag period between the administration of biologically active chromium and its optimal effects on insulin action *in vivo* (8).

9.2 Deficiency and toxicity

Chromium-deficient rats exhibit a glucose intolerance similar to clinical diabetes mellitus. Other deficiency signs in animals (2) include impaired growth, elevated serum cholesterol and triglycerides, increased incidence of aortic plaques, corneal lesions and decreased fertility and sperm count.

Signs of chromium deficiency have been found in three women who were receiving long-term total parenteral nutrition with infusates low in chromium. Jeejeebhoy et al. (9) found that a patient receiving total parenteral nutrition for

$3\frac{1}{2}$ years exhibited impaired glucose tolerance and glucose utilization, weight loss, neuropathy, elevated plasma free fatty acids, depressed respiratory quotient and abnormalities in nitrogen metabolism. All were alleviated by chromium supplementation. A woman given total parenteral nutrition for 5 months developed severe glucose intolerance, weight loss and a metabolic encephalopathy-like confusional state; all were found to be reversible by chromium supplementation (10). Brown et al. (11) found that chromium supplementation reversed the development of an unexplained hyperglycaemia and glycosuria during administration of a total parenteral nutrition regimen of several months' duration. All subjects in these three studies exhibited impaired glucose tolerance or hyperglycaemia, with glycosuria and a refractiveness to insulin, which should therefore be considered definite signs of chromium deficiency.

Trivalent chromium has such a low toxicity that deleterious effects of excessive intake of this form of chromium do not readily occur. Hexavalent chromium is much more toxic than the trivalent form; oral administration of 50 $\mu g/g$ diet has been found to induce growth depression together with liver and kidney damage in experimental animals (12). Apart from acute intoxication, chromium toxicity through oral ingestion is apparently not of practical importance for humans.

9.3 Epidemiology of deficiency and toxicity

Countries in which refined foods predominate in the diet are likely to have an elevated occurrence of chromium deficiency, since appreciable losses of chromium occur in the refining of certain foods (2). In addition, infants and children with protein–energy malnutrition may be susceptible to chromium deficiency (13).

Chromium toxicity as a result of oral ingestion is very unlikely. Chromium toxicity usually occurs in an industrial environment where concentrations in the air are high, or contact with the skin is frequent.

9.4 Assessment of status

Tissue chromium stores apparently do not readily equilibrate with blood chromium; thus fasting plasma or serum chromium concentrations are probably not good indices of chromium status (13, 14). However, some reports suggest that concentrations of chromium much lower than the normal value of 0.14–0.15 ng/ml for serum or 0.26 or 0.28 ng/ml for plasma (15) might indicate the presence of a severe chromium deficiency. Elevated serum chromium may be a useful indicator of excessive exposure to chromium. Serum from tannery workers exposed to trivalent chromium had a median chromium concentration of 0.49 ng/ml, whereas that of non-exposed subjects was 0.15 ng/ml (16). Median urinary chromium was four times as high in these tannery workers as in controls. High urinary levels may be a good indicator of exposure to excessive amounts of chromium.

Supplementation of the diet with chromium has been shown to improve glucose tolerance in children with protein–energy malnutrition, in some diabetics, and in some people with marginally elevated blood glucose (14). Thus, an abnormal glucose tolerance may indicate a low chromium status, and an improvement in glucose tolerance after chromium supplementation may be a valid indicator of chromium deficiency.

9.5 Absorption and bioavailability

Intestinal absorption of trivalent chromium is low, varying between approximately 0.5% and 2.0% depending on dietary intake (17, 18). Preliminary findings (19) led to the suggestion that biologically active chromium (glucose tolerance factor) is more readily absorbed than trivalent chromium. However, later studies indicate that this may not be the case (5). Some evidence suggests that, while organic chromium may be readily absorbed, it is quickly passed through the body without being utilized (20).

The mechanism of absorption of chromium from the intestine has not been clearly identified, but it apparently involves processes other than simple diffusion. It has been claimed that numerous dietary factors, including oxalate, iron and high dietary intakes of simple carbohydrates, change the bioavailability or absorption of chromium (5, 6). It has also been found that chromium absorption is elevated by chemically induced diabetes and depressed by aging (21).

9.6 Dietary intake

The daily intake of chromium can vary widely depending on the proportions of various food groups in the diet. Processed meats, whole grain products, pulses and spices (22) are the best sources of chromium, while dairy products and most fruits and vegetables contain only small amounts (22).

The high dietary intakes of chromium generally reported before 1980 are apparently questionable, since the chromium analyses on which they were based were flawed by contamination and by analytical problems. Recent reports indicate that many diets in the United States supply less than 50 μg of chromium/day. Thus in one study the content of the self-selected diets of 10 men and 22 women collected by the duplicate portion method on a daily basis for 7 consecutive days was determined (17); the daily intake for the men was $33 \pm 3\,\mu g$ (mean $\pm$ SEM) with a range of 22–48 μg, and for the women $25 \pm 1\,\mu g$ with a range of 13–36 μg. In another study, 18 lactating women collected diet samples for 3 consecutive days 2 months after parturition. These diets supplied $41 \pm 4\,\mu g$ of chromium/day (mean $\pm$ SEM); control women consumed $27 \pm 2\,\mu g$/day (23). A total of 22 diets designed by nutritionists contained $13.3 \pm 5.2\,\mu g$ of chromium (mean $\pm$ SD)/1000 kcal (22). Diets consumed by 23 healthy, well-nourished, active elderly volunteers supplied 37.1 μg of chromium/day (range 15–55 μg/day) (24). Diets in some other countries apparently supply similar amounts of chromium. Thus the self-selected diets of 84 Canadian women supplied 55.5 ± 33.5 (mean $\pm$ SD) μg of chromium/day (range 11–157 μg/day) (25). The distribution of the findings was non-Gaussian; the median daily intake was 47 μg of chromium. The self-selected diets of 22 apparently healthy elderly English people supplied 24.5 μg of chromium/day (range 13.6–47.7 μg/day) (26). These values were similar to those calculated for diets in Finland (27), but lower than those found in Spain (28) and Sweden (29).

9.7 Safe range of population mean intakes

The available data are too limited to make it possible to determine the basal and normative requirements for chromium. However, glucose-intolerant subjects consuming less than 20 μg of chromium/day for 14 weeks responded to chromium supplementation (i.e. glucose metabolism variables improved); healthy subjects did not (30). Intakes of 24.5 μg and 37 μg of chromium/day were apparently adequate to maintain health in elderly people (24, 26). This suggests that, for chromium, the average basal requirement is less than 20 μg/day, and that the mean population intake to meet basal needs may be close to 25 μg/day. It is reasonable to derive a normative estimate of the requirement for chromium since there is evidence of a storage reserve of this element. A 30% increase above the basal requirement might be appropriate. Thus, *the minimum population mean intake likely to meet normative needs for chromium might be approximately 33 μg/day.*

The relatively non-toxic nature of chromium as found in food indicates that the tolerable limit for chromium is quite high. Findings that supplements of 125–200 μg of chromium/day, in addition to the usual dietary intake, can in some cases reverse hypoglycaemia and impaired glucose tolerance, and improve both circulating insulin levels and the lipid profile, suggest that the upper limit of the safe range of population mean intakes could be above 250 μg/day. However, until more is known about chromium, it seems appropriate that supplementation of this element should not exceed this amount.

9.8 Recommendations for future studies

More detailed information about the metabolic roles and modes of action of chromium is needed. Such information may suggest additional biochemical or other criteria for use in assessing the adequacy of chromium status and thus permit a wider investigation of the nutritional significance of this element.

References

1. Anderson RA. Recent advances in the role of chromium in human health and diseases. In: Prasad AS ed. *Essential and toxic trace elements in human health and disease.* New York, Alan R. Liss, 1988: 189–197.
2. Anderson RA. Chromium. In: Smith K ed. *Trace minerals in foods.* New York, Marcel Dekker, 1988: 231–247.
3. Mertz W. Chromium—an overview. In: Shapcott D, Hubert J eds. *Chromium in nutrition and metabolism.* Amsterdam, Elsevier/North Holland Biomedical Press, 1979: 1–14.
4. Mertz W et al. Present knowledge of the role of chromium. *Federation proceedings,* 1974, 33: 2275–2280.
5. Offenbacher EG, Pi-Sunyer FX. Chromium in human nutrition. *Annual review of nutrition,* 1988, 8: 543–563.
6. Stoecker BJ. Chromium. In: Brown ML, ed. *Present knowledge in nutrition,* Washington, DC, International Life Sciences Institute, 1990: 287–293.
7. Okada S, Ohba H, Taniyama M. Alterations in ribonucleic acid synthesis by chromium(III). *Journal of inorganic biochemistry,* 1981, 15: 223–231.
8. Tuman RW, Doisy RJ. Metabolic effects of the glucose tolerance factor (GTF) in normal and genetically diabetic mice. *Diabetes,* 1977, 26: 820–826.
9. Jeejeebhoy KN et al. Chromium deficiency, glucose intolerance, and neuropathy reversed by chromium supplementation in a patient receiving long-term parenteral nutrition. *American journal of clinical nutrition,* 1977, 30: 531–538.
10. Freund H, Atamian S, Fischer JE. Chromium deficiency during total parenteral nutrition. *Journal of the American Medical Association,* 1979, 241: 496–498.
11. Brown RO et al. Chromium deficiency after long-term total parenteral nutrition. *Digestive diseases and sciences,* 1986, 31: 661–664.
12. MacKenzie RD et al. Chronic toxicity studies. II. Hexavalent and trivalent chromium administered in drinking water to rats. *AMA archives of industrial health,* 1958, 18: 232–234.
13. Saner G. The metabolic significance of dietary chromium. *Nutrition international,* 1986, 2: 213–220.
14. Borel JS, Anderson RA. Chromium. In: Frieden E, ed. *Biochemistry of the essential ultratrace elements.* New York, Plenum Press, 1984: 175–199.
15. Offenbacher EG et al. Rapid enzymatic pretreatment of samples before determining chromium in serum and plasma. *Clinical chemistry,* 1986, 32: 1383–1386.
16. Randall JA, Gibson RS. Serum and urine chromium as indices of chromium status in

tannery workers. *Proceedings of the Society of Experimental Biology and Medicine,* 1987, **185**: 16–23.

17. Anderson RA, Kozlovsky AS. Chromium intake, absorption and excretion of subjects consuming self-selected diets. *American journal of clinical nutrition,* 1985, **41**: 1177–1183.

18. Offenbacher EG et al. Metabolic chromium balances in men. *American journal of clinical nutrition,* 1986, **44**: 77–82.

19. Mertz W, Roginski EE. Chromium metabolism: the glucose tolerance factor. In: Mertz W, Cornatzer WE, eds. *Newer trace elements in nutrition.* New York, Marcel Dekker, 1971: 123–153.

20. Anderson M, Riley D, Rotruck J. Chromium(III) tris-acetylacetonate: an absorbable, bioactive source of chromium. *Federation proceedings,* 1980, **39**: 787.

21. Craft NE, Polansky MM, Anderson RA. The effect of age, sex, diet, and diabetes on chromium absorption. *Federation proceedings,* 1984, **43**: 471.

22. Anderson RA et al. Dietary chromium intake. In: *Abstracts of the 14th International Congress of Nutrition.* Seoul, 1989: 488.

23. Anderson RA et al. Elevated chromium intake, absorption and urinary excretion of lactating women. *FASEB journal,* 1988, **2**: A1092.

24. Offenbacher EG, Rinko CJ, Pi-Sunyer FX. The effects of inorganic chromium and brewer's yeast on glucose tolerance, plasma lipids, and plasma chromium in elderly subjects. *American journal of clinical nutrition,* 1985, **42**: 454–461.

25. Gibson RS, Scythes CA. Chromium, selenium, and other trace element intakes of a selected sample of Canadian premenopausal women. *Biological trace element research,* 1984, **6**: 105–116.

26. Bunker VW et al. The uptake and excretion of chromium by the elderly. *American journal of clinical nutrition,* 1984, **39**: 797–802.

27. Koivistoinen P. Mineral element composition of Finnish foods: N, K, Ca, Mg, P, S, Fe, Cu, Mn, Zn, Mo, Co, Ni, Cr, F, Se, Si, Rb, Al, B, Br, Hg, As, Cd, Pb, and ash. *Acta agriculturae scandinavica,* Suppl. 22, 1980.

28. Barberá R, Farré R, Lozano A. Oral intake of cadmium, lead, cobalt, chromium, nickel, manganese, and zinc in the Spanish diet, estimated by a duplicate meal study. *Journal of micronutrient analysis,* 1989, **6**: 47–57.

29. Abdulla M, Behbehani A, Dashti H. Dietary intake and bioavailability of trace elements. *Biological trace element research,* 1989, **21**: 173–178.

30. Polansky MM et al. Beneficial effects of supplemental chromium (Cr) on glucose, insulin and glucagon of subjects consuming controlled low chromium diets. *FASEB journal,* 1990, **4**: A777.

B

Trace elements that are probably essential

10.
Manganese

The following account is based principally upon three recent reviews (1–3).

10.1 Biochemical function

Manganese is both an activator and a constituent of several enzymes. Those activated by manganese are numerous and include hydrolases, kinases, decarboxylases and transferases, but most of these enzymes can also be activated by other metals, especially magnesium. This does not apply, however, to the activation of glycosyltransferases nor possibly to that of xylosyltransferase. Manganese metalloenzymes include arginase, pyruvate carboxylase, glutamine synthetase, and manganese superoxide dismutase.

10.2 Deficiency and toxicity

Manganese deficiency has been produced in many species of animals, but not, so far, in humans. Signs of manganese deficiency include impaired growth, skeletal abnormalities, disturbed or depressed reproductive function, ataxia of the newborn, and defects in lipid and carbohydrate metabolism.

Unequivocal evidence of manganese deficiency in humans has not so far been reported, but a possible case of such deficiency was described by Doisy (4). A man fed a semipurified formula diet found to be low in manganese (0.35 mg/day) lost weight and suffered depressed growth of hair and nails, dermatitis and hypocholesterolaemia, but responded to being fed a mixed hospital diet; supplementation with manganese alone was not tried.

Another possible case of manganese deficiency in humans was reported by Friedman et al. (5). Men fed a diet containing only 0.11 mg of manganese/day for 39 days exhibited decreased serum cholesterol and a fleeting dermatitis (miliaria crystallina). Calcium, phosphorus and alkaline phosphatase activity in blood increased. However, because short-term manganese supplementation (10 days) did not reverse these changes, the suggestion that the syndrome was attributable to manganese deprivation was not substantiated.

Other possible signs of manganese deprivation have been reported (1, 3). A diabetic patient who was not responsive to insulin injections responded to oral manganese with decreased blood glucose concentrations. In addition, whole-blood manganese concentrations have been reported to be low in patients with certain types of epilepsy.

Manganese is often considered to be among the least toxic of the trace elements when administered orally. Thus, reported cases of human toxicity caused by oral ingestion of large amounts of manganese are few. The most common form of manganese toxicity is the result of chronic inhalation of large amounts of airborne manganese in mines, steel mills and some chemical industries (6). The major signs of manganese toxicity in animals are depressed growth, depressed appetite, impaired iron metabolism and altered brain function (1). Signs of toxicity in Chilean manganese miners were first manifested in the form of severe psychiatric abnormalities, including hyperirritability, violent acts and hallucinations; these changes were called manganic madness (6). As the disease progressed, there was a permanent crippling neurological disorder of the extrapyramidal system with morphological lesions similar to those of Parkinson disease (6).

10.3 Epidemiology of deficiency and toxicity

The natural incidence of effects attributable to abnormal manganese nutrition is apparently exceedingly low. It has been suggested that the high incidence of cartilage disorders in children in some geographical areas may be the result of low intakes of manganese (7).

10.4 Assessment of status

Keen et al. (3, 8) have suggested that the blood manganese concentration may be useful in assessing status because low blood concentrations in manganese-deficient rats reflected low concentrations of manganese in soft tissue. This suggestion is supported by the finding that whole-blood manganese concentrations are elevated with excessive manganese intake in humans (9). Normal whole-blood manganese in humans is apparently about 8.4 μg/l (9).

Urinary manganese may also be an indicator of manganese status. Young men who were fed 0.11 mg of manganese/day for 39 days exhibited a sharp drop in urinary manganese excretion, namely from about 8.6 μg/day to about 0.9 μg/day (5). Upon repletion with 1.53–2.55 mg of manganese/day for 10 days, urinary manganese excretion increased to about 4.0 μg/day. These changes, however, may merely reflect recent diet history.

Further investigation might show that both the activity of manganese superoxide dismutase and the ratio of manganese superoxide dismutase to copper–zinc superoxide dismutase could serve as indicators of manganese status, since these two variables, when measured in the livers of rats, were responsive to manipulations of dietary manganese intake (10).

10.5 Absorption and bioavailability

For many species, including humans, it has been assumed that manganese absorption is independent both of body manganese status and of dietary manganese content. This assumption has had to be extensively revised in the light of recent work with rats (11). For example, it was shown that the efficiency of absorption declined from 29% to 2% as dietary manganese increased from 1.5 to 100 $\mu g/g$, direct evidence that both true absorption and endogenous faecal excretion vary markedly in homoeostatic response to dietary manganese. Thus, the often-cited hypothesis that manganese homoeostasis is regulated mainly by a variable excretion via the digestive tract may have to be discarded.

In the rat, intestinal manganese absorption is a rapidly saturable process probably mediated by a high-affinity, low-capacity active transport system (12). In patients with varying iron stores and subjected to duodenal perfusion with manganese, the rate of manganese absorption was found to increase in iron deficiency. The enhanced manganese absorption was inhibited by iron (6). Apparently, the mechanisms involved in the absorption of manganese are very similar to those involved in that of iron.

Dietary fibre is believed to have the greatest negative effect on manganese bioavailability (2), but this hypothesis is in conflict with the results of a balance study in which 12 men consumed two diets containing different amounts of dietary fibre in natural foods for 6 weeks each in a crossover design (13) and the overall manganese balance was found not to be significantly affected by such differences in fibre content.

10.6 Dietary intake

Diets high in unrefined cereals, nuts, leafy vegetables and tea will be high in manganese; diets high in refined grains, meats and dairy products will be low. Such differences are typified by the finding that Indian diets high in foods of plant origin supplied an average of 8.3 mg of manganese/day (14), whereas highly refined hospital diets in the United States supplied a range of less than 0.36–1.78 mg of manganese/day (15). Most other reported mean intakes of manganese throughout the world fall between those values. For example, the mean daily manganese intake of adults consuming self-selected diets was 3.1, 2.7 and 2.9 mg in Canada, New Zealand and the United States, respectively (16–18). A mean intake of 5.1 mg/day has been reported for adults in the United Kingdom (19).

10.7 Requirement and tolerable intakes

Average basal or normative requirements for manganese cannot be established because the data required for this purpose are not available. Attempts to produce manganese deficiency by feeding diets providing as little as 0.74 mg/day (5) or 1.0 mg/day (20) resulted in neither conclusive nor marked effects on the health of adults. The threshold toxicity level is also unknown. *Thus, a safe range of mean population intakes for manganese cannot be proposed.*

However, Friedman et al. (5) suggested that the minimal requirement for manganese based on obligatory losses in young men consuming a semipurified manganese-deficient formula diet was 0.74 mg/day. Another study done in the same laboratory (21) found negative retention of manganese at dietary intakes of 1.21, 2.06 and 2.89 mg/day, but positive retention at 2.65 and 3.79 mg/day. Based on regression analysis of intake versus balance, an intake of 3.5 mg/day was recommended. This value is difficult to reconcile with the fact that many dietary intakes are close to 2.5–3.0 mg/day, yet no evidence that manganese deficiency is a problem has appeared. Data like these were used to set a safe and adequate intake of 2.0–5.0 mg/day for adults in the United States (22). Whether the lower limit of the safe range of population mean intakes for manganese is in this range remains to be determined.

10.8 Recommendations for future studies

The essentiality of manganese for animals is established beyond question but instances of nutritional deficiency in human subjects have not been unequivocally identified. A legacy of analytical problems has also hindered both the identification of subjects exposed to dietary deficiency of manganese and the circumstances under which a low availability of the element from the diet can be expected. The continuing scrutiny of the experimental evidence of the pathological effects of deficiency is recommended with a view to subsequent epidemiological studies under circumstances that indicate that the dietary intake of available manganese may be low.

References

1. Hurley LS, Keen CL. Manganese. In: Mertz W, ed. *Trace elements in human and animal nutrition,* 5th ed., Vol 1. San Diego, Academic Press, 1987: 185–223.
2. Johnson PE, Nielsen FH. Copper, manganese, cobalt, and magnesium. *Advances in meat research,* 1990, 6: 275–299.
3. Keen CL, Lönnerdal B, Hurley LS. Manganese. In: Frieden E, ed. *Biochemistry of the essential ultratrace elements.* New York, Plenum Press, 1984: 89–132.

4. Doisy EA Jr. Micronutrient controls of biosynthesis of clotting proteins and cholesterol. *Trace substances in environmental health,* 1972, **6**: 193–199.

5. Friedman BJ et al. Manganese balance and clinical observations in young men fed a manganese-deficient diet. *Journal of nutrition,* 1987, **117**: 133–143.

6. Mena I. Manganese. In: Bronner F, Coburn JW, eds. *Disorders of mineral metabolism.* New York, Academic Press, 1981: 233–270.

7. Fincham JE, van Rensburg SJ, Marasas WFO. Mseleni joint disease—a manganese deficiency? *South African medical journal,* 1981, **60**: 445–447.

8. Keen CL et al. Whole blood manganese as an indicator of body manganese. *New England journal of medicine,* 1983, **308**: 1230.

9. Cotzias GC, Miller ST, Edwards J, Neutron activation analysis: the stability of manganese concentrations in human blood and serum. *Journal of laboratory and clinical medicine,* 1966, **67**: 836–849.

10. Zidenberg-Cherr S et al. Superoxide dismutase activity and lipid peroxidation in the rat: developmental correlations affected by manganese deficiency. *Journal of nutrition,* 1983, **113**: 2498–2504.

11. Weigand E, Kirchgessner M, Helbig U. True absorption and endogenous fecal excretion of manganese in relation to its dietary supply in growing rats. *Biological trace element research,* 1986, **10**: 265–279.

12. Garcia-Aranda JA, Wapnir RA, Lifshitz F. *In vivo* intestinal absorption of manganese in the rat. *Journal of nutrition,* 1983, **113**: 2601–2607.

13. Kelsay JL et al. Mineral balances of men fed a diet containing fibre in fruits and vegetables and oxalic acid in spinach for six weeks. *Journal of nutrition,* 1988, **118**: 1197–1204.

14. Soman SD et al. Daily intake of some major and trace elements. *Health physics,* 1969, **17**: 35–40.

15. Gormican A. Inorganic elements in foods used in hospital menus. *Journal of the American Dietetic Association,* 1970, **56**: 397–403.

16. Wolf WR. Assessment of inorganic nutrient intake from self-selected diets. In: Beecher GR, ed. *Human nutrition research.* Totowa, NJ, Allanheld, Osmun, 1981: 175–196 (Beltsville Symposia in Agricultural Research, No. 4).

17. Gibson RS, Scythes CA. Trace element intakes of women. *British journal of nutrition,* 1982, **48**: 241–248.

18. Guthrie BE, Robinson MF. Daily intakes of manganese, copper, zinc and cadmium by New Zealand women. *British journal of nutrition,* 1977, **38**: 55–63.

19. Buss DH. Essential trace elements in the UK diet. *Chemistry and industry,* 1983, **13**: 493–498.

20. Johnson PE, Lykken GI. Manganese and calcium balance and absorption in women fed two levels of Ca and Mn. *FASEB journal,* 1989, **3**: A760.

21. Freeland-Graves JH et al. Metabolic balance of manganese in young men consuming diets containing five levels of dietary manganese. *Journal of nutrition,* 1988, **118**: 764–773.

22. National Research Council. *Recommended dietary allowances,* 10th ed., Washington, DC, National Academy of Sciences, 1989.

11.
Silicon

Silicon, the second most abundant element in the earth's crust, is not found free in nature, but occurs chiefly as the oxide and silicates. Asbestos, tremolite, the feldspars, clays and micas are but a few of the silicate minerals.

The essential function of silicon has been independently demonstrated by two groups of researchers in two species of experimental animals (1, 2). Growth stimulation of rats following administration of silicon was observed only when low-silicon (<5 μg of silicon/g of diet) synthetic rations based on crystalline amino acids were fortified with 250–500 μg of silicon/g of diet. However, regardless of dietary composition, all other experiments in which silicon deficiency has been induced have demonstrated the importance of the element for the normal development of connective tissue and bone in chickens and rats. Deficiency always produced deformities of skull and peripheral bones, characterized by poorly formed joints, defective endochondral bone growth and reduced contents of articular cartilage, hexosamine, collagen and water (3).

Silicon's mode of action is related to the formation of bone, possibly by the following two mechanisms: (1) by facilitating the formation of glycosaminogly-can and collagen components of the bone matrix through its role as a constituent of the enzyme prolylhydroxylase (4); (2) by a structural role for silicon as a component of glycosaminoglycans and glycosamino–protein complexes in which it is believed to occur as silanolate in mucopolysaccharides, linking different polysaccharides in the same polysaccharide chain, or linking acid mucopolysaccharides to protein. The postulated structures of such links have still to be identified (5).

Silicon can be detected in small areas of ossifying bone during the early stages of mineralization. The silicon content of young osteoid tissue increases markedly, together with that of calcium, but at more advanced stages of bone formation, when calcification sets in, the silicon content decreases again to trace levels (6). The element is located within the mitochondria of the osteoblast.

It has been shown that silicon concentrations in human arteries decrease with increasing age and with the onset of atherosclerosis, and that a combination of large intravenous and oral doses of silicon reduces the incidence and severity of atherosclerosis in cholesterol-fed rabbits (7). Several reports have independently confirmed a decline in silicon with age in some animal tissues, but its causes and possible relevance to the aging process remain unknown (3).

The general manifestations of silicon toxicity are collectively described as silicosis. As with other essential elements, certain chemical forms of silicon are toxic if inhaled or ingested in large amounts. The carcinogenic effects of asbestos fibres have caused serious public health problems where some forms of asbestos have been used extensively in construction projects in the past (8). Urolithiasis from the consumption of high-silicon forages is well known in cattle and sheep in several areas of the world. In contrast, few cases of siliceous calculi have been reported in human beings (9).

Foods of plant origin contain more silicon than those of animal origin. Whole grasses and cereals may contain 3–6% as silica. The silicon intake of adults in Finland (10), the United Kingdom, and the USA (11) varies between 21 and 49 mg/day. Fruits and most animal products contribute little silicon, whereas most foods of vegetable origin contain the element in amounts roughly proportional to their fibre content (8). The factors governing the biological availability of silicon have not been adequately defined.

In conclusion, while silicon has been shown to play an essential role in the development of bone in two species of experimental animal, for which a requirement of 100–250 µg/g of diet has been suggested, no data are available from which human requirements for silicon can yet be estimated.

References

1. Schwarz K, Milne DB. Growth-promoting effects of silicon in rats. *Nature*, 1972, **239**: 333–334.
2. Carlisle EM. Silicon: an essential element for the chick. *Science*, 1972, **178**: 619–621.
3. Carlisle EM. Silicon. In: Mertz W, ed. *Trace elements in human and animal nutrition*, 5th ed., Vol. 2. Orlando, Academic Press, 1986: 373–390.
4. Carlisle EM, Berger JW, Alpenfels WF. A silicon requirement for prolyl hydroxylase activity. *Federation proceedings*, 1981, **40**: 886.
5. Schwarz K. Significance and functions of silicon in warm-blooded animals. Review and outlook. In: Bendz G, Lindquist I, eds. *Biochemistry of silicon and related problems*. New York, Plenum Press, 1978: 207–230.
6. Carlisle EM. Silicon: a possible factor in bone calcification. *Science*, 1970, **167**: 279–280.
7. Loeper J, Loeper J, Fragny M. The physiological role of silicon and its antiatheromatous action. In: Bendz G, Lindquist I, eds. *Biochemistry of silicon and related problems*. New York, Plenum Press, 1978: 281–306.
8. National Research Council. Silicon. In: *Geochemistry and the environment*. Vol. II. *The relation of other selected trace elements to health and disease*. Washington, DC, National Academy of Sciences, 1977: 54–72.

9. Herring LC. Observations on the analysis of ten thousand urinary calculi. *Journal of urology*, 1962, **88**: 128–129.
10. Varo P, Koivistoinen P. Mineral element composition of Finnish foods. XII. General discussion and nutritional evaluation. *Acta agriculturae scandinavica*, 1980, Suppl. **22**: 165–171.
11. Kelsay JL, Behall KM, Prather ES. Effect of fiber from fruits and vegetables on metabolic response of human subjects. II. Calcium, magnesium, iron and silicon balances. *American journal of clinical nutrition*, 1979, **32**: 1876–1880.

12.
Nickel

12.1 Biochemical function

The four typical nickel-containing enzymes found in plants and micro-organisms, namely urease, hydrogenase, methylcoenzyme M reductase and carbon-monoxide dehydrogenase, have been comprehensively described in a number of reviews (1–4). Evidence that nickel functions similarly in animals or humans is awaited with interest.

12.2 Deficiency and toxicity

The reported signs of nickel deprivation in the chick, cow, goat, pig, rat and sheep are numerous (4–8). Unfortunately, recent studies indicate that many of them may have been misinterpreted, and claimed responses to repletion may have been manifestations of pharmacological actions of nickel (9, 10). However, certain signs are apparently specifically attributable to nickel deficiency. If the nickel deficiency is severe, growth and haematopoiesis are depressed, especially in animals with a marginal iron status, or in methyl-depleted animals. Iron utilization is impaired, and the trace element profiles of femur and liver change.

As a result of excellent homoeostatic regulation, nickel salts exert their toxic action mainly by gastrointestinal irritation and not by inherent toxicity. However, an oral dose of nickel as nickel sulfate as low as 0.6 mg, given with water to fasting subjects, produced a positive skin reaction in some nickel-sensitive individuals (11).

12.3 Epidemiology of deficiency and toxicity

Discussion of the epidemiology of nickel deficiency must await clarification of the effects of such deficiency in human subjects. Contact dermatitis is the most important clinical effect of excessive nickel exposure. The prevalence of sensitization to nickel in the general population is not known, but 5% (11/212) of patients in one study exhibited nickel sensitivity when tested before hip replacement operations (12). There thus appears to be a large population who may benefit from abstinence from foods or drinking-water with a high nickel content.

12.4 Assessment of status

Serum concentrations above 1.0 μg of nickel/litre probably indicate a chronically excessive intake of nickel. However, high serum nickel can also reflect a recent intake of a large dose of highly available nickel. Between 8% and 50% of nickel ingested in drinking-water after an overnight fast was absorbed by humans, resulting in marked hypernickelaemia (*11, 13, 14*). Because nickel deficiency has not been seen, status indicators of a low intake of nickel have not received much attention.

12.5 Absorption and bioavailability

When ingested in water after an overnight fast (*13, 14*) or in very small quantities (*15*), a very high percentage of nickel is absorbed, sometimes up to 50% of the dose, but usually 20–25%. However, a number of foodstuffs and simple substances, including milk, coffee, tea, orange juice, ascorbic acid and ethylenediaminetetra-acetate depress this high absorption (*13*). Foods included in a typical Guatemalan meal or a North American breakfast reduced the absorption of nickel to 1% or less (*13, 14*). Thus, most nickel in food remains unabsorbed by the gastrointestinal tract, and typically less than 10% of nickel ingested with food is absorbed (*5*). However, nickel absorption is enhanced by iron deficiency, pregnancy and lactation. For example, pigs absorbed over 19% of nickel ingested from day 21 of pregnancy until parturition (*6*).

Foulkes & McCullen (*16*) suggested that nickel crosses the basolateral membrane through passive leakage or diffusion, perhaps in the form of an amino acid, or other low molecular weight complex. In the light of the absorption characteristics of nickel in water and food (see above), this hypothesis is probably correct.

12.6 Dietary intake

Total dietary nickel intakes of humans vary greatly with the amounts and proportions of food of animal (low-nickel) or plant (high-nickel) origin consumed, and with the amount of refined or processed foods in the diet. Approximately half the total daily intake of nickel is usually derived from the consumption of bread, cereals and beverages. Recent reports indicate that diets often provide less than 150 μg daily. Examples of reported intakes (μg/day) are:

United Kingdom, 140–150 for adults and 14–250 for children (17); United States, 69–162 (18); and Denmark, mean 130, range 60–260 (19).

12.7 Requirement and tolerable intakes

Average basal and normative requirements and a safe range of population intakes for nickel cannot be established because of the scarcity of data. For this reason, a safe range of population mean intakes for nickel is not proposed here. However, available information indicates that most monogastric animals have a nickel requirement of less than 200 µg/kg of diet (1, 15, 20). Thus, if animal data are extrapolated to humans, it is reasonable to suggest a basal nickel requirement of less than 100 µg daily for adults. The finding that an oral dose as low as 600 µg nickel as nickel sulfate given with water to fasting subjects produced a positive skin reaction in some nickel-sensitive individuals (11) suggests that the threshold level for toxicity can be quite low in specific situations, and could thus be set at less than 600 µg/day.

References

1. Thauer RK. Nickelenzyme in Stoffwechsel von methanogenen Bakterien. [Nickel enzymes in the metabolism of methanogenic bacteria.] *Biological chemistry Hoppe-Seyler*, 1985, **366**: 103–112.
2. Hausinger RP. Nickel utilization by microorganisms. *Microbiological reviews*, 1987, **51**: 22–42.
3. Walsh CT, Orme-Johnson WH. Nickel enzymes. *Biochemistry*, 1987, **26**: 4901–4906.
4. Nielsen FH. Possible future implications of nickel, arsenic, silicon, vanadium, and other ultratrace elements in human nutrition. In: Prasad AS, ed. *Clinical, biochemical, and nutritional aspects of trace elements*. New York, Alan R. Liss, 1982, 379–404.
5. Nielsen FH. Nickel. In: Frieden E, ed. *Biochemistry of the essential ultratrace elements*. New York, Plenum Press, 1984: 293–308.
6. Kirchgessner M, Roth-Maier DA, Schnegg A. Progress of nickel metabolism and nutrition research. In: Howell J McC, Gawthorne JM, White CL, eds. *Trace element metabolism in man and animals—TEMA 4*. Canberra, Australian Academy of Science, 1981: 621–624.
7. Anke M et al. Nickel—an essential element. In: Sunderman FW Jr. et al., eds. *Nickel in the human environment*. Lyon, International Agency for Research on Cancer, 1984: 339–365 (IARC Scientific Publications Series, No. 53).
8. Spears JW. Nickel as a "newer trace element" in the nutrition of domestic animals. *Journal of animal science,* 1984, **59**: 823–835.
9. Nielsen FH et al. Nickel influences iron metabolism through physiologic, pharmacologic, and toxicologic mechanisms in the rat. *Journal of nutrition*, 1984, **114**: 1280–1288.

10. Nielsen FH. The importance of diet composition in ultratrace element research. *Journal of nutrition*, 1985, **115**: 1239–1247.

11. Cronin E. Di Michiel AD, Brown SS. Oral challenges in nickel-sensitive women with hand eczema. In: Brown SS, Sunderman FW Jr, eds. *Nickel toxicology*. New York, Academic Press, 1980: 149–152.

12. Deutman R et al. Metal sensitivity before and after total hip arthroplasty. *Journal of bone and joint surgery*, 1977, **59A**: 862–865.

13. Solomons NW et al. Bioavailability of nickel in man. Effects of foods and chemically-defined dietary constituents on the absorption of inorganic nickel. *Journal of nutrition*, 1982, **112**: 39–50.

14. Sunderman FW Jr et al. Nickel absorption and elimination in human volunteers. In: Hurley LS et al. eds. *Trace elements in man and animals — TEMA 6*. New York, Plenum Press, 1987: 427–428.

15. Kirchgessner M, Reichlmayr-Lais A, Maier R. Ni retention and concentrations of Fe and Mn in tissues resulting from different Ni supply. In: Mills CF, Bremner I, Chesters JK, eds. *Trace elements in man and animals — TEMA 5*. Farnham Royal, CAB International, 1985: 147–151.

16. Foulkes EC, McMullen DM. On the mechanism of nickel absorption in the rat jejunum. *Toxicology*, 1986, **38**: 35–42.

17. Smart GA, Sherlock JC. Nickel in foods and the diet. *Food additives and contaminants*, 1987, **4**: 61–71.

18. Pennington JAT, Jones JW. Molybdenum, nickel, cobalt, vanadium, and strontium in total diets. *Journal of the American Dietetic Association*, 1987, **87**: 1644–1650.

19. Veien NK, Andersen MR. Nickel in Danish food. *Acta dermato-venereologica*, 1986, **66**: 502–509.

20. Nielsen FH. The ultra trace elements. In: Smith KT ed. *Trace minerals in foods*. New York, Marcel Dekker, 1988, 357–428.

13.
Boron

13.1 Biochemical function

Little is known of the biochemical function of boron in human and animal tissues. Because boron affects steroid hormone metabolism in humans (1, 2) and animals (3, 4), and because the response of experimental animals to boron deficiency seems to be enhanced by nutritional stressors that induce secondary hyperparathyroidism (i.e. magnesium deficiency (5) and aluminium toxicity (6)), it would not be surprising to find that boron affects major mineral metabolism via a regulatory role involving a hormone.

13.2 Deficiency and toxicity

The signs of boron deficiency in animals vary in nature and severity as the dietary content of aluminium, calcium, cholecalciferol, magnesium, methionine and potassium is varied (3, 4, 6, 7). Variables affected by dietary boron include plasma and organ calcium and magnesium concentrations, plasma alkaline phosphatase, and bone calcification. Two studies showing a response to boron deprivation in humans have been reported. The first, on postmenopausal women housed in a metabolic unit, indicated that a low boron diet (0.25 mg/2000 kcal) elevated urinary excretion of calcium and magnesium, and depressed serum concentrations of 17β-estradiol and ionized calcium (1, 8). The second, in which five men, nine postmenopausal women (five on estrogen therapy) and one premenopausal woman were fed a low-magnesium, marginal-copper diet, showed that plasma ionized calcium and serum 25-hydroxy-cholecalciferol were lower and serum calcitonin and osteocalcin were higher during boron depletion (0.23 mg/2000 kcal) than during boron repletion (2). Brain function was affected in these 15 adults; electroencephalograms indicated that they were less mentally alert during boron depletion than during boron repletion (9). In these experiments (1, 2) the first 21 days of depletion were not included in the statistical analyses because there were no apparent changes in variables of interest. Peace et al. (10) also failed to find any significant effects in postmenopausal women fed a low-boron diet (0.33 mg/day) for 21 days.

Boron has a low toxicity when administered orally. Chronic toxicity signs have been described for the cow, dog, pig and rat (11). In pigs, high boron levels were found to affect calcium metabolism detrimentally, and the animals exhibited osteoporosis associated with a reduction in parathyroid activity (12).

The signs of chronic boron toxicity in humans have not been clearly defined. Two infants whose pacifiers were dipped into a preparation of borax and honey over a period of several weeks exhibited scanty hair, patchy dry erythema, anaemia and seizure disorders (13). The seizures stopped and the other abnormalities were alleviated when the use of the borax and honey preparation was discontinued.

13.3 Epidemiology of deficiency and toxicity

Consumption of foods of plant origin, and thus of boron, is often higher in countries with a lower incidence of osteoporosis. However, no comprehensive epidemiological studies establishing relationships between boron status and osteoporosis have yet been conducted. Because signs of chronic boron toxicity have not been clearly defined, it remains uncertain whether there are areas in the world where the population may be affected by it.

13.4 Assessment of status

The finding that boron may be nutritionally important for humans is so recent that there has been no opportunity to investigate possible indicators of an inadequate boron status. Also, because boron is not a particularly toxic element, indicators of chronic excessive boron intake are not well defined. However, elevated blood boron and urinary excretion of boron are indicators of acute and possibly chronic excessive intake of boron by both animals and humans (11). The normal concentration of boron in blood is apparently between 0.1 and 0.2 μg/ml (11).

13.5 Absorption and bioavailability

The boron of foods, sodium borate and boric acid is apparently rapidly absorbed and excreted largely in the urine (11, 14). Very little is known about the mechanism whereby boron is absorbed from the gastrointestinal tract, nor about its transport in the body. Boron is distributed throughout the tissues and organs of animals and humans at concentrations mostly between 0.05 and 0.6 μg/g fresh weight, and several times these concentrations in bones (11).

13.6 Dietary intake

The daily intake of boron by humans can vary widely depending on the proportions of various food groups in the diet (14). Foods of plant origin, especially fruits, leafy vegetables, nuts and legumes are rich sources. Wine, cider and beer are also high in boron. Meat, fish and dairy products are poor sources.

The possible variation in daily boron intake is exemplified by the study carried out by Gormican (15), who found that the boron content of hospital menus was much higher in summer than winter. Some examples of boron supplied daily (in mg) by the various institutional menus in summer and winter respectively were: general diet, 1.58 and 1.15; "mechanical soft" diet, 1.06 and 0.60; low-sodium diet, 1.46 and 0.47; "40-g protein" diet, 0.94 and 0.56; "1000-calorie" diet, 1.27 and 0.47; and "1500-calorie" diet, 0.79 and 0.51. Analyses of composites of "total diet", drawn from four different cities in the USA in 1965 showed that boron content ranged from 2.07 to 5.32 mg/4200 kcal (16), with a mean of 3.11 mg/4200 kcal and a CV of 18–31% (mean 25%). More recent data suggested that boron intake from the "total diet" (as defined by the United States Food and Drug Administration) could be 1.52 ± 0.38 (SD) mg/day. Type A school lunches in the USA were found to provide an average of 0.5 mg of boron/735 kcal and to range from < 0.12 to 1.31 mg boron/735 kcal (17). One-day diet composites collected by 22 Canadian premenopausal women consuming self-selected omnivorous diets contained 1.33 ± 0.13 (SEM) mg of boron (18). Compared with the above, the calculated average daily boron intake of English people is relatively high and variable, namely 2.8 ± 1.5 mg (19).

13.7 Safe range of population mean intakes

Human studies indicating that subjects consuming about 0.25 mg of boron/day can be responsive to boron supplementation (1, 2, 8, 9) suggest that the basal requirement for boron must be higher than this. A recent study indicated that about 1 μg of boron/g of dry diet meets the needs of most or all chicks (4). If it is assumed that adult humans consume 500 g of a mixed diet daily (dry basis), a boron concentration of 1 μg/g would result in an intake of 0.5 mg/day. As indicated previously, the CV of usual boron intakes seems to be about 25%. If it is assumed that the variance attributable to the quantity of food and to specific food selection is of comparable magnitude (total relative variance = 0.25^2), the CV for each component would be about 17.5. Thus, an individual mean basal requirement for adults may be about 0.375 mg/day (0.5/1.35). It is tentatively suggested that the minimum mean population intake that meets basal needs could be about 0.75 mg/day for adults (0.375/0.5).

The body probably has a storage reserve of boron because there is evidence that more than 21 days are required to induce changes in humans by feeding a low-boron diet. Thus, a normative requirement should be probably set for this element; however, there are no data from which to derive such a requirement. If it is assumed arbitrarily that the increment above the basal requirement is approximately 30%, the mean population intake to meet the normative needs of adults would be 1.0 mg of boron/day. This would be in line with the range of intakes reported in the preceding section for populations that apparently have no recognizable signs of boron deficiency.

Because the chronic toxicity of boron has rarely been studied or recognized, setting a threshold toxicity level is difficult. Overt signs of toxicity in animals generally occur only after the dietary boron concentration exceeds 100 $\mu g/g$. The richest food sources of boron, such as nuts and dried fruits, generally supply 15–30 $\mu g/g$ (11). A diet high in these foods plus wine (8.5 μg boron/g) is not necessarily unusual; thus a daily intake of 10–20 mg of boron/day can be achieved. If 20 mg of boron/day is assumed to be the threshold level for toxicity and the CV is 25%, an upper limit for the mean population intake would be 13 mg/day.

To summarize, an acceptable safe range of population mean intakes for boron for adults could well be 1.0–13 mg/day.

13.8 Recommendations for future studies

The functions of boron in mammalian tissues are unknown. Its physiological roles and the pathological effects of boron deficiency should be investigated more fully with a view to assessing the nutritional significance of dietary boron. The geochemical distribution of low-boron regions is well known and this information should be exploited in any future epidemiological studies.

References

1. Nielsen FH et al. Effect of dietary boron on mineral, estrogen, and testosterone metabolism in postmenopausal women. *FASEB journal*, 1987, **1**: 394–397.
2. Nielsen FH, Mullen LM, Gallagher SK. Effect of boron depletion and repletion on blood indicators of calcium status in humans fed a magnesium-low diet. *Journal of trace elements in experimental medicine*, 1990, **3**: 45–54.
3. Hunt CD, Nielsen FH. Interaction between boron and cholecalciferol in the chick. In: Howell J McC, Gawthorne JM, White CL, eds. *Trace element metabolism in man and animals*. Canberra, Australian Academy of Science, 1981: 597–600.
4. Hunt CD. Boron homeostasis in the cholecalciferol-deficient chick. *Proceedings of the North Dakota Academy of Sciences*, 1988, **42**: 60.
5. Nielsen FH et al. Magnesium and methionine deprivation affect the response of rats to boron deprivation. *Biological trace element research*, 1988, **17**: 91–107.
6. Nielsen FH et al. Dietary magnesium, manganese and boron affect the response of rats to high dietary aluminum. *Magnesium*, 1988, **7**: 133–147.
7. Nielsen FH, Zimmerman TJ, Shuler TR. Dietary potassium affects the signs of boron and magnesium deficiency in the rat. *Proceedings of the North Dakota Academy of Sciences*, 1988, **42**: 61.

8. Nielsen FH et al. Effects of dietary boron, aluminum and magnesium on serum alkaline phosphatase, calcium and phosphorus, and plasma cholesterol in postmenopausal women. In: Hurley LS et al., eds. *Trace elements in man and animals—TEMA 6.* New York, Plenum Press, 1988: 187–188.

9. Penland JG. Effects of dietary boron on the brain electrophysiology of healthy adults. *American journal of clinical nutrition* (in press).

10. Peace H et al. No effect of boron on bone mineral excretion and plasma sex steroid levels in healthy postmenopausal women. In: Momcilović B, ed. *Trace elements in man and animals—TEMA 7.* Zagreb, University of Zagreb, 1991: 38.

11. Nielsen FH. Other elements: Sb, Ba, B, Br, Cs, Ge, Rb, Ag, Sr, Sn, Ti, Zr, Be, Bi, Ga, Au, In, Nb, Sc, Te, Tl, W. In: Mertz W, ed. *Trace elements in human and animal nutrition,* 5th ed., Vol. 2. Orlando, FL, Academic Press, 1986: 415–463.

12. Franke J et al. Boron as an antidote to fluorosis? Part I: Studies on the skeletal system. *Fluoride,* 1985, **18**: 187–197.

13. Gordon AS, Prichard JS, Freedman MH. Seizure disorders and anemia associated with chronic borax intoxication. *Canadian Medical Association journal,* 1973, **108**: 719–721.

14. Nielsen FH. The ultratrace elements. In: Smith KT, ed. *Trace minerals in foods.* New York, Marcel Dekker, 1988: 357–428.

15. Gormican A. Inorganic elements in foods used in hospital menus. *Journal of the American Dietetic Association,* 1970, **56**: 397–403.

16. Zook EG, Lehmann J. Total diet study: content of ten minerals—aluminum, calcium, phosphorus, sodium, potassium, boron, copper, iron, manganese, and magnesium. *Journal of the Association of Official Analytical Chemists,* 1965, **48**: 850–855.

17. Murphy EW, Page L, Watt BK. Trace minerals in Type A school lunches. *Journal of the American Dietetic Association,* 1971, **58**: 115–122.

18. Clarke WB, Gibson RS. Lithium, boron, and nitrogen in 1-day diet composites and a mixed-diet standard. *Journal of food composition and analysis,* 1988, **1**: 209–220.

19. Hamilton EI, Minski MJ. Abundance of the chemical elements in man's diet and possible relations with environmental factors. *Science of the total environment,* 1972/73, **1**: 375–394.

14.
Vanadium

14.1 Biochemical function

Recently, in a number of reviews (*1–6*), the possibility has been considered that vanadium might play a role in the regulation of Na^+/K^+-exchanging ATPase, phosphoryl-transfer enzymes, adenylate cyclase and protein kinases. The possible role of the vanadyl ion as an enzyme cofactor, and its roles in hormone, glucose, lipid, bone and tooth metabolism have also been discussed. No specific biochemical function has yet been identified for vanadium in higher animals. However, the recent discovery in lower forms of life of vanadium-activated enzymes lends credence to the view that vanadium has similar roles in higher animals. Vanadium-dependent enzymes in lower organisms include nitrogenase in bacteria (*7*), which reduces molecular nitrogen to ammonia, and iodoperoxidase and bromoperoxidase in algae (*8, 9*) and lichens (*10*), which catalyse the oxidation of halide ions by hydrogen peroxide, thus facilitating the formation of a carbon–halogen bond. Haloperoxidases, such as thyroid peroxidase, play essential roles in higher animals, and it was recently shown that vanadium deprivation in rats affected the response of thyroid peroxidase to changing dietary iodine (*11*).

14.2 Deficiency and toxicity

Most of the deficiency signs reported for vanadium are questionable (*3*). However, Anke and coworkers (*12*) recently reported some reasonably well substantiated deficiency signs in goats which, when fed only 10 ng of vanadium/g of diet, as opposed to 2 µg of vanadium/g of diet, exhibited a higher abortion rate and produced less milk during the first 56 days of lactation. There was a high mortality among kids from vanadium-deprived goats. Serum creatinine and β-lipoprotein were elevated and serum glucose was depressed in these goats. In addition, skeletal deformations were seen in the forelegs, and forefoot tarsal joints were thickened.

Uthus & Nielsen (*11*) reported that, when compared with 1 µg of vanadium/g of diet, vanadium deprivation (2 ng vanadium/g of diet) increased both the thyroid weight and thyroid weight/body weight ratio of rats, and tended to decrease growth.

Vanadium is a relatively toxic element. A variety of signs of vanadium toxicity exist because they vary both with species and with dosage. Some of the more consistent signs include depressed growth, elevated organ vanadium, diarrhoea, depressed food intake and death. Signs of excessive vanadium intake in humans include gastrointestinal disturbances and green tongue (13, 14).

14.3 Epidemiology of deficiency and toxicity

The only epidemiological study in which an association between vanadium intake and a human disorder is reported is that of Masironi (15), in which an association between low intakes and cardiovascular disease was found.

Toxic effects resulting from the intake of large amounts of vanadium in the diet are unlikely. Toxicity usually occurs only as the result of industrial exposure to high levels of airborne vanadium.

14.4 Assessment of status

Serum vanadium may be a good indicator of exposure to high dietary vanadium. Cornelis et al. (16) found that human serum vanadium was in the range 0.016–0.939 ng/ml, most values being below 0.15 ng/ml. Thus, serum vanadium values above 1.0 ng/ml probably indicate excessive exposure. No good indicator of low vanadium status in humans has been established.

14.5 Absorption and bioavailability

Most ingested vanadium is apparently not absorbed and is excreted via the faeces (2, 4). A comparison of the very low concentrations of vanadium normally present in urine with the estimated daily intake and faecal levels of the element indicates that less than 5% of vanadium ingested is absorbed. Byrne & Kosta (17) estimated that no more than 1% of vanadium normally ingested in diet is absorbed. The results of animal studies are, in general, in agreement with these conclusions. However, two studies on rats indicated that a much greater amount of vanadium (greater than 10%) can be absorbed from the gastrointestinal tract under some conditions (18, 19).

The V^{5+} ion is absorbed 3–5 times as effectively as V^{4+}. Thus, the effect of other dietary components on the form of the vanadium present in the stomach, and the speed with which it is transformed into V^{4+}, probably markedly affect the percentage of ingested vanadium absorbed. This is supported by the finding that a number of substances, including ethylenediaminetetra-acetate, ascorbic acid, chromium, protein, ferrous iron, chloride and aluminium hydroxide (*3, 4*) can reduce vanadium toxicity.

14.6 Dietary intake

The daily dietary intake of vanadium is of the order of a few tens of μg and may vary widely (*17*). Nine institutional diets supplied 12.4–30.1 μg of vanadium/day (*20*), and intake averaged 20 μg. Ten diets in the United Kingdom Total Diet Study were found to supply an average of 13 μg of vanadium/day (*21*). Estimation of the daily intakes of vanadium for eight age–sex groups suggested a range of 6.2–18.3 μg in the United States Food and Drug Administration's Total Diet Study (*22*). Myron et al. (*20*) found that beverages, fats and oils, and fresh fruits and vegetables contained the least vanadium, ranging from 1 to 5 ng/g. Whole grains, seafood, meats and dairy products generally contained 5–30 ng/g. Byrne & Kosta (*17*) obtained similar results. Only a few food items, including spinach, parsley, mushrooms and oysters, contain relatively large amounts of vanadium.

14.7 Requirement and tolerable intakes

Average basal and normative requirements for vanadium cannot be set because the data required to do so are not available, nor can a safe range of population mean intakes for vanadium be proposed. However, the diets used in animal deprivation studies contained only 2–25 ng of vanadium/g and there was often no significant clinical effect. Vanadium deficiency has not been identified in humans although many diets supply less than 30 μg daily and most about 15 μg daily. This suggests that a dietary intake of 10 μg daily probably meets any postulated basal vanadium requirement. A daily intake of 10 mg of vanadium produced signs of overt vanadium toxicity in humans (*13, 14*). Much smaller amounts of vanadium (10–100 times the amount normally present in the diet) were found to have pharmacological effects on animals and humans. The threshold toxicity level may be much lower than 10 mg of vanadium/day.

References

1. Nielsen FH. Ultratrace elements in nutrition. *Annual review of nutrition*, 1984, 4: 21–41.
2. Nielsen FH. The ultratrace elements. In: Smith KT, ed. *Trace minerals in foods*. New York, Marcel Dekker, 1988: 357–428.
3. Nechay BR et al. Role of vanadium in biology. *Federation proceedings*, 1986, 45: 123–132.
4. Nielsen FH. Vanadium. In: Mertz W, ed. *Trace elements in human and animal nutrition*, 5th ed., Vol. 1. San Diego, Academic Press, 1987: 275–300.

5. Boyd DW, Kustin K. Vanadium: a versatile biochemical effector with an elusive biological function. *Advances in inorganic biochemistry*, 1984, **6**: 311–365.

6. Nechay BR. Mechanisms of action of vanadium. *Annual review of pharmacology and toxicology*, 1984, **24**: 501–524.

7. Smith BE et al. Biochemistry of nitrogenase and the physiology of related metabolism. *Philosophical transactions of the Royal Society of London, series B: biological sciences*, 1987, **317**: 131–146.

8. Vilter H. Peroxidases from Phaeophyceae: a vanadium (V)-dependent peroxidase from *Ascophyllum nodosum*. *Phytochemistry*, 1984, **23**: 1387–1390.

9. Krenn BE, Plat H, Wever R. The bromoperoxidase from the red alga *Ceramium rubrum* also contains vanadium as a prosthetic group. *Biochimica et biophysica acta*, 1987, **912**: 287–291.

10. Plat H, Krenn BE, Wever R. The bromoperoxidase from the lichen *Xanthoria parietina* is a novel vanadium enzyme. *Biochemical journal*, 1987, **248**: 277–279.

11. Uthus EO, Nielsen FH. The effect of vanadium, iodine, and their interaction on thyroid status indices. In: Anke M et al., eds. *Proceedings of the Sixth International Trace Element Symposium*, Vol. 1. Jena, Friedrich-Schiller-Universität, 1989: 44–49.

12. Anke M et al. New research on vanadium deficiency in ruminants. In: Anke M et al., eds. *5. Spurenelement-Symposium: new trace elements*. Jena, Friedrich-Schiller-Universität, 1986: 1266–1275.

13. Somerville J, Davies B. Effect of vanadium on serum cholesterol. *American heart journal*, 1962, **64**: 54–56.

14. Dimond EG, Caravaca J, Benchimol A. Vanadium: excretion, toxicity, lipid effect in man. *American journal of clinical nutrition*, 1963, **12**: 49–53.

15. Masironi R. Trace elements and cardiovascular diseases. *Bulletin of the World Health Organization*, 1969, **40**: 305–312.

16. Cornelis R et al. The ultratrace element vanadium in human serum. *Biological trace element research*, 1981, **3**: 257–263.

17. Byrne AR, Kosta L. Vanadium in foods and in human body fluids and tissues. *Science of the total environment*, 1978, **10**: 17–30.

18. Bogden JD et al. Balance and tissue distribution of vanadium after short-term ingestion of vanadate. *Journal of nutrition*, 1982, **112**: 2279–2285.

19. Wiegmann TB, Day HD, Patak RV. Intestinal absorption and secretion of radioactive vanadium ($^{48}VO_3^-$) in rats and effect of $Al(OH)_3$. *Journal of toxicology and environmental health*, 1982, **10**: 233–245.

20. Myron DR et al. Intake of nickel and vanadium by humans. A survey of selected diets. *American journal of clinical nutrition*, 1978, **31**: 527–531.

21. Evans WW, Read JI, Caughlin D. Quantification of results for estimating elemental dietary intakes of lithium, rubidium, strontium, molybdenum, vanadium and silver. *Analyst*, 1985, **110**: 873–877.

22. Pennington JAT, Jones JW. Molybdenum, nickel, cobalt, vanadium and strontium in total diets. *Journal of the American Dietetic Association*, 1987, **87**: 1640–1650.

C

Potentially toxic elements, some possibly with essential functions

15.
Fluoride

Fluorine in the form of fluoride occurs in nature ubiquitously and enters the body as a variable constituent of both drinking-waters and foods. The total intake of adults is usually within the range 0.2–2.0 mg of fluoride/day but higher intakes are not uncommon where the fluoride content of drinking-water is high. The fluoride content of natural waters may range from less than 0.1 mg/litre to more than 20 mg/litre. In the USA and in Central Europe generally, the fluoride content of natural waters is at the lower end of the range. In Asian countries and in many African countries, levels of fluoride in waters are typically towards the higher limit of the distribution. Some industrial fumes and dusts from chemical or smelting plants contribute significantly to environmental fluoride. The total ingestion of fluoride from all sources is taken into consideration when safe levels are derived. Body fluoride status depends on a multiplicity of factors, including the fluoride content of natural drinking-water, the total amount ingested daily, the duration of ingestion and the efficiencies of intestinal absorption and renal excretion. Since rises in environmental temperature increase water consumption, seasonal fluctuations occur in total fluoride ingestion and retention.

15.1 Absorption

Fluoride dissolved in drinking-water is frequently absorbed with an efficiency exceeding 90%. Absorption of dietary fluoride is in the range 30–60%, varies from region to region and is influenced by dietary composition. A recent Indian study has suggested that the fluoride of fluoridated toothpaste is absorbed by children but further confirmatory evidence is needed to determine the extent of fluoride absorption from this source. Most ingested fluoride is absorbed from the upper intestines. In children receiving fluoride supplements in infant formulae (0.5 mg of fluoride/day) and after weaning (1.0 mg of fluoride/day), the relatively high systemic retention of fluoride has been reflected in the form of mild to moderate dental mottling (1). About 80% of absorbed fluoride is excreted daily (2).

15.2 Biochemical function

The complex and frequently indirect relationships between low fluoride intakes and increased susceptibility to dental caries have been reviewed elsewhere (3). Fluoride is reported to be required for the transformation of osteocalcium phosphate to apatite, the chief mineral component of skeletal tissue. Higher fluoride contents increase the crystallinity of apatite and decrease its solubility in acid. Although the exact biological roles of fluoride in humans have not been established, animal experiments have suggested that it may be a structurally important constituent of bone collagen and of the glycosamino-glycans of the vascular system, the skin and other tissues. A single study reported by Schwartz & Milne (4) suggested that the growth of young rats was retarded if they were kept on low intakes of dietary fluoride (3–25μg of fluoride/100 kcal). This growth retardation was reversed by supplementation of the diet with fluoride. Diets low in fluoride content (< 0.3 mg of fluoride/kg dry matter) offered to goats during pregnancy and lactation and to the kids during postnatal growth reduced by 16% the 4-year life expectancy of the latter. This effect was not apparent if dietary fluoride was in the range 1.5–2.5 mg/kg (5).

15.3 Tissue fluoride

Ingested fluoride accumulates in bone tissue. The fluoride content of human bones varies from 300 to 7000 μg/g of dry tissue depending on total fluoride exposure. Studies carried out in India suggest that the body fluoride burden of individuals exposed to higher levels of environmental fluoride may be 2–3 times higher than normal, judging from the fluoride content of bone dry matter (6). Bone fluoride is a good indicator of lifetime exposure of the body to the element.

Blood levels of fluoride are almost negligible among people living in low-fluoride environments. However, when drinking-water contained 3 μg of fluoride/ml, blood fluoride concentrations of 0.6 μg of fluoride/ml were reported from Algeria (7). A significantly higher range of values for blood fluoride is seen in people living in areas of endemic fluorosis. Saliva normally contains 0.02 μg of fluoride/ml. Fluoride is actively secreted in milk (8) and human milk has been reported to contain 7 μg of fluoride/litre when environmental fluoride was 1 μg/ml in drinking-water. At lower levels of drinking-water fluoride, a concentration of 5 μg/litre of fluoride was reported in human milk. Transplacental transfer of fluoride is known to occur (9).

15.4 Balance studies

There is significant individual variability in the metabolic handling of fluoride (10). Retention is also influenced by diet. Millet-based diets promoted significantly greater retention of fluoride than rice-based diets in normal healthy active populations of young adults given 11 mg of elemental fluorine as sodium fluoride (*11*). Individuals living in endemic, high-fluoride areas have been shown to have positive fluoride balances, but these change to negative ones when they are withdrawn from environmental exposure. However, they continue to excrete abnormally large quantities of fluoride long after their removal from such areas.

15.5 Toxicity

The toxicity of ingested fluoride is well documented (*12*). The range of intakes compatible with human health is relatively narrow. Dental tissue usually shows the earliest signs of toxicity, mottling of tooth enamel being a well known manifestation of excess fluoride. Long-term exposure to high levels of fluoride leads to dental destruction. As drinking-water fluoride increases above 1 mg of fluoride/l, a variety of clinical symptoms of toxicity may develop. The blood concentration of fluoride increases from the value for normal blood fluoride of 0.04 μg/ml to values as high as 0.5–8.0 μg/ml, which have been reported in patients exhibiting clinical signs of fluorosis.

The term *fluorosis* covers a wide spectrum of clinical manifestations related to fluoride toxicity. Fluoride is a cumulative toxin. In the body, ionic fluoride rarely exists in blood; most ingested fluoride is trapped by bone tissue. In bone, fluoride accumulates in the lattice of bone crystal, where it stimulates new bone formation locally. The newly formed bone outgrowths (exostoses) lead to clinical syndromes including radiculopathy, myelopathy and peripheral neuropathy.

Target-specific effects of excess fluoride have been described. Secondary and tertiary hyperparathyroidism have been described in humans (*13*) and experimental animals (*14, 15*) exposed to excess fluoride, which also induces calcification of soft tissues, such as ligaments, tendons, membranes and periarticular attachments (*16*). In toxic amounts, fluoride interferes with calcium metabolism; increased bone accretion rate, increased bone resorption rate and increased total body turnover of calcium have all been reported.

Fluoride in excess also interferes with collagen synthesis in bone (*17*). In laboratory animals, toxic amounts of fluoride have been shown to reduce ^{14}C-labelled proline incorporation into the hydroxyproline of bone collagen.

Ingestion of large amounts of fluoride (5–40 mg/day) in drinking-water produces severe forms of skeletal deformity. These include kyphosis, fixed spine and other joint deformities, and the dramatic skeletal manifestations of the disease genu valgum. Endemic genu valgum has been reported from endemic fluorosis areas in India (*18*), Kenya, the United Republic of Tanzania (*19*) and

189

other African countries. In China, skeletal fluorosis due to ingestion of excess fluoride, particularly from fluoride-containing food, has been reported (20, 21). Concurrent dietary inadequacy of calcium seems to predispose to the osteomalacial form of skeletal fluorosis. The radiological features of fluoride toxicity range from osteosclerosis, osteoporosis and osteomalacia (21; for review, see reference 23) to those of secondary hyperparathyroidism (13, 24, 25). Hormonal involvement in the etiology of genu valgum is suggested by a male-to-female ratio of 10 : 1 in the preadolescent incidence of the disease. An increased urinary hydroxyproline output in endemic genu valgum results from an increased breakdown of bone; this bone loss is reflected as radiological osteoporosis. Urinary fluoride is elevated in chronic fluorosis, including genu valgum. Kenhardt bone disease is a form of chronic fluoride toxicity (26).

The crippling bone deformities of genu valgum have been reported to develop by adolescence when the cumulative intake of fluoride in water from birth was estimated to be > 10 mg. Analysis of bone samples has shown a significantly lower content of copper in the bone ash in this condition (27).

15.5.1 Interactions with calcium

Biological interactions between fluoride and calcium are known to occur. Particularly severe clinical forms of fluoride toxicity are reported among population groups whose calcium nutritional status is poor. While exposure to toxic levels of fluoride produces osteosclerotic forms of fluorosis in those whose dietary intakes of calcium are adequate, osteomalacia develops in subjects exposed to fluoride whose calcium intake is low. The primary lesion in the bone in the latter is a form of osteomalacia in which the presence of fluoride inhibits calcification of newly formed excess osteoid. The clinical manifestation of this lesion is the enlargement of the ends of the shafts of long bones but without any increase in bone density. In vivo, calcium turnover studies with radiolabelled calcium-47 in subjects with endemic genu valgum showed increased whole-body turnover of calcium (28), increased bone accretion and resorption rates, but a decrease in the renal elimination of calcium. Under the influence of fluoride, there is an attempt to retain calcium when dietary calcium is at the lower end of its range.

15.6 Intake

In assessments of intakes of fluoride and their relation to tolerable levels, account should be taken of fluoride ingestion through water and food, and as a result of environmental contamination from both natural and industrial sources. Enormous variation exists in water consumption patterns both in the same individual and from one individual to another. Age, occupation, environmental temperature, perspiration and food habits all determine water intake, and consequently may markedly influence fluoride intake.

15.6.1 Infants

The fluoride intakes of infants and small children are usually negligible. Human milk normally supplies 4.8–6.8 μg/l, but median intakes from breast milk in a six-country study ranged from 3 to 74 μg of fluoride/day in 3-month-old infants (29). In a comparative assessment, infant formulae dissolved in distilled water were found to supply 30 μg/l. However, the fluoride content of formula milk can increase, depending on that of the water used for its reconstitution. Fruit juices can supply as much as 90 μg of fluoride/l. Computed values of the fluoride intake of infants range from 3 μg/day during the first month of life to 50 μg/day at 5–6 months of age in breast-fed infants, at which time supplementary foods are usually introduced. Bergmann et al. calculated the total fluoride intake of German infants from food, water, air and supplements; mean estimates were 0.35 mg of fluoride at 1 month of age, 0.44 mg at 6 months and 0.46 mg at 1 year of age (30). Their work also suggests that prenatal maternal exposure to fluoride sufficient to maintain maternal urinary fluoride above 0.5 mg/l has a positive influence on the postpartum weight gain of infants in areas where drinking-water fluoride is normally low (0.02–0.16 mg/l) and maternal urinary fluoride typically less than 0.3 mg/l (31). The results of this interesting study have yet to be independently confirmed.

15.6.2 Children and adults

In Germany, where natural waters generally have a low fluoride content, it has been estimated that the mean total daily intake of children is 0.25 mg, increasing to 1.0–1.25 mg when fluoride supplements have been given. The corresponding estimates for adults were 0.51 and 1.51 mg, respectively (30).

In the USA, the daily intakes of infants, 2-year-old children and young adults were 0.23 mg, 0.21 mg and 0.86 mg, respectively, where water contained less than 0.3 mg/l of fluoride (32,33). In areas where water fluoride was more than 0.7 mg/l, the corresponding values were 0.42 mg, 0.62 mg and 1.85 mg, respectively (32, 34, 35). Japanese men and women consume, on average, 1.34 mg and 1.12 mg of fluoride/day, respectively. This greater intake probably reflects the high fluoride content of the volcanic geological parent materials from which the soils and aquifers in this region are derived. In hot climates, total fluoride intakes are frequently high because significantly more water is consumed than in cooler climates. In parts of India where skeletal fluorosis is endemic, water fluoride is often in the range 2–11 mg/l (*36*) and intakes between 6 and 30 mg/day are possible.

15.7 Safe levels

Although fluoride should probably be regarded as essential, there is no evidence so far from human studies that overt clinical signs of fluoride deficiency exist. No specifically diagnostic clinical or biochemical parameters have been related to fluoride inadequacy. The Expert Consultation was therefore unable to specify a minimum desirable intake. However, in view of the toxicity associated with excessive fluoride ingestion from a variety of sources, recommendations for maximum safe intakes are required. For this purpose, dental mottling may be taken as a definitive indication of toxicity.

There are indications that susceptibility to the dental mottling of fluorosis is increased by generalized malnutrition (*37*). In the absence of malnutrition dental mottling has been reported very occasionally when the fluoride content of drinking-water has exceeded 0.8 mg/l. However, it is rarely significant from the age of 4 years onwards unless fluoride intake from the diet plus drinking-water exceeds 2 mg/l or the intake from water alone exceeds 1.5 mg/day. These and higher intakes of fluoride are readily revealed by increases in urinary fluoride concentration to mean values greater than 1 mg/l for a 24-hour sample (*38*).

Total intakes at 1, 2 and 3 years of age should, if possible, be limited to 0.5, 1.0 and 1.5 mg/day respectively, with not more than 75% in the form of the highly soluble fluorides of drinking-water.

Because of the higher per capita water consumption in countries with high environmental temperatures, intakes of fluoride from water will be higher than in temperate countries. This must be taken into account when deriving regionally applicable estimates for safe upper limits of fluoride consumption from drinking-water and the diet. Adult intakes exceeding 5 mg of fluoride per day from all sources probably pose a significant risk of skeletal fluorosis.

Since the margins of safety are small, efforts should be made to reduce the intake of fluoride from drinking-water in areas where excess fluorides are present. If alternatives exist, irrigation waters low in fluoride should be used in preference to high-fluoride waters.

15.8 Recommendations for future studies

- Claims that a low fluorine status may prejudice postnatal growth should be further investigated.

● Existing measures to regulate the exploitation of water reserves for human consumption or crop irrigation are failing to prevent massive outbreaks of fluorosis in humans and their livestock from the inadvertent use of water from fluoride-rich aquifers. Liaison between WHO, FAO and the International Union of Geological Sciences should facilitate the investigation of the predictive value of geological data in avoiding such problems.

References

1. Aasenden R, Peebles TC. Effects of fluoride supplementation from birth on human deciduous and permanent teeth. *Archives of oral biology*, 1974, **19**: 321–326
2. Bagga OP. Urinary fluoride excretion in endemic fluorosis. *Fluoride*, 1979, **12**: 72–75.
3. Murray JJ, Rugg-Gunn AJ, Jenkin GN. *Fluoride in caries prevention*, 3rd ed. London, Butterworth-Heinemann, 1991.
4. Schwarz K, Milne DB. Fluorine requirement for growth in the rat. *Bioinorganic chemistry*, 1972, **1**: 331–338.
5. Anke M, Groppel B, Krause U. Fluorine deficiency in goats. In: Momcilovic B, ed. *Trace elements in man and animals—TEMA7*. Zagreb, University of Zagreb, 1991: 26–28.
6. Jolly SS et al. Human fluoride intoxication in Punjab. *Fluoride*, 1971, **4**: 94–97.
7. Elsair J et al. Fluoride content of blood, nails and hair in endemic skeletal fluorosis. *Fluoride*, 1982, **15**: 43–47.
8. Spak CJ, Hardell LI, DeChateau P. In: Mertz W, ed. *Trace elements in human nutrition*, 5th ed., Vol. 1. San Diego, Academic Press, 1987: 374.
9. Feltman R, Kosel G. In: Mertz W, ed. *Trace elements in human nutrition*, 5th ed., Vol. 1. San Diego, Academic Press, 1987: 382.
10. Jolly SS. Fluoride balance studies in endemic fluorosis. *Fluoride*, 1976, **9**: 138–147.
11. Lakshmaiah N, Srikantia SG. Fluoride retention in humans on sorghum and rice-based diets. *Indian journal of medical research*, 1973, **65**: 543.
12. Takamaori T. Recent studies on fluorosis. *Fluoride*, 1971, **4**: 154.
13. Makhni SS et al. The parathyroid in human fluorotic syndrome. *Fluoride*, 1980, **13**: 17.
14. Faccini JM, Care AD. The effect of sodium fluoride on the ultrastructure of parathyroid glands of the sheep. *Nature*, 1965, **207**: 1399–1401.
15. Makhni SS, Singh P, Thapar GS. Long-term effect of fluoride administration—an experimental study. 1. Radiological aspects. *Fluoride*, 1977, **10**: 82–86.
16. Franke J et al. Industrial fluorosis. *Fluoride*, 1975, **8**: 58–61.
17. Susheela AK, Mukherjee D. Fluoride poisoning and the effect on collagen biosynthesis of osseous and nonosseous tissues of the rabbit. *Toxicological European research*, 1981, **111**: 99–104.
18. Krishnamachari KAVR, Krishnaswamy K. Genu Valgum and osteoporosis in an area of endemic fluorosis. *Lancet*, 1973, **ii**: 877–879.

19. Christie DP. The spectrum of radiographic bone changes in children with fluorosis. *Radiology*, 1980, **138**: 85–90.

20. Daijei Huo. X-ray analysis of 34 cases of food borne skeletal fluorosis. *Fluoride*, 1981, **14**: 51–55.

21. Zan-dao W, Lin-ye Z, Ri-chuan B. Endemic food borne fluorosis in Guizhou, China. *Chinese journal of preventive medicine*, 1979, **13**: 148–151.

22. Krishnamachari KAVR. Osteomalacia in fluoride toxicity. *Fluoride*, 1982, **15**: 1.

23. Krishnamachari KAVR. Fluorine. In: Mertz W, ed. *Trace elements in human and animal nutrition*, 5th ed., Vol. 1. San Diego, Academic Press, 1987: 365–415.

24. Teotia SPS, Teotia M. Secondary hyperparathyroidism in patients with endemic skeletal fluorosis. *British medical journal*, 1973, **1**: 637–640.

25. ShivaKumar B, Krishnamachari KAVR. Circulating levels of immunoreactive parathyroid hormone in endemic genu valgum. *Hormone and metabolic research*, 1976, **8**: 317–319.

26. Jackson WPU. Further observations on the Kenhardt Bone Disease and its relation to osteoporosis. *South African medical journal*, 1962, **36**: 932–936.

27. Krishnamachari KAVR. Trace elements in serum and bone in endemic genu valgum. *Fluoride*, 1982, **15**: 25–31.

28. Nuissinyaiou BS, Krishnamachari KAVR, Vijayasarathy C. ^{47}Ca turnover in endemic fluorosis and endemic genu valgum. *British journal of nutrition*, 1979, **41**: 7–14.

29. Iyengar GV. *Elemental composition of human and animal milk*. Vienna, International Atomic Energy Agency, 1982 (Tec-doc-269).

30. Bergmann KE et al. Fluoridgesamtaufnahme im ersten Lebensjahr. [Total fluoride intake in the first year of life.] *Deutsche zahnärztliche Zeitschrift*, 1983, **38**: 145–147.

31. Bergmann RL, Bergmann KE. Fluoride nutrition in infancy—is there a biological role of fluoride for growth? In: Chandra RK, ed. *Trace elements in nutrition of children*, II. New York, Raven Press, 1991: 105–117 (Nestlé Nutrition Workshop Series, Vol. 23).

32. Singer L, Ophaug R. Total fluoride intake of infants. *Pediatrics* 1979, **63**: 460–466.

33. Singer L, Ophaug RH, Harland BF. Dietary fluoride intakes of 15–19 year-old male adults residing in the United States. *Journal of dental research*, 1985, **64**: 1302–1305.

34. Ophaug RH, Singer L, Harland BF. Dietary fluoride intake of 6-month and 2-year-old children in four dietary regions of the United States. *American journal of clinical nutrition*, 1985, **42**: 701–707.

35. Taves DR. Dietary intakes of fluoride ashed (total fluoride) v. unashed (inorganic fluoride) analysis of individual foods. *British journal of nutrition*, 1983, **49**: 295–301.

36. Krishnamachari KAVR. Further observations on the syndrome of endemic genu valgum of South India. *Indian journal of medical research*, 1976, **64**: 284–291.

37. Murray MM, Wilson DC. Fluorosis and nutrition in Morocco; dental studies in relation to environment. *British dental journal*, 1948, **84**: 97–100.

38. *Appropriate uses of fluorides for human health*. Geneva, World Health Organization, 1986: 3–32.

16.

Lead, cadmium and mercury

Apart from those communities exposed to high levels of pollution by industrial effluents or emissions rich in heavy metals, it is evident that, for most individuals, food and diet are the most important sources of these potentially toxic elements. Thus, Bennett (1), modelling the routes of human exposure to the heavy metals, presented data illustrating that the proportion of heavy metal intake normally accounted for by the content of these elements in food and drinking-water amounts to approximately 80% for cadmium, 40% for lead and 98% for mercury.

The principal causes and consequences of human exposure to dietary sources of lead, cadmium and mercury are briefly considered here. The effects of acute intoxication arising from industrial or other accidental exposure are not considered; information on such effects is available elsewhere (2–6). Claims arising from studies on experimental animals that very low dietary concentrations of lead and cadmium may be essential are examined briefly. Physiological and dietary variables having a general influence on pathological responses to changes in heavy metal intake are considered before the effects of individual elements are discussed. Such variables have a profound effect on the health risks associated with chemical evidence of heavy metal contamination of the diet or environment.

Trends in human exposure to these and other dietary contaminants have been reported in documents produced by the Joint UNEP/FAO/WHO Food Contamination Monitoring Programme (GEMS/Food).

16.1 Variables influencing tolerance

16.1.1 Stage of physiological development

During gestation and lactation, both lead and methylmercury can be transferred from mother to progeny via the placenta or breast milk. Quite apart from the intrinsically higher absorption of lead, cadmium and mercury from liquid diets (to be considered later), the immaturity of the digestive tract of infants and young children promotes higher absorption of these elements than is the case with older subjects. The immature kidney also excretes these elements less readily. Thus a greater proportion of the administered dose is liable to accumulate in the body of young children than in older children or adults. Incomplete development of the blood–brain barrier also reduces the capacity to restrict the accumulation of such metals by the brain in young children. Both the immediate consequences of such accumulation and the possibility that they may disturb the maturation of tissues such as the central nervous system have led to strong suspicions that vulnerability to the effects of heavy metal exposure is particularly high at early stages of growth and development (7).

There are particularly strong indications that infants and young children should be considered high-risk groups if environmental exposure to lead is excessive (8,9). Studies on young children with a reasonably stable exposure history (10–12) show that they absorb and retain substantially more ingested lead than adults, namely 40–50% as compared with 10–50%. Comparisons of lead metabolism in immature and adult experimental animals show identical phenomena (13), and also indicate differing metal distributions in the young, where retention in the brain is at least 10 times greater (14, 15) than in adults. Adverse effects of lead on health, including effects on haem synthesis and the function of the central nervous system occur at lower blood levels in infants and children than in adults. Lower standards for permissible lead exposure have therefore been adopted for young than for adult subjects (13, 16).

Evidence of a progressive accumulation of cadmium in the kidney with increasing age suggests that cadmium exposure will adversely affect health particularly in older age groups. However, cadmium absorption is also higher in children than in adults (14). Furthermore, the body burden of cadmium increases steeply during the first years of life (17), suggesting that absorption or retention is higher during these early stages of development. Cadmium, in contrast to lead and methylmercury, is not transported readily into the fetus but is retained in the placenta, where it restricts the transfer of elements such as zinc and copper essential for brain function and mental development (18, 19).

Methylmercury readily crosses the placenta into the fetus and passes into the neonate via maternal milk. It is readily incorporated into the central nervous system at early stages of development. Epidemiological evidence from instances of accidental exposure to methylmercury indicates that perinatal exposure is particularly harmful to the developing infant and presents a substantially greater hazard than exposure in adulthood. Studies on experimental animals also show that inorganic (mercuric) mercury is absorbed and retained in the brain more readily during perinatal periods of exposure (20).

16.1.2 Nutrition

Most available data relate to the interaction of heavy metals with dietary macromolecules (21). Absorption of lead is substantially greater by fasted than by fed subjects (22). Increasing the intervals between meals increases the efficiency of lead absorption (23). Such data are in line with evidence showing an inverse relationship between lead uptake and the quantity of food and digesta in the gut. Of the many dietary interactions influencing lead uptake or retention (13), those with calcium and iron are particularly important. Phosphate and vitamin D metabolites are also important, but their effects are not as fully characterized epidemiologically (24).

Mahaffey et al. (25) showed that a statistically significant inverse relationship existed between dietary calcium intake and blood lead, as indicated by the results of the Second National Health and Nutrition Examination Survey in the United States (NHANES-2). Data from this substantial study are consistent with others for infants (10), children (26) and adult volunteers (27). Recent epidemiological data also show higher lead blood levels in women from geographical areas where dietary calcium intakes are low than in women where such intakes are traditionally higher (28). Iron status has also been shown to be inversely related to blood lead, iron deficiency being associated with higher blood lead levels (29, 30). Other reports show that a corresponding inverse relationship exists between iron status and lead uptake in children at risk (31).

Iron status and the absorption and retention of cadmium also appear to be inversely related. Cadmium uptake was enhanced in elderly people with low body iron stores (32). This enhanced absorption or retention of cadmium by subjects with a low iron status places rapidly growing infants and women in the reproductive phase of life at particular risk as both of these groups are inclined to develop such a status. Nutritional inadequacies probably aggravate the pathological consequences of an enhanced cadmium intake resulting from the pollution of rice and drinking-water in the etiology of "itai-itai" disease (33–35) (see p. 205). Exacerbation of this manifestation of cadmium toxicity by interactions between cadmium and other trace elements (36), vitamin D, calcium and dietary protein (34) have all been invoked to explain the increased severity of this syndrome during periods of food shortage.

Dietary variables are also likely to influence the tolerance of humans for methylmercury, and such variability must be taken into account when evaluating the toxic levels of organic mercurials (37). Experiments on animal models suggest that dietary selenium may reduce the toxic effects of methylmercury. The finding that communities such as Peruvian coastal villagers, Korean fishermen and Samoan cannery workers exhibit no clinical signs of methylmercury poisoning despite their high body burdens of mercury (38) may well reflect the usually adequate or high levels of selenium intake of fish-eating communities. The possibility that high dietary fibre, by modifying methylating activity in the lower gut, might influence the conversion of inorganic mercury into methylmercury and thus enhance risks of toxicity is being investigated (39).

197

16.1.3 Liquid diets

The absorption and retention of lead, cadmium and mercury are greatly enhanced in experimental animals given liquid diets as their only source of food (*40*). This phenomenon, which is also found with milk diets, only occurs if the total diet is in liquid form, and is not seen with mixed feeding. While it is suspected that the high neonatal absorption of metals from infant feeds is partly attributable to the immaturity of the gastrointestinal tract, the early reliance of infants on liquid milk or milk substitutes will also play a part (*41*). Although based almost exclusively on the results of studies on experimental animal models and not yet adequately quantified, there are strong grounds for the belief that such effects may influence the risks to health of infants receiving milk or its liquid substitutes in environments contaminated with lead, cadmium or mercury.

16.1.4 Other variables

Experimental studies on animal models and the limited data so far available from human studies indicate that the accumulation of heavy metals in the body and the manifestations of heavy metal toxicity are influenced by a wide range of factors other than their concentration in the diet (*21, 37, 42*). Developmental and nutritional variables, as discussed in sections 16.1.1 and 16.1.2, must be considered when evaluating the health effects of heavy metals on populations exposed to contaminated diets or environments.

Investigations of the nutritional status and nutrient intake of the populations under investigation should be an integral part of any protocol for studies of the effects of heavy metal exposure. Particular attention should be paid to observations on the youngest age groups. Such data may well indicate the extent to which dietary manipulation might be expected to confer some protection against the health effects of heavy-metal exposure.

16.2 Entry into food chains

Geological and soil conditions and the extent to which these are modified by human activities, such as the disposal of mine and other industrial or urban wastes, irrigation and agricultural practices, can have a significant influence on the lead, cadmium and mercury contents of foods of plant or animal origin.

Lead is widely distributed in rocks and soils, the highest concentrations being found in localities in which it has accumulated by geochemical mineralization and particularly where lead-rich ores have been mined and the waste has been dispersed on land used for cultivation or grazing. Other methods of industrial or urban waste disposal and the presence of road traffic can also increase soil lead and, since its phytotoxicity is low, such high-lead areas often remain unsuspected. Acid soil conditions increase lead uptake.

Bread, cereals and beverages account, typically, for about 35% of the daily intake of lead, the remainder being derived from a variety of food types. Mean dietary intakes of children have been reported to be in the range 9–278 μg of lead/day and for adults 20–282 μg/day. Atypically high dietary intakes (e.g. > 500 μg of lead/day) were found in one Indian investigation.

High contents of cadmium in soils and crops are usually associated with its presence in shales and other sedimentary rocks in association with minerals rich in both cadmium and zinc. Local surface distribution of mine wastes from mineral-rich deposits often increases crop cadmium levels. Soil distribution of urban wastes and sludges is also responsible for significant increases in the normally low (< 0.15 μg/g) cadmium content of most food crops.

Cereals and other vegetables normally account for about 50% of cadmium intake which, in children, is typically in the range 2–25 μg/day and in adults 10–50 μg/day. The highest values within these ranges were all reported from countries noted for extensive industrial activities involving the processing of cadmium-rich ores or other raw materials.

Biological accumulation of cadmium occurs in molluscs, in crustacea and in kidney tissues. The influence of high-cadmium environmental anomalies on the dietary intake of cadmium is substantially increased if the diet contains such food items.

Biological concentration in specific food types also markedly influences the dietary intake of mercury and in addition, may enhance its toxicity. Mercury derived from natural sources is probably greater than that from industrial emissions by a factor of at least 10, most being in the form of inorganic compounds. Typical total dietary intakes reported were in the range 2–6 μg of mercury/day for children and 2–140 μg/day for adults, the mercury of fish and foods of marine origin accounting for about 40% and fruit and vegetables 20%. The contribution from fish is markedly greater in some communities and this, coupled with its biotransformation to toxic organic mercury in marine ecosystems, increases the significance of environmental anomalies in mercury distribution irrespective of their precise causes.

Many of the factors influencing the significance of the diet as a source of lead, cadmium and mercury are considered in more detail elsewhere (1–6, 43).

16.3 Toxicity of lead

The toxic effects of lead involve several organs and are the consequence of a variety of biochemical defects (44). The risks form a continuum, ranging from overt, clinical manifestations of toxicity to covert biochemical effects. The nervous system of infants and children is particularly sensitive to lead toxicity (45). Adults exposed occupationally or accidentally to excessively high levels exhibit peripheral neuropathology and/or chronic nephropathy. However, the critical or most sensitive effect for adults in the general population may be the development of hypertension (46). Defects in haem synthesis provide biochemical indications of lead exposure in the absence of clinically detectable effects, but anaemia in the absence of other effects attributable to such exposure is uncommon.

16.3.1 Neurological, neurobehavioural and developmental effects in children

Clinically overt lead encephalopathy may occur in children with high exposure to lead, probably at blood levels of 80 μg/dl or higher. Early symptoms of lead encephalopathy include lethargy, vomiting, irritability, loss of appetite and dizziness, progressing to obvious ataxia and a reduced level of consciousness which may lead to coma and death. Children who recover from lead encephalopathy often have sequelae such as mental retardation, epilepsy and optic neuropathy with blindness in some cases (47). At lower levels of exposure, cross-sectional epidemiological studies have provided evidence of intelligence quotient (IQ) decrements of approximately 5 points at average blood lead levels of 50–70 μg/dl, 4 points at 30–50 μg/dl, and 1–2 points at 15–30 μg/dl (48). Recent cross-sectional studies designed to obviate many of the problems of earlier epidemiological investigations have produced further evidence of a lead–IQ relationship with no apparent threshold (49), at blood lead levels down to less than 10 μg/dl. Although the results of these and of recent studies show some inconsistencies, the United States Environmental Protection Agency has concluded that lead produces impairments in neurobehavioural development at blood levels of 10–15 μg/dl and possibly lower (48). Reports that subnormal cognitive ability at age 4–5 years was related to prenatal lead exposure, as judged by umbilical cord-blood lead, provide additional support for these conclusions (50, 51). A maternal blood lead level of 10–15 μg/dl or possibly lower may result in measurable impairment of nervous system development in the unborn child (48).

16.3.2 Haematological effects

The anaemia of lead poisoning results from two basic defects: shortened erythrocyte life span and impairment of haem synthesis. The shortened life span of the red blood cell is probably the consequence of the increased mechanical fragility of the cell membrane. A negative exponential relationship exists between the activity of the enzyme δ-aminolevulinate dehydratase and blood lead. Coproporphyrinogen oxidase activity decreases, resulting in increased coproporphyrin concentrations and a decrease in the activity of ferrochelatase, which normally catalyses the incorporation of ferrous ion into the porphyrin ring structure. The excess protoporphyrin resulting from the inhibition of ferrochelatase takes the place of haem in the haemoglobin molecule and, as the red blood cells containing protoporphyrin circulate, zinc is chelated at the centre of the molecule at the site usually occupied by iron. Erythrocytes containing zinc-protoporphyrin are intensely fluorescent and may be used as biochemical indicators of lead toxicity. Depressed haem synthesis is probably the stimulus for increasing the activity of δ-aminolevulinate synthase, the first step in haem synthesis. This markedly increases the circulating blood levels and urinary excretion of δ-aminolevulinic acid. Lead retention also increases haem oxygenase activity, and thus increases bilirubin formation. These changes in enzyme activity induced by lead are dose-related. Anaemia only occurs in very marked lead toxicity. The changes in enzyme activities, particularly of δ-aminolevulinate dehydratase in peripheral blood, and in the excretion of δ-aminolevulinic acid in urine correlate very closely with actual blood lead and serve as early biochemical indicators of lead exposure (44).

16.3.3 Renal effects

The toxicological effects of lead on the kidney are of two types: reversible renal tubular dysfunction, occurring mostly in children with acute exposure to lead and usually associated with overt central nervous system effects, and irreversible chronic interstitial nephropathy characterized by vascular sclerosis, tubular cell atrophy, interstitial fibrosis and glomerular sclerosis. Chronic lead nephropathy is most common after prolonged industrial exposure. In the early stages of excessive exposure, morphological and functional changes in the kidney are confined to the renal tubules and are pronounced in proximal tubular cells. The suggestion made more than 100 years ago that a relationship exists between chronic lead exposure and gouty nephropathy has recently been supported by the results of studies showing that gout patients with renal disease exhibit greater increments in urinary lead after administration of edetate than do renal patients without gout. Lead reduces uric acid excretion (52).

16.3.4 Effect on blood pressure

Epidemiological studies indicate an association between an elevated body burden of lead and increased blood pressure in adults. The data as a whole provide highly convincing evidence of a small but statistically significant association between blood lead levels and increased blood pressure in adult men, the strongest association being for men aged 40–59 and particularly for systolic pressure. Virtually all analyses show positive associations for the 40–59 age group that remain or become significant ($P < 0.05$) when allowance is made for geographical differences in lead exposure. Quantitatively, the relationship holds good across a wide range of blood lead levels down to as low as 7 µg/dl for middle-aged men. Systolic blood pressure increases by about 0.200–0.400 kPa (1.5–3.0 mmHg) for every doubling of blood lead concentration in adult males, but by less than 0.133–0.267 kPa (1.0–2.0 mmHg) in adult females (46).

16.3.5 Other effects

Lead is classified as a category 2B carcinogen by the International Agency for Research on Cancer (53); evidence of carcinogenicity is adequate in animals but inadequate in humans. The induction of renal adenocarcinoma by lead in rats and mice is dose-related but has not been reported at levels below that producing nephrotoxicity (54). Lead compounds stimulate the proliferation of renal tubular epithelial cells (55), and similar effects have been noted in rat livers.

Severe lead toxicity causes sterility, abortion and neonatal mortality and morbidity. Gametotoxic effects occur in both male and female experimental animals, but the potential for such effects in humans is unknown.

16.3.6 Biochemical signs of intoxication

Direct measurement of lead in blood is currently the most useful indicator of the risk of toxic effects. Urinary lead is variable and is not a useful indicator of toxicity. Lead in shed teeth of paediatric populations provides an index of cumulative exposure to lead (56).

Lead chelatable with sodium calcium edetate represents lead removed from soft tissue (57). Both WHO (16) and the Centers for Disease Control in the United States (58) regard chelatable lead as the most useful index of the toxicologically active lead burden in children and adults, but its determination requires an invasive procedure that should not be performed without other evidence of an increase in lead exposure, e.g. increased blood lead.

Measurement of lead by the recently developed X-ray fluorescence technique provides a method of assessing lead in long bones (59, 60).

The effects of lead on haem metabolism provide at least three biochemical indicators of low-level lead effects, including the linear inhibition of δ-aminolevulinate dehydratase in peripheral red blood cells at levels of lead in blood exceeding as little as 10 μg/dl in children or 20 μg/dl in adults. However, the enzyme is more difficult to measure than blood lead and is no more informative (61). On a group basis, elevation of δ-aminolevulinic acid in urine serves as a useful indicator of lead exposure once blood lead is greater than 40 μg/dl, but blood lead is not a sufficiently sensitive index of low-level lead exposure.

Measurement of erythrocyte zinc-protoporphyrin provides a simple index of the effect of lead on haem metabolism when blood lead begins to exceed 15 μg/dl (62); however, it is also elevated with iron deficiency, so that codetermination of iron status is required. This, together with the lack of sensitivity once blood lead is below 15 μg/dl, restricts the usefulness of this approach to the assessment of low-level lead exposure.

16.3.7 Maximum tolerable intakes

The Joint FAO/WHO Expert Committee on Food Additives provisionally recommends that the weekly intake of lead should not exceed 25 μg/kg of body weight per week for adults, children and infants (2, 3). A recent review of 38 reports of dietary intakes of lead from a variety of national sources (63) showed that intake was highly variable. Thus the mean intake of adults was in the range 20–514 μg/day. Data from 26 countries indicated that the dietary intake of adults was in the range 2–64 μg/kg per week; for infants and children in 14 countries, the corresponding figure was 2–24 μg/kg per week (14).

Contamination of foods by lead from the soldered seams of cans is gradually decreasing with the wider introduction of lacquered cans and lead-free solders. Glazed ceramic cooking or storage utensils can contribute appreciably to the lead content of acid foods and beverages. Contamination of water for drinking or cooking by lead from piping can be appreciable and may often exceed tolerable intakes for children or infants unless the water is neutral or alkaline in pH. Soils overlying lead containing mine deposits or subject to industrial or urban pollution can contain up to 4000 mg of lead/kg instead of the normal 0.1–20 mg/kg. The lead content of vegetable and cereal food crops reflects such anomalies if low soil pH promotes its absorption. As already mentioned, the phytotoxicity of lead is low and thus such crops may show no external signs of their high lead content.

16.4 Toxicity of cadmium

The risks to health arising from cadmium are greatest when inhalation of cadmium from occupational sources results directly in lung damage.

The effects of less acute exposure to dietary or environmental sources usually reflect the toxic action of a high body burden on the kidney and possibly the skeleton. Cadmium retention in body tissues is related to the formation of cadmium-metallothionein, a cadmium–protein complex of low molecular weight. The synthesis of metallothionein is induced by the essential metals copper and zinc in liver and kidney, but also by cadmium, which may replace these metals or share the protein with them. Cadmium is present in most organs, but the highest concentrations are found in kidney, where it accumulates with age in proportion to the total body cadmium burden. The toxicity of cadmium has been reviewed in detail (4, 64, 65).

16.4.1 Kidney damage

The effects of cadmium on the kidney take the form of renal tubular dysfunction and subsequent pathological changes. The former is reflected by failure to resorb substances normally, and results in proteinuria, aminoaciduria, glucosuria and decreased renal tubular absorption of phosphate. Cadmium excretion and low molecular weight proteinuria are early indicators of renal cadmium damage (66).

The predominant feature of cadmium-induced proteinuria is the presence in urine of β_2-microglobulin. However, other low molecular weight proteins have also been identified in the urine of workers occupationally exposed to high levels of calcium, including retinol-binding protein, lysozyme, ribonuclease and immunoglobulin light chains. High molecular weight proteins, such as albumin and transferrin, in the urine suggest that damage to the kidney glomerulus has also occurred. The pathogenesis of the glomerular lesion is not currently understood (67).

The critical concentration of cadmium in the renal cortex, based on the occurrence of tubular dysfunction in 10% of the population, is about 200 μg/g. Liver and kidney cadmium levels increase simultaneously until the average renal cortex cadmium concentration is about 300 μg/g and the average liver concentration about 60 μg/g. Daily intakes in food of 140–260 μg cadmium per day for more than 50 years or workroom air exposures of 50 μg/m^3 for more than 10 years have produced renal dysfunction (68). An epidemiological study of the dose–response relationship for cadmium intake from rice, based on retrospective analytical data and assessments of β_2-microglobulin output as a measure of renal tubular dysfunction, have suggested that the total lifetime cadmium intake likely to produce an adverse health effect is approximately 2000 mg for both men and women (69). The mechanistic aspects of the initiation of renal damage by cadmium have been considered in a recent review (70).

16.4.2 Skeletal damage

Individuals with severe cadmium nephropathy may have renal calculi and exhibit excessive urinary loss of calcium. With chronic exposure, urinary calcium may eventually decline to become less than normal. Associated skeletal changes probably related to calcium loss include osteomalacia and osteoporosis. Bone changes associated with intense skeletal pain are features of a syndrome previously mentioned (itai-itai disease) seen in postmenopausal multiparous women living in the Fuchu area of Japan before and during the Second World War. Other features of the syndrome included severe body deformities and chronic renal disease. Excess cadmium exposure has been implicated in the pathogenesis of itai-itai disease, but anomalies of vitamin D supply or metabolism and perhaps other nutritional deficiencies may also have been involved.

Nogawa et al. (71) reported that serum 1,25-dihydroxyvitamin D levels were lower than normal in itai-itai disease patients and in cadmium-exposed subjects with renal damage. Decreases in serum 1,25-dihydroxyvitamin D levels were closely related to serum concentrations of parathyroid hormone and β_2-microglobulin, and to the percentage tubular reabsorption of phosphate, suggesting that cadmium-induced bone effects were mainly due to a disturbance in vitamin D and parathyroid hormone metabolism. Friberg et al. (65) suggested that cadmium in the proximal tubular cells depresses cellular functions, including depressed conversion of 25-hydroxyvitamin D to 1,25-dihydroxyvitamin D. This is likely to decrease calcium absorption and bone mineralization and thus lead to osteomalacia.

16.4.3 Pulmonary damage

Inhalation of cadmium causes irritation and possibly an acute inflammatory reaction of the lungs. Long-term exposure produces chronic bronchitis and increased susceptibility to infections, bronchiectasis and emphysema. Such pulmonary effects are dose-related and are of concern principally in cases of industrial exposure. Other pulmonary irritants, particularly cigarette smoke, a significant source of cadmium, may exacerbate its toxic effects (72).

16.4.4 Biochemical signs of intoxication

The most important measure of excessive cadmium exposure is increased cadmium excretion in urine. In populations not exposed to excessive cadmium, urinary cadmium excretion is small and relatively constant, usually of the order of only 1 or 2 μg/day, or less than 1 μg of cadmium/g of creatinine. With excessive exposure (e.g. in some cadmium workers), increases in urinary cadmium may not occur until all the available cadmium-binding sites of metallothionein are saturated. Increased urinary cadmium reflects recent exposure, an increased body burden and, in particular, an elevation of renal cadmium.

Urinary cadmium measurement thus provides a good index of excessive cadmium exposure. Nogawa et al. (66) determined the urinary concentration of cadmium corresponding to a number of other compositional anomalies of urine. Tubular proteinuria (excretion of β_2-microglobulin) occurred at a 1% prevalence rate with a urinary cadmium concentration of 3.2 μg/g of creatinine, i.e. at a slightly lower urinary cadmium level than other signs of renal tubular dysfunction. The presence of retinol-binding protein may provide a more practical and reliable test of proximal tubular function than β_2-microglobulinuria because sensitive immunological analytical methods are now available for it and it is more stable in urine. Urinary excretion of N-acetyl-β-D-glucosaminidase activity may prove to be an even more sensitive indicator of cadmium-induced renal tubular dysfunction (73). Changes in the urinary excretion of low molecular weight proteins are mainly observed in workers excreting more than 10 μg of cadmium/g of creatinine (68, 72).

16.4.5 Maximum tolerable intakes

The Joint FAO/WHO Expert Committee on Food Additives (2, 4) recommends that 7 μg of cadmium/kg of body weight should be regarded, provisionally, as the maximum tolerable weekly intake of cadmium. For a 65-kg man, this corresponds to a dietary intake of 65 μg/day. Of 35 dietary studies reviewed by this Committee, only one, from a cadmium-contaminated area of Japan, reported mean daily intakes exceeding this figure. A survey of dietary intakes of cadmium in 24 countries indicated that adult intakes varied from 0.9 to 7 μg/kg per week; the corresponding range for infants or children from 10 countries was 1.9–9.9 μg/kg per week (74). Representative mean intakes of cadmium were in the range 10–60 μg/day for adults and 5–20 μg/day for children. Concentrations of cadmium in most foods are typically less than 0.15 mg/kg. Notable exceptions are shellfish and kidneys, the former containing typically 1–2 mg of cadmium/kg and the latter 0.5 mg/kg. The cadmium content of vegetable and cereal crops is influenced by the soils on which they are grown if these are polluted by cadmium-rich industrial or urban wastes or are derived from geological parent materials containing the zinc–cadmium ore, sphalerite.

WHO has recently set the upper guideline value for cadmium in drinking-water at 3 μg/l (75).

16.5 Toxicity of mercury

The toxicological features of mercury reflect its three forms: elemental, and inorganic and organic compounds (5, 6, 76). Inorganic compounds may contain mercury in oxidation states $+1$ or $+2$.[1] The gastrointestinal absorption of inorganic compounds from food is less than 15% in mice and was about 7% in a study on human volunteers. Absorption of methylmercury is of the order of 90–95%.

Kidneys retain the greatest concentrations of mercury following exposure to its inorganic compounds or vapour, whereas organic mercury has a greater affinity for the brain, and particularly the posterior cortex. However, mercury from mercury vapour tends to accumulate in the central nervous system more readily than inorganic mercury compounds.

Excretion of mercury in urine and faeces varies with the form of mercury, size of dose and time after exposure. Faecal excretion predominates initially after exposure to inorganic mercury, renal excretion increasing with time. About 90% of methylmercury is excreted in faeces after acute or chronic exposure, and the proportion changes only slowly with time.

Current understanding of the metabolism of mercury is based principally on the results of experimental animal studies (see references 6 and 76). All forms of mercury cross the placenta to the fetus. Fetal uptake of elemental mercury by rats is 10–40 times higher than uptake after exposure to inorganic compounds. Concentrations of mercury in the fetus after exposure to alkyl mercury compounds are twice those found in maternal tissues. Methylmercury levels in fetal red blood cells are 30% higher than in maternal red cells. The positive fetal–maternal gradient and increased concentration of mercury in red blood cells enhance the fetal toxicity of mercury, particularly following exposure to alkyl mercury. Although maternal milk may contain only 5% of the mercury concentration of maternal blood, neonatal exposure to mercury may be greatly augmented by breast-feeding. Methylmercury, the most toxic form of the element, causes the greatest risk to health from environmental or dietary exposure. Many effects produced by short-chain alkyl mercury compounds are unique in terms of mercury toxicity but are diagnostically non-specific. Most evidence of the clinical signs, symptoms and neuropathology of overt methylmercury toxicity has been obtained from studies of epidemics in Iraq and Japan (6, 76) and of populations eating mercury-contaminated fish (77) as well as from cases of occupational exposure (78).

The major risks to human health arise from the neurotoxic effects of mercury in adults (79) and its toxicity to the fetus if women are exposed to methylmercury during pregnancy (80). The brain is the critical organ. A genotoxic effect resulting in chromosomal aberrations has also been demonstrated in methylmercury-exposed populations.

---

[1] Corresponding to the obsolete terms mercurous and mercuric, respectively.

207

Its neurotoxic effects include: paraesthesia, a numbness and tingling sensation around the mouth, lips and extremities, particularly the fingers and toes; ataxia, a clumsy stumbling gait; difficulty in swallowing and articulating; neurasthenia, a generalized sensation of weakness, fatigue and inability to concentrate; loss of vision and hearing; spasticity and tremor; and, finally, coma and death.

The pathological effects of chronic low-level dietary exposure to inorganic dietary forms of mercury have not been extensively studied. Acute exposure to soluble salts of mercury(II) has been reported to cause extensive damage to the gastrointestinal tract and circulatory collapse. Compounds of mercury(I) are less toxic. Calomel, i.e. dimercury(I) chloride, has a long history of use in medicine. When used as a teething powder for children, it is now known to be responsible for acrodynia or "pink disease". Children develop fever, vasodilation, hypersecretion of sweat, a pink-coloured rash, swelling of the spleen and lymph nodes, and hyperkeratosis and swelling of fingers. The effects are independent of dose and are thought to be a hypersensitivity reaction (81).

16.5.1 Signs of intoxication

The biochemical indices of mercury toxicity are limited to measurements of mercury in body fluids and tissues and the monitoring of their relationship to clinical signs (80).

The critical effect in adults is paraesthesia. It has been estimated that the average long-term daily intake associated with adverse health effects in the most susceptible individual is 300 μg/day for an adult or 4.3 μg of mercury/kg of body weight per day. Psychomotor retardation is the critical effect in prenatal exposure. The infant may appear normal at birth but there is a 12-month or longer delay in learning to walk and talk and an increased incidence of seizures.

The "threshold" level of exposure at which the occurrence of critical effects exceeds background occurs at a lower dose when exposure is prenatal than during adulthood. Epidemiological studies on dose–effect relationships in prenatal exposure have now been conducted in Canada, Iraq and New Zealand. From these, it has been calculated (78) that the lowest level at which adverse effects attributable to psychomotor retardation are observed corresponds to maternal hair concentrations during pregnancy of 10–20 mg/kg. If it is assumed that the relationship between intake and body burden of methylmercury is the same in pregnant and non-pregnant women, this hair value would correspond to an intake of 800–1700 ng of mercury/kg per day, and to a maternal red blood cell level of 40–80 μg/l. At higher levels of exposure *in utero*, the child may develop ataxic motor disturbance and mental symptoms similar to those occurring in a child with cerebral palsy of unknown etiology. Postnatal poisoning may result from the transfer of methylmercury via breast milk. Symptoms of this type of poisoning are similar to those in the adult.

16.5.2 Maximum tolerable intakes

The Joint FAO/WHO Expert Committee on Food Additives (82, 83) provisionally recommends that total mercury intake should not exceed 5 µg/kg of body weight per week with not more than 3.3 µg/kg per week as methylmercury. Of 26 national dietary surveys recently reviewed by IAEA (63), none showed mean dietary intakes approaching this figure. Other sources report mean intakes of mercury from diet and water of 0.2–3.1 µg/kg of body weight per week for infants and 0.5–2.0 µg/kg for adults (74). Typically, 1% of the total intake of inorganic mercury is derived from drinking-water and 84% from the diet; fish can account for between 20% and 85% of total mercury, mostly as methylmercury.

With the exception of the accidental consumption of cereal grains dressed with organomercurials, the potential threat posed by terrestrial pollution with mercury compounds is appreciably less than that arising from the alkylation of mercury by aquatic components of the food chain. Mercury contamination of the marine environment is rapidly reflected by increased intakes of readily absorbable methylmercury derived from the tissues of predatory fish. Such considerations make difficult the toxicological interpretation of data on dietary mercury contents if evidence of its form is not available.

16.6 Possible essentiality of lead and cadmium

Nutritional essentiality has been difficult to demonstrate for elements of high atomic numbers. None of the 39 elements of atomic number exceeding 53 (iodine) has so far been shown to have any biological role in animals (84). However, although a toxic element may nevertheless be essential, there is no functional relationship between toxicity and biological role. Essentiality and toxicity are unrelated and, for the known essential elements, toxicity is a matter of dose. Investigation of the possible essentiality of elements normally regarded as "toxic" has become feasible only with the development of experimental environments and animal management regimens that rigorously exclude adventitious contaminants.

16.6.1 Lead

The toxic effects of lead have now been demonstrated at very low levels, and there is some suggestion that there may be no level of exposure below which lead is harmless. Any demonstration of the essentiality of lead must therefore relate to very small amounts. Since some lead is present in almost all plant and animal tissue, the experimental achievement of low levels and the demonstration of a biological requirement have posed formidable challenges.

Schwarz reduced the lead content of a basal diet for rats to approximately 0.2 mg/kg and was able to show that the addition of 1.0–2.5 mg lead/kg produced a consistent positive growth response (84). Reichlmayr-Lais & Kirchgessner (85) found that rats fed lead-depleted diets (10–30 µg of lead/kg) over several generations showed growth depression as compared with controls. Depleted rats also had microcytic anaemia and an impaired ability to absorb iron (86). Other studies suggest that the growth changes in offspring may be attributable to changes in the composition of the milk of the lead-depleted mothers, especially in relation to trace elements. Reduced activities of Na^+/K^+-exchanging ATPase and (Ca, Mg)-ATPase in red cell membranes could be a further reason for the microcytic anaemia (87) that develops after lead depletion.

A subsequent experiment showed that absolute lead retention in growing rats increased in association with dietary lead up to 0.225 µg/kg but decreased thereafter. Homoeostasis did not occur until the dietary lead concentration fell below 5 mg/kg (88). More recently, Kirchgessner and co-workers (89) found that newborn pigs fed lead-depleted diets (30 ± 15 µg/kg) showed significantly less growth than control animals supplemented with 850 ± 10 µg/kg. The lipid contents of carcasses of lead-depleted animals killed after 58 days were lower than those of control animals. The conclusion reached after a review of the earlier studies by an Expert Committee of the United States Environmental Protection Agency was that the evidence was not sufficient to establish the nutritional essentiality of lead for rats (90). A requirement for lead for the function of an enzyme or an essential metabolic pathway has not yet been demonstrated. In addition it has been questioned whether the effects observed at very low exposures were a consequence of inadvertent changes in diet constituents associated with the preparation of the diets low in lead (91). Until further studies have been undertaken, no minimum levels of dietary lead can be recommended.

16.6.2 Cadmium

Three independent investigations reported during the period 1976–1977 are occasionally cited as evidence that cadmium at low concentrations in diet or drinking-water may be required to maximize the growth of experimental animals. The growth of rats maintained on semisynthetic diets increased by up to 8% as dietary cadmium was increased from 12.5 to 50 or 100 µg/kg (92). In another study, with rats given a low-cadmium basal diet (0.014 mg/kg), trends, not statistically analysed, towards a higher growth rate were noted in animals given supplements providing 16–30 μg of cadmium/day in drinking-water (93). Finally, brief details have been reported of a study in which the growth of goats before and during pregnancy was markedly restricted when dietary cadmium was held below 20 μg/kg rather than 250 μg/kg feed (94). Further evidence, accompanied by adequate statistical verification of the data, is needed before cadmium can be regarded as physiologically essential.

References

1. Bennet EG. Modelling exposure routes of trace metals from sources to man. In: Nriagu JO ed. *Changing metal cycles and human health.* Berlin, Springer-Verlag, 1984: 345–356.
2. *Evaluation of certain food additives and contaminants. Forty-first report of the Joint FAO/WHO Expert Committee on Food Additives.* Geneva, World Health Organization, 1993 (WHO Technical Report Series, No. 837).
3. Lead (evaluation of health risks to infants and children). In: *Toxicological evaluation of certain food additives and contaminants.* Geneva, World Health Organization, 1987: 223 (WHO Food Additives Series, No. 21).
4. Cadmium. In: *Toxicological evaluation of certain food additives and contaminants.* Geneva, World Health Organization, 1989: 163–219 (WHO Food Additives Series, No. 24).
5. *Mercury.* Geneva, World Health Organization, 1976: 131 (Environmental Health Criteria 1).
6. *Methylmercury.* Geneva, World Health Organization, 1990: 144 (Environmental Health Criteria 101).
7. *Infancy and early childhood, principles for evaluating health risks from chemicals.* Geneva, World Health Organization, 1986 (Environmental Health Criteria 59).
8. Goyer RA, Mahaffey KR. Susceptibility to lead toxicity.*Environmental health perspectives,* 1972, 2: 73–80.
9. Lin-Fu JS, Vulnerability of children to lead exposure and toxicity: parts one and two. *New England journal of medicine,* 1973, 289: 1229–1233.
10. Ziegler EE et al. Absorption and retention of lead by infants. *Pediatric research,* 1978, 12: 29–34.
11. Alexander FW, Delves HT, Clayton BE. The uptake and excretion by children of lead and other contaminants. In: Barth D et al., eds. *Proceedings of an International Symposium.* Luxembourg, Commission of the European Communities, 1973: 319–331.
12. Alexander FW, Clayton BE, Delves HT. Mineral and trace metal balances in children receiving normal and synthetic diets. *Quarterly journal of medicine,* 1974, 43: 89–111.
13. *Air quality criteria for lead.* Research Triangle Park, NC, US Environmental Protection Agency, 1986 (Report NO. EPA-600/8-83/028cF).

14. Kostial K et al. The influence of age on metal metabolism and toxicity. *Environmental health perspectives*, 1978, **25**: 81–86.

15. Kostial K. The absorption of heavy metals by the growing organisms: experimental experience with animals. In: Schmidt EHF, Hildebrandt A, eds. *Health evaluation of heavy metals in infant formula and junior food*. Berlin, Springer-Verlag, 1983: 99–104.

16. *Lead*. Geneva, World Health Organization, 1977 (Environmental Health Criteria 3).

17. Henke G, Sachs HW, Bohn G. Cadmium: Bestimmungen in Leber und Nieren von Kindern und Jugendlichen durch Neutronaktivierungsanalyse. [Cadmium: determinations in the liver and kidneys of children and adolescents by neutron-activation analysis.] *Archives of toxicology*, 1970, **26**: 8–16.

18. Baranski B. Effect of maternal cadmium exposure on postnatal development and tissue cadmium, copper and zinc concentrations in rats. *Toxicology*, 1986, **59**: 255–260.

19. Davis GK, Mertz W. Copper. In: Mertz W, ed. *Trace elements in human and animal nutrition*, 5th ed., Vol. 1. San Diego, Academic Press, 1987: 301–364.

20. Jugo S. Metabolism of toxic heavy metals in growing organisms: review. *Environmental research*, 1977, **13**: 36–46.

21. Kargačin B, Kostial K. Toxic metals: influence of macromolecular dietary components on metabolism and toxicity. In: Rowland I, ed. *Nutrition, toxicity and cancer*. Palm Beach, FL, CRC Press, 1991:

22. Rabinowitz MB, Kopple JD, Wetherill GW. Effect of food intake and fasting on gastrointestinal lead absorption in humans. *American journal of clinical nutrition*, 1980, **33**: 1784–1788.

23. James ZHM, Hilburn ME, Blair YA. Effects of meal and meal times on uptake of lead from the gastrointestinal tract of humans. *Human toxicology*, 1985, **4**: 401–407.

24. Mushak P. Gastrointestinal absorption of lead in children and adults: overview of biological and biophysico-chemical aspects. In: *Proceedings: Symposium on the Bioavailability and Dietary Uptake of Lead*. Chapel Hill, NC, 1991:

25. Mahaffey KR, Gartside PS, Glueck CJ. Blood lead levels and dietary calcium intake in 1- to 11-year old children: The Second National Health and Nutrition Examination Survey, 1976–1980, *Pediatrics*, 1986, **78**: 257–262.

26. Johnson NE, Tenuta K. Diets and blood lead levels of children who practice pica. *Environmental research*, 1979, **18**: 369–376.

27. Heard MJ, Chamberlain AC. Effect of minerals and food on uptake of lead from the gastrointestinal tract in humans. *Human toxicology*, 1982, **1**: 411–415.

28. Kostial K et al. Dietary calcium and blood lead levels in women. *Biological trace element research*, 1990, **28**: 10–14.

29. Mahaffey KR, Annest JL. Association of erythrocyte protoporphyrin with blood lead level and iron status in the Second National Health and Nutrition Examination Survey, 1976–1980. *Environmental research*, 1986, **41**: 327–338.

30. Marcus A, Schwartz J. Dose–response curves for erythrocyte protoporphyrin vs. blood lead: effects of iron status. *Environmental research*, 1987, **44**: 221–227.

31. Yip R, Norris TN, Anderson AS. Iron status of children with elevated blood lead concentrations. *Journal of pediatrics*, 1981, **98**: 922–925.
32. Bunker VW et al. The intake and excretion of lead and cadmium by the elderly. *American journal of clinical nutrition*, 1984, **39**: 803–809.
33. Friberg L et al. *Cadmium in the environment. III. A toxicological and epidemiological appraisal.* Washington, DC, Environmental Protection Agency, 1975 (Report No. EPA-650/2-75-049).
34. Friberg L et al. *Cadmium in the environment,* 2nd ed. Cleveland, OH, CRC Press, 1978.
35. Tsuchiya K. *Cadmium studies in Japan: a review,* Amsterdam, North Holland, 1978.
36. Murata I et al. Cadmium enteropathy, renal osteomalacia ("Itai-itai" disease in Japan). *Bulletin de la Société Internationale de Chirurgie*, 1970, **1**: 1–6.
37. Elsenhans B, Schumann K, Forth W. Toxic metals. Interaction with essential metals. In: Rowland I, ed. *Nutrition, toxicity and cancer.* London, CRC/Telford Press, 1991.
38. Thrower SJ, Anderwartha KA. Glutathione peroxidase response in tissues of rats fed diets containing fish protein concentrate prepared from shark flesh of known mercury and selenium content. *Bulletin of environmental contamination and toxicology*, 1981, **26**: 77–84.
39. Rowland IR et al. Are developmental changes in methylmercury metabolism and excretion mediated by the intestinal microflora? In: Clarkson TW, Nordberg GF, Sager PR, eds. *Reproductive and developmental toxicity of metals.* New York, Plenum Press, 1983: 745–758.
40. Kostial K. Specific features of metal absorption in suckling animals. In: Clarkson TW, Nordberg GF, Sager PR, eds. *Reproductive and developmental toxicity of metals.* New York, Plenum Press, 1983: 727–744.
41. Quarterman J. Lead. In: Mertz W, ed. *Trace elements in human and animal nutrition,* 5th ed., Vol. 2. Orlando, FL, Academic Press, 1986: 281–317.
42. Bremner I. Cadmium toxicity. Nutritional influences and the role of metallothioneins. *World review of nutrition and diet*, 1978, **32**. 165–197.
43. Nriagu JO, ed. *Changing metal cycles and human health.* Berlin, Springer-Verlag, 1984 (Life Science Research Report 28).
44. *Lead effects on cardiovascular function, early development and stature: an addendum to U.S. EPA Air Quality Criteria for Lead.* Research Triangle Park, NC, US Environmental Protection Agency, 1986.
45. Needleman HL, Gatsonis CA. Low-level lead exposure and the I.Q. of children. A meta-analysis of modern studies. *Journal of the American Medical Association*, 1990, **263**: 673–678.
46. Tyroler HA. Epidemiology of hypertension as a public health problem: an overview as background for evaluation of blood lead–blood pressure relationship. *Environmental health perspectives*, 1988, **78**: 3–7.
47. Perlstein MA, Attala R. Neurologic sequelae of plumbism in children. *Clinical pediatrics*, 1966, **5**: 292–298.
48. *Supplement to the 1986 EPA Air Quality Criteria for Lead Volume (Addendum*

pages A1-A67). Washington, DC, US Environmental Protection Agency, 1989 (Report No. EPA/600/8-89/049A).

49. Grant LD, Davis JM. Effects of low-level lead exposure on paediatric neuro-behavioural development: current findings and future directions. In: Smith MA, Grand LD, Sors EI, eds. *Lead exposure and child development: an international assessment.* Lancaster, Kluewer Academic Publishers, 1989: 49–115.

50. McMichael AJ et al. Port Pirie cohort study: environmental exposure to lead and children's abilities at the age of four years. *New England journal of medicine,* 1988, **319**: 468–475.

51. Bellinger D, Leviton A, Sloman J. Antecedents and correlates of improved cognitive performance in children exposed *in utero* to low levels of lead. *Environmental health perspectives,* 1990, **89**: 5–11.

52. Goyer RA, Rhyne B. Pathological effects of lead. *International review of experimental pathology,* 1973, **12**: 1–77.

53. *Overall evaluations of carcinogenicity: an updating of IARC Monographs Volumes 1–42.* Lyon, International Agency for Research on Cancer, 1987: 230–232 (IARC Monographs on the Evaluation of the Carcinogenic Risk of Chemicals to Humans, Supplement No. 7).

54. *Evaluation of the potential carcinogenicity of lead and lead compounds.* Washington, DC, US Environmental Protection Agency, 1989 (Report No. EPA 600/8-89/045A).

55. Choie DR, Richter GW. Cell proliferation in rat kidneys after prolonged treatment with lead. *American journal of pathology,* 1972, **68**: 359–370.

56. Grandjean P, Hansen ON, Lyngbye G. Analysis of lead in circumpulpal dentine of deciduous teeth. *Annals of clinical and laboratory science,* 1984, **14**: 270–275.

57. Chisholm JJ Jr, Barltrop D. Recognition and management of children with increased lead absorption. *Archives of disease in childhood,* 1979, **54**: 249–262.

58. *Preventing lead poisoning in young children.* Atlanta, GA, Centers for Disease Control, 1985 (Report No. 99–2230).

59. Hu H, Milder FL, Burger DE. X-ray fluorescence measurements of lead burden in subjects with low level community lead exposure. *Archives of environmental health,* 1990, **45**: 335–341.

60. Weeden RD. *In vivo* tibial XFR measurement of bone lead. *Archives of environmental health,* 1990, **45**: 69–71.

61. Mushak P. Biological monitoring of lead exposure in children: overview of selected biokinetic and toxicologic issues. In: Smith MA, Grant LD, Sors AI, eds. *Lead exposure and child development: an international assessment.* Lancaster, Kluewer Academic Publishers, 1989: 120–129.

62. Piomelli S et al. Threshold for lead damage to heme synthesis in children. *Proceedings of the National Academy of Sciences,* 1982, **79**: 3335–3339.

63. Parr RM et al. *Human dietary intakes of trace elements: a global literature survey mainly for the period 1970–1991. I. Data listings and sources of information.* Vienna, International Atomic Energy Agency, 1992 (NAHRES-12).

64. *Cadmium.* Geneva, World Health Organization, 1992 (Environmental Health Criteria 134).

65. Friberg et al., ed. *Cadmium and health: a toxicological and epidemiological appraisal*, Vol. II, *Effects and responses*. Boca Raton, FL, CRC Press, 1986.

66. Nogawa K, Kobayashi E, Honda R. A study of the relationship between cadmium concentrations in urine and renal effects of cadmium. *Environmental health perspectives*, 1979, **28**: 161–168.

67. Bernard A et al. Renal excretion of proteins and enzymes in workers exposed to cadmium. *European journal of clinical investigation*, 1979, **9**: 11–22.

68. Thun MJ et al. Nephropathy in cadmium workers: assessment of risk from airborne occupational exposure to cadmium. *British journal of industrial medicine*, 1989, **46**: 689–697.

69. Nogawa K et al. A dose-response analysis of cadmium in the general environment with special reference to total cadmium intake limit. *Environmental research*, 1989, **48**: 7–16.

70. Goyer RA et al. Non-metallothionein-bound cadmium in the pathogenesis of cadmium nephropathy in the rat. *Toxicology and applied pharmacology*, 1989, **101**: 232–244.

71. Nogawa K et al. Mechanism for bone disease found in inhabitants environmentally exposed to cadmium: decreased serum 1,25-dihydroxyvitamin D level. *International archives of occupational and environmental health*, 1987, **59**: 21–30.

72. Oberdörster G. Pulmonary toxicity and carcinogenicity of cadmium. *Journal of the American College of Toxicology*, 1989, **8**: 1251–1263.

73. Kawada T, Koyama H, Suzuki S. Cadmium, NAG activity and β-2-microglobulin in the urine of cadmium pigment workers. *British journal of industrial medicine*, 1989, **46**: 52–55.

74. Jelinek CF. *Assessment of dietary intake of chemical contaminants*. Nairobi, United Nations Environment Programme, 1992.

75. *Guidelines for drinking-water quality*, 2nd ed. *Volume 1. Recommendations*. Geneva, World Health Organization, 1993.

76. Berlin M. Mercury. In: Friberg L, Nordberg GF, Vouk VB, eds. *Handbook on the toxicology of metals*, 2nd ed. New York, Elsevier/North Holland, 1986: 387–445.

77. Swedish Expert Committee. Methyl mercury in fish — a toxicologic-epidemiologic evaluation of risks. Report from an expert group. *Nordisk hygienisk tidskrift*, 1971, **4** (Suppl. 4), 1–364.

78. *Recommended health-based limits in occupational exposure to heavy metals. Report of a WHO Study Group*. Geneva, World Health Organization, 1980: 116 (WHO Technical Report Series, No. 647).

79. Bakir F et al. Methyl mercury poisoning in Iraq. *Science*, 1973, **181**: 230–241.

80. Cox C et al. Dose-response analysis of analysis of infants prenatally exposed to methyl mercury: an application of a single compartment model to single strand hair analysis. *Environmental research*, 1989, **49**: 318–332.

81. Matheson DS, Clarkson TW, Gelfand EW. Mercury toxicity (acrodynia) induced by long-term injection of gamma globulin. *Journal of pediatrics*, 1980, **97**: 153–155.

82. *Evaluation of certain food additives and the contaminants mercury, lead and cadmium. Sixteenth report of the Expert Committee*. Rome, Food and Agriculture Organization of the United Nations, 1972 (FAO Nutrition Meetings Report Series,

No. 51) Geneva, World Health Organization, 1972 (WHO Technical Report Series, No. 505).

83. *Evaluation of certain food additives and contaminants. Twenty-second report of the Joint FAO/WHO Expert Committee on Food Additives.* Geneva, World Health Organization, 1978 (WHO Technical Report Series, No. 631).

84. Schwarz K. Essentiality versus toxicity of metals. In: Brown SS, ed. *Clinical chemistry and chemical toxicology of metals.* New York, Elsevier/North Holland, 1977: 3–22.

85. Reichlmayr-Lais AM, Kirchgessner M. Depletionsstudien zur Essentialität von Blei an Wachsenden Ratten. [Depletion studies on the essential nature of lead in growing rats.] *Archiv für Tierernährung,* 1981, **31**: 731–737.

86. Reichlmayr-Lais AM, Kirchgessner M. Hematologische Veränderungen bei alimentarem Bleimangel. [Haematological changes in alimentary lead deficiency.] *Biological trace element research* 1981, **3**: 279–285.

87. Reichlmayr-Lais AM, Eder K, Kirchgessner M. Lead deficiency: newer results. In: Momcilović B, ed. *Trace elements in man and animals—TEMA 7.* Zagreb, University of Zagreb, 1991: 11-21–11-22.

88. Kirchgessner M, Reichlmayr-Lais AM, Stokl KN. Retention of lead in growing rats with varying dietary lead supplements. *Journal of trace elements and electrolytes in health and disease,* 1988, **2**: 149–152.

89. Kirchgessner M, Plass DL, Reichlmayr-Lais AM. Lead deficiency in swine. In: Momcilović B, ed. *Trace elements in man and animals — TEMA 7.* Zagreb, University of Zagreb, 1991: 11-20–11-21.

90. Grant LD. *Independent peer review of selected studies by Drs Kirchgessner and Reichlmayr-Lais concerning the possible nutritional essentiality of lead.* Research Triangle Park, NC, US Environmental Protection Agency, 1983 (Report No. EPA-600/8-83-028A).

91. Needleman HL. The hazard to health of lead exposure at low dose. In: Nriagu JO, ed. *Changing metal cycles and human health.* Berlin, Springer-Verlag, 1984: 311–322.

92. Schwarz K, Spallholz J. Growth effects of small cadmium supplements in rats maintained under trace element controlled conditions. *Federation proceedings,* 1976, **35**: 255.

93. Perry HM, Erlanger M, Perry EF. Elevated systolic pressure following chronic low-level cadmium feeding. *American journal of physiology,* 1977, **232**: H114–H121.

94. Anke M et al. The biochemical role of cadmium. In: Kirchgessner M, ed. *Trace element metabolism in man and animals.* Weihenstephan, Arbeitskreis fur Tierernährung, 1978: 540–548.

17.

Arsenic

Arsenic occurs in the trivalent and pentavalent forms in foods, water and the environment, and is widely distributed geologically as a component of about 245 different minerals. Unweathered soils may contain 0.1–40 mg of arsenic/kg; the amount of arsenic in the biomass of the earth has been estimated at 30 million tonnes (1). Industrial production is approximately 50 000 tonnes/ year; the main uses are in agricultural chemicals, such as pesticides, herbicides, cotton desiccants and wood preservatives, and as additives to animal feeds, as well as in pharmaceutical products, all of which have a direct impact on the environment (2).

Although arsenic compounds are best known historically for their toxicity, their pharmacological action is also well documented. Less well documented is the increasing evidence of the essential function fulfilled by very low dietary arsenic intakes in four species of experimental animals. The biological effects of arsenic depend markedly on the chemical form in which the element is presented, inorganic compounds being more toxic than most organic ones. Most living organisms convert the former by methylation into a large variety of less toxic organoarsenic compounds, which are then excreted. Cacodylic acid and methanearsonic acid are typical urinary excretion products in humans, whereas organic compounds containing arsenobetaine, dimethylarsenoribo-sides or arsenolipids are metabolites of aquatic organisms (3). These compounds contribute substantial amounts of arsenic to human diets containing fish and other seafood.

The major cause of concern in connection with arsenic is the potential toxicity of its compounds to humans. Acute poisoning, characterized by nausea, vomiting, diarrhoea and severe abdominal pain, is relatively rare. Chronic toxicity, on the other hand, is known to occur as a result of exposure to natural sources in some countries (4), or from accidental contamination of foods (5). Consumption of water containing 0.8 mg of arsenic/l over extended periods of time and a dietary intake of approximately 3 mg or arsenic/day for 2–3 weeks have been identified as causes of arsenic intoxication. However, the toxicity of arsenic compounds depends so greatly on their chemical nature that general estimates of safe intakes cannot be made with confidence.

Epidemiological studies have associated long-term exposure to airborne arsenic in industrial plants processing arsenic compounds with an increased incidence of bronchial cancer. Chronic exposure to excessive levels in drinking-water or in arsenic-containing drugs is associated with an increased incidence of keratinization and pigmentation of the skin, together with an increased risk of skin cancer (6). There is no evidence to suggest that normal dietary intakes of arsenic increase the risk of cancer. There is, in addition, no experimental evidence from studies on animal models to suggest that dietary arsenic is carcinogenic. The role of arsenic as a potential carcinogen has been reviewed by the International Agency for Research on Cancer (7).

A substantial number of organic arsenicals, most of them derivatives of phenylarsonic acid, are used as feed additives in poultry and swine production. At dietary concentrations in the range of a few g/kg they increase weight gain, possibly by protecting against enteric diseases and by increasing the efficiency of feed utilization for reasons as yet unknown (2). Whether treatment with arsenicals such as Fowler's solution (potassium arsenite solution) or the consumption of arsenic produces any beneficial effects is difficult to prove. On the other hand, the antisyphilitic activity of arsphenamine, much used before the advent of modern antibiotics, is well documented.

The beneficial effects of substantially lower intakes of arsenic have been demonstrated in three independent studies involving four animal species offered basal diets providing less than 1μg of arsenic/g (for reviews, see refs 8–10). Rats, chickens, minipigs and goats raised on low-arsenic diets (< 35 ng of arsenic/g) exhibited reduced growth rates during early life. In goats, the most closely investigated species, reproductive performance is also impaired, as a result of decreased conception rates, increased abortion frequency, greatly increased maternal mortality (especially during lactation) and reduced viability of newborn kids. Cardiomyopathy, associated with a derangement of cardiac mitochondrial structure, may be the cause. Several biochemical changes accompanying the signs of arsenic deficiency have been described, but the fundamental mode and site of action of the element are not yet known.

Most foods and feeds of terrestrial origin contain less than 1 μg of arsenic/g dry weight; the levels present in those of marine origin are substantially higher, ranging up to 80 μg/g (2). Dietary intake is therefore greatly influenced by the amount of seafood in the diet. Based on recent surveys in several countries, the daily arsenic intake of adults is estimated to be < 200 μg, and often below 100 μg/day (11). It is unlikely that the arsenic intake from uncontaminated diets poses a risk of toxicity. Extrapolation from animal experiments suggests that human adult intakes in the range 12–25 μg/day are probably adequate to meet any possible requirement (9).

In contrast to dietary intake, contaminated drinking-water can be a significant source of arsenic at near toxic and toxic levels. The arsenic concentration in the oceans and in uncontaminated rivers, lakes and ground-waters varies from non-detectable levels to a few μg/l. Much higher concentrations, at the mg/l level, are present in hot springs and waters in contact with natural arsenic deposits or exposed to industrial contamination (2). The consumption of such waters is associated with subacute toxicity and an increased risk of cancer of the skin and possibly of other sites.

Because inorganic arsenic is known to be carcinogenic in humans, there is understandable concern to limit human exposure to excessive environmental concentrations of the element. However, the metabolism and effects of arsenic can differ markedly, depending on the chemical nature of the arsenic source; these differences partly account for the provisional nature of the recommended safe exposure limit for adults of 15 μg/kg of body weight per week (12). Since experimental arsenic deficiency has been produced in four species, the element may have an essential function. If a human requirement for arsenic does exist, it is probably close to 20 μg/day for adults and is easily met by most diets.

References

1. Kovalskij VVM. *Geochemische Ökologie, Biogeochemie. [Geochemical ecology, biogeochemistry.]* Berlin, Deutscher Landwirtschaftsverlag, 1977.
2. Arsenic. In: *Mineral tolerances of domestic animals.* Washington, DC, National Academy of Sciences, 1980: 40–53.
3. Nissen P, Benson AA. Arsenic metabolism in freshwater and terrestrial plants. *Physiologia plantarum*, 1982, 54: 446.
4. Borgono, JM, Greiber R. Epidemiological study of arsenicism in the city of Antofagasta. *Trace substances in environmental health*, 1973, 5: 13–24.
5. Mizuta N et al. An outbreak of acute arsenic poisoning caused by arsenic-contaminated soy-sauce (shoyu): a clinical report of 220 cases. *Bulletin of Yamaguchi Medical School*, 1956, 4: 131–150.
6. National Research Council. *Diet and health, implications for reducing chronic disease risk.* Washington, DC, National Academy of Sciences, 1989.
7. Case reports and epidemiological studies. In: *Some metals and metallic compounds.* Lyon, International Agency for Research on Cancer, 1980: 101–112 (IARC Monographs on the Evaluation of the Carcinogenic Risk of Chemicals to Humans, Vol. 23).
8. Schwarz K. Essentiality versus toxicity of metals. In: Brown SS, ed. *Clinical chemistry and chemical toxicology of metals.* New York, Elsevier/North Holland, 1977: 3–22.
9. Anke M, Krause U, Groppel B. The effect of arsenic deficiency on growth, reproduction, life expectancy and disease symptoms in animals. *Trace substances in environmental health*, 1987, 21: 533–550.

10. Nielsen FH. Ultratrace elements in nutrition. *Annual review of nutrition*, 1984, **4**: 21–41.

11. Parr RM, Crawley H. *Dietary intake of minor and trace elements: a global survey.* Vienna, International Atomic Energy Agency, 1990: 1–3.

12. *Evaluation of certain food additives and contaminants. Thiry-third Report of the Joint FAO/WHO Expert Committee on Food Additives.* Geneva, World Health Organization, 1989 (WHO Technical Report Series, No. 776).

18.
Aluminium

Aluminium is among the most plentiful elements in the earth's crust, accounting for 8% of the total. Exposure to aluminium increased markedly as its production increased rapidly in the 20th century, reaching approximately 15 million tonnes in the early 1980s. Human exposure to aluminium may also have increased since both the solubility and the bioavailability to plants and aquatic life of environmental aluminium may have been increased by acid rain and industrial emissions. Aluminium is an extremely versatile metal with a wide variety of uses, e.g. in packing and building materials, paint pigments, insulating materials, abrasives, cosmetics, food additives and antacids. This results in a wide range of human contacts with the metal and a consequent potential impact on human populations. Factors influencing exposure to aluminium and its tolerance by human subjects have been extensively reviewed by the Joint FAO/WHO Expert Committee on Food Additives (1).

There is no substantiated evidence that aluminium has any essential function in animals or humans. However, while goats given low-aluminium semisynthetic rations (162 μg/kg) for 4 years failed to exhibit any adverse effects on feed intake, growth, reproduction or milk production, they did have a significantly reduced life expectancy, as compared with that of control goats receiving 25 mg/kg (2). These results await independent confirmation.

The main concern with respect to aluminium and health is its potential toxicity if exposure is excessive. Dialysis encephalopathy in a large number of patients with renal failure undergoing chronic dialysis was shown by Alfrey et al. (3) to be attributable to the high aluminium content of some water used for the preparation of dialysates. Aluminium levels in the brain and in other tissues of affected subjects were consistently elevated. Excess aluminium also affects the skeleton by markedly reducing bone formation, resulting in osteomalacia. A further pathological manifestation of aluminium toxicity is a microcytic hypochromic anaemia not associated with iron deficiency. Such problems have practically disappeared since the use of aluminium-free de-ionized water for dialysis became routine (3).

The toxicological aspects of orally consumed aluminium are less well defined. The element is poorly absorbed from the intestines; the small amounts absorbed from normal diets are excreted by healthy kidneys, so that no accumulation occurs. At an estimated daily intake of 3–14 mg from typical Western diets (4), a mean of 86 μg/day was excreted in the urine of healthy subjects (5). While there is no evidence that aluminium accumulates in the organism at these intakes, the habitual use of gram quantities of aluminium compounds results in a positive balance and accumulation (6). The risk of aluminium toxicity is greatly increased in persons with impaired kidney function (3).

Aluminium interacts with a number of other elements, including calcium, fluorine, iron, magnesium, phosphorus and strontium, and, when ingested in excess, can reduce their absorption (7). Because of this property, it has been used therapeutically to treat fluorosis and to reduce phosphorus absorption in uraemic patients. These interactions are unlikely to present health risks at typical dietary intakes, estimated at 3–14 mg/day. Water would add from less than 100 μg to 1 mg/l, depending on its pH, and the use of aluminium cooking utensils with acidic foods may increase intake.

By far the most important contribution to aluminium intake comes from antacid medications that can provide several grams of the metal per day. These amounts do interfere with the absorption of other elements; they also may lead to a gradual accumulation of aluminium in the skeleton.

Locally increased concentrations of aluminium occur in the brain of patients with Alzheimer dementia, but whether the metal has a causative role in the pathogenesis of this disease has not been established.

It has been provisionally suggested that the tolerable weekly intake of aluminium may be approximately 7 mg/kg of body weight (1, 8). Milk, milk products and cereal products account, typically, for about 60% of the total dietary intake of aluminium (9). Mean intakes in the range 3–14 mg of aluminium/day have been reported.

In conclusion there is no known risk to healthy people from typical dietary intakes of aluminium. Risks arise only from the habitual consumption of gram quantities of aluminium antacids over long periods of time; they are markedly increased in persons with impaired kidney function. Long-term intravenous application always results in serious toxicity.

References

1. Aluminium. In: *Toxicological evaluation of certain food additives and contaminants.* Cambridge, Cambridge University Press, 1989: 113–153 (WHO Food Additives Series, No. 24).
2. Anke M et al. Aluminiummangelerscheinungen beim Tier. [Manifestations of aluminium deficiency in animals.] In: Anke M et al., ed. *Mengen-und Spurenelemente, 10. Arbeitstagung. [Major and trace elements, 10th working meeting.]* Jena, Universität Jena, 1990: 505–515.

3. Alfrey AC. Aluminium. In: Mertz W, ed. *Trace elements in human and animal nutrition*, 5th ed, Vol. 2. Orlando, FL, Academic Press, 1986: 399–413.
4. Greger JL, Baier MJ. Excretion and retention of low or moderate levels of aluminium by human subjects. *Food chemistry and toxicology*, 1983, **21**: 473–476.
5. Recker RR et al. Evidence for aluminium absorption from the gastrointestinal tract and bone deposition by aluminium carbonate ingestion with normal renal function. *Journal of laboratory and clinical medicine*, 1977, **90**: 810–815.
6. Gorsky JE et al. Metabolic balance of aluminium studied in six men. *Clinical chemistry*, 1979, **25**: 1739–1743.
7. Lotz M, Zisman E, Bartter FC. Evidence for a phosphorus-depletion syndrome in man. *New England journal of medicine*, 1968, **278**: 409–415.
8. *Evaluation of certain food additives and contaminants. Thirty-third Report of the Joint FAO/WHO Expert Committee on Food Additives.* Geneva, World Health Organization, 1989 (WHO Technical Report Series, No. 776).
9. Pennington JAT. Aluminium content of foods and diets. *Food additives and contaminants*, 1988, **5**: 161–232.

19.
Lithium

Lithium, the lightest alkali metal, with a relative atomic mass of 6.94, occurs in soils at concentrations of <10 to >100 $\mu g/g$. Concentrations in plants vary widely $(0.4->1000$ $\mu g/g)$, depending on species and on the type of soil in which the plant is grown. Concentrations in human and animal tissues are much lower; values of 2–200 ng/g wet weight have been reported. Intake from typical diets in the USA has been estimated to be 60–70 $\mu g/day$; the mean intake from Turkish diets was 102 and from Finnish diets 35 $\mu g/day$ (1).

Lithium exhibits two dose-dependent types of biological activity. The first of these, its pharmacological action, exploited in the treatment of manic-depressive psychoses, is exhibited when intakes are sufficient to raise plasma lithium to 7–10 $\mu g/ml$. It is toxic at slightly higher levels. In addition, there is evidence from experimental animal studies that it has an essential functional role which is maintained even when blood plasma lithium falls below 1 ng/ml (2).

Lithium salts have been used worldwide as an effective treatment for manic-depressive episodes ever since their introduction by Cade, more than 40 years ago (3). Effective dosages, 250–500 mg of lithium/day in an adult, require close monitoring, because the margin of safety is not wide and effects on the thyroid and excessive weight gains are not uncommon. Lithium affects many metabolic pathways and organ functions at therapeutic and toxic intakes, but its basic function and mode of action are still unknown (4, 5).

The low therapeutic dose of 250 mg/day is equivalent to approximately 625 mg/kg of dry diet, a concentration that produces chronic toxicity in experimental animals, as shown by reduced feed consumption in pigs, rats and chickens. Dietary lithium at 100 mg/kg reduced the weight gain of ruminants, while 500 mg/kg increased mortality in pigs.

An essential function for lithium at very low levels of intake has been postulated independently by two groups of investigators using goats (6) or rats (7). Lithium deficiency resulted in reduced birth weight and reduced weight gain at 0–6 months of age. As compared with normal controls, lithium-depleted females exhibited higher abortion rates and suffered higher postpartum mortality. In contrast, no growth depression was observed in rats raised for three

224

generations on severely lithium-deficient rations, but the survival of the litters and reproductive efficiency were significantly reduced. Tissue lithium concentrations were found to reflect dietary lithium supply, except in some endocrine and exocrine glands and areas of the brain, in which near-normal concentrations were maintained even after prolonged depletion (8).

Epidemiological studies in the USA have shown negative correlations between lithium in drinking-water and mortality, especially from heart disease (9), and admission rates to mental hospitals (10).

In summary lithium at high, near toxic doses effectively controls the symptoms of manic-depressive disorders. Toxicity from dietary lithium is unknown, the intake from dietary sources being approximately 100 μg/day or less and, typically, less than 0.1% of the therapeutic or potentially toxic doses. Lithium may have essential functions in experimental animals but it is not known whether there is a human requirement.

References

1. Iyengar GV, Clarke WB, Downing RG. Determination of boron and lithium in diverse biological matrices using neutron activation-mass spectrometry (NA-MS). *Fresenius' journal of analytical chemistry*, 1990, **338**: 562–566.
2. Mertz W. Lithium. In: Mertz W, ed. *Trace elements in human and animal nutrition*, 5th ed., Vol. 2. Orlando, FL, Academic Press, 1986: 391–397.
3. Cade JFJ. Lithium salts in the treatment of psychotic excitement. *Medical journal of Australia*, 1949, **2**: 349.
4. Schou M. Special review: lithium in psychiatric therapy and prophylaxis. *Journal of psychiatric research*, 1968, **6**: 67.
5. Schou M. Possible mechanisms of action of lithium salts: approaches and perspectives. *Biochemical Society transactions*, 1973, **1**: 81.
6. Anke M, Groppel B, Kronemann H. Significance of newer essential trace elements (like Si, Ni, As, Li, V) for the nutrition of man and animals. In: Brätter P, Schramel P, eds. *Trace element analytical chemistry in medicine and biology*, Vol. 3. Berlin, De Gruyter, 1984: 421–464.
7. Pickett EE. Evidence for the essentiality of lithium in the rat. In: Anke M et al., eds. *Spurenelementsymposium 4-Lithium*. [*Trace element symposium 4-lithium*.] Jena, Friedrich-Schiller Universität, 1983: 66–70.
8. Burt J. *The essentiality of lithium in the rat* [PhD Thesis]. Columbia, MO, University of Missouri, 1982.
9. Voors AW. Minerals in the municipal water and atherosclerotic heart death. *American journal of epidemiology*, 1971, **93**: 259–266.
10. Dawson EB, Moore TD, McGanity WJ. Mathematical relationship of drinking water, lithium, and rainfall to mental hospital admission. *Diseases of the nervous system*, 1972, **31**: 811–820.

20.
Tin

20.1 Biochemical function

Tin has no known biochemical function. However, Schwarz et al. (1) have described several properties of tin which suggest that it could have a function in the tertiary structure of proteins or other biosubstances. In industry, organotin compounds are used as catalysts for polymerization, transesterification and olefin condensation reactions. The $Sn^{2+} \rightarrow Sn^{4+}$ potential of -0.154 V is well within the physiological range and is close to the oxidation–reduction potential of many flavin enzymes.

20.2 Claimed deficiency and toxicity

Early studies of tin deficiency were flawed and thus did not conclusively establish the essentiality of tin (2). However, a recent study by Yokoi et al. (3) on rats presents reasonable evidence in support of the view that tin is essential. When compared with those fed 2 μg of tin/g of diet, rats fed 17 ng of tin/g of diet exhibited poor growth, decreased efficiency of food utilization, alopecia, depressed response to sound, and changes in mineral concentrations in various organs.

Signs of chronic exposure to excessive intakes of inorganic tin include growth depression and anaemia (4, 5). Tin toxicity also modifies the activities of several enzymes, and it has been claimed that it interferes with the metabolism of zinc, copper and calcium and alters the tissue concentrations of several elements (6–8).

As compared with inorganic tin, organotin compounds are appreciably toxic (9, 10) and attack the central nervous system. The resulting myelino-pathies and spongy degeneration of the brain lead to limb incoordination and ataxia, and may result in complete paralysis and death.

20.3 Epidemiology of deficiency and toxicity

Signs of tin deficiency in humans have yet to be described. Instances of tin intoxication after oral ingestion are usually associated with elevated intakes through food contaminated by corrosion of tin-lined cans. The conclusion reached in most studies to date is that the usual environmental exposure poses little threat of toxicity.

20.4 Assessment of status

Methods of assessing low or excessive tin status have neither been established nor studied. Elevated tin concentrations in blood, faeces and urine indicate that exposure to elevated amounts of dietary tin has occurred (11). A urinary loss of over 100 μg of tin/day might indicate an excessive intake of dietary tin.

20.5 Absorption and bioavailability

When fed at relatively high amounts, tin is poorly absorbed and retained by humans, and is excreted mainly in the faeces. It appears that the lower the dietary intake of tin, the higher the percentage that is absorbed. When the dietary intake of tin was 49.7 mg/day, the apparent absorption of tin was 3%; in contrast, it was 50% when the dietary intake of tin was 0.11 mg/day (11). An earlier study (12) showed that faecal excretion of tin was high and approximated dietary intakes when the diet provided 9–190 mg of tin/day.

20.6 Dietary intake

Most fresh and frozen foods probably contain less than 1 μg of tin/g (13). The major source of dietary tin is canned foods. Since their tin content can vary greatly, the same applies to dietary intake (14). Some recent data on the dietary intake of tin by humans include 1.0–2.3 mg/kg of diet (15) in the United Kingdom and 0.65 mg/day (16) in the Netherlands.

20.7 Requirement and tolerable intakes

Average basal and normative requirements and a safe range of population intakes cannot be set for tin because of a lack of data. However, if it is assumed that animal data can be extrapolated to humans, the tin-deprivation studies of Yokoi et al. (3) suggest that the dietary content of tin should be above 17 ng of tin/g; for human adults, this will be equivalent to about 8 μg of tin daily.

Schäfer & Femfer (17) have suggested that biochemical effects attributable to excess tin can be detected when dietary tin is 30 μg/g or higher, equivalent to about 15 mg daily for adults. Schroeder & Balassa (18) found that 5 μg/ml in drinking-water was not detrimental to the growth and longevity of mice; however, it was slightly toxic to rats (19). These estimates contrast markedly with the views of the Joint FAO/WHO Expert Committee of Food Additives, which suggested a provisional tolerable weekly intake for tin of 14 mg/kg of body weight (20).

References

1. Schwarz K, Milne DB, Vinyard E. Growth effects of tin compounds in rats maintained in a trace element-controlled environment. *Biochemical and biophysical research communications*, 1970, **40**: 22–29.

2. Nielsen FH. Ultratrace elements in nutrition. *Annual review of nutrition*, 1984, **4**: 21–41.

3. Yokoi K, Kimura M, Itokawa Y. Effect of dietary tin deficiency on growth and mineral status in rats. *Biological trace element research*, 1990, **24**: 223–231.

4. de Groot AP, Feron VJ, Til HP. Short-term toxicity studies on some salts and oxides of tin in rats. *Food and cosmetics toxicology*, 1973, **11**: 19–30.

5. Fritsch P, De Saint Blanquat G, Derache R. Etude nutritionnelle et toxicologique, chez le rat, d'un contaminant alimentaire: l'étain. [Nutritional and toxicological study of a food contaminant in the rat: tin.] *Toxicology*, 1977, **8**: 165–175.

6. Yamaguchi M, Saito R, Okada S. Dose-effect of inorganic tin on biochemical indices in rats. *Toxicology*, 1980, **16**: 267–273.

7. Johnson MA, Greger JL. Tin, copper, iron, and calcium metabolism of rats fed various dietary levels of inorganic tin and zinc. *Journal of nutrition*, 1985, **115**: 615–624.

8. Radar JI et al. Dietary tin at low levels decreases tissue copper and zinc in weanling rats. *FASEB journal*, 1989, **3**: A1074.

9. Barnes JM, Stoner HB. The toxicology of tin compounds. *Pharmacological reviews*, 1959, **11**: 211–231.

10. Piver WT. Organotin compounds: industrial applications and biological investigation. *Environmental health perspectives*, 1973, **4**: 61–79.

11. Johnson MA, Greger JL. Effects of dietary tin on tin and calcium metabolism of adult males. *American journal of clinical nutrition*, 1982, **35**: 655–660.

12. Calloway DH, McMullen JJ. Fecal excretion of iron and tin by men fed stored canned foods. *American journal of clinical nutrition*, 1966, **18**: 1–6.

13. Sherlock JC, Smart GA. Tin in foods and the diet. *Food additives and contaminants*, 1984, **1**: 277–282.

14. Greger JL. Tin and aluminium. In: Smith KT, ed. *Trace minerals in foods*. New York, Marcel Dekker, 1988: 291–323.

15. Evans WH, Sherlock JC. Relationships between elemental intakes within the United Kingdom total diet study and other adult dietary studies. *Food additives and contaminants*, 1987, **4**: 1–8.

16. Van Dokkum W et al. Minerals and trace elements in total diets in The Netherlands. *British journal of nutrition*, 1989, **61**: 7–15.

17. Schäfer SG, Femfer U. Tin—a toxic heavy metal? A review of the literature. *Regulatory toxicology and pharmacology*, 1984, **4**: 57–69.

18. Schroeder HA, Balassa JJ. Arsenic, germanium, tin and vanadium in mice: effects on growth, survival and tissue levels. *Journal of nutrition*, 1967, **92**: 245–252.

19. Schroeder HA et al. Germanium, tin and arsenic in rats: effects on growth, survival, pathological lesions, and life span. *Journal of nutrition*, 1968, **96**: 37–45.

20. *Evaluation of certain food additives and contaminants. Thirty-third report of the Joint FAO/WHO Expert Committee on Food Additives.* Geneva, World Health Organization, 1989 (WHO Technical Report Series, No. 776).

D

Conduct and interpretation of trace-element investigations

21.
Analytical methodology

A large body of data exists for most trace elements in biological media. However, such data are often of limited value because of inherent analytical inaccuracies (1) and may be regarded with scepticism by some. When ostensibly conflicting analytical data continue to appear, this is the consequence primarily of failure to appreciate the technical limitations of the procedures used. There is therefore an urgent need to re-establish the credibility of trace-element analysis by generating accurate data and thus restore the confidence of many users. The development of a reliable element database for this purpose is a multidisciplinary task involving the drawing up of well defined protocols, and the use both of adequately tested methods for sampling and handling biomaterials, and of appropriate analytical procedures.

In recent years, increased understanding of the problems of sample contamination and of the need for better conditions of sample storage has increased the ability to identify the sources of errors but has only partially improved the quality of analytical data. Past errors in the selection of techniques are the direct responsibility of the analyst concerned, who should have established, quantitatively, their detection and quantification limits (2, 3) and have validated the working range of the proposed analytical technique for a given matrix. This may be accomplished either by the use of appropriate certified reference materials or, if these are not available, by replacing them with suitably prepared calibration standards. Despite the range of techniques available, few laboratories in the world carry out reliable trace-element determinations, and even fewer are capable of achieving over long periods even an accuracy and precision of 10–20% in analysing biomaterials. Errors arising from the improper use of analytical methodologies can be detected when data for the same test material from different laboratories are pooled, as illustrated, often alarmingly, by the results of IAEA analytical intercomparisons (4, 5). Inconsistencies are widespread and are found for several elements at low concentration levels, as demonstrated by a comparison of literature data (1, 6–8). For a number of trace elements, namely aluminium, antimony, arsenic, caesium, chromium, cobalt, mercury, manganese, molybdenum, nickel, silver, tin and vanadium, recent investigations show orders of magnitude decreases in reported concentrations in tissues and body fluids in comparison with earlier results (1,4,6,7). For example, data for chromium in serum have varied by a factor of 5586 (high, 782 ng/ml; low, 0.14 ng/ml), for molybdenum by one of 443 (high, 257 ng/ml; low, 0.58 ng/ml) and for manganese by one of 63.5 (high, 34.3 ng/ml; low, 0.54 ng/ml) (6).

21.1 Biomedical specimens

The investigation of trace-element relationships in biological systems is a multidisciplinary task involving two crucial parameters, namely biological insight and analytical awareness in planning the studies. The analyst should be associated with the investigation from its inception since it is difficult to interpret the analytical results obtained from samples over which the analyst had no control during sampling. The analyst must cooperate with those familiar with the biological considerations governing the selection of the correct specimens to enable the problem in question to be solved. The need for a multidisciplinary approach in biological trace-element research is effectively illustrated by the development of rigorous multidisciplinary techniques for sampling blood platelets for trace-element analysis (9).

21.1.1 Sample quality

Two major considerations govern the quality of biomedical samples. Of these, the first relates to the routine analytical precautions required to prevent the extraneous contamination of the sampled materials, and the conditions for their storage and preservation if the analyses are not to be completed within a short time, and the second to the physiological variables governing the biochemical characteristics of specimens liable to be affected by presampling factors (see below) (10).

21.1.2 Presampling factors

Presampling factors are essentially events associated with biological phe-nomena which influence sample composition, including biological variations (e.g. genetic factors, long- and short-term physiological influences and seasonal changes), postmortem changes (e.g. cell swelling, imbibition and autolysis), both intrinsic and artefactual alterations (e.g. haemolysis, and changes due to stress-induced redistribution of body water) and internal "contaminations" (e.g. arising from medication, implants, unusual diets) (11). Minimizing the effect of intrinsic variables which influence the trace-element content of clinical specimens is important but not easy. The understanding and documentation of the influence of such factors on element content are of crucial importance.

21.1.3 Extraneous contamination

The significance of the errors introduced by the extraneous contamination of samples is inversely related to the concentration of the analyte. For example, analyses for aluminium, chromium, lead and manganese are more susceptible to errors introduced by airborne and other contaminants than are those for certain other elements. Thus, analytical grade ethylenediaminetetra-acetic acid contains up to 50 ng of chromium/g and 300 ng of zinc/g (12). About 4 mg are needed as anticoagulant per ml of blood; even if it is assumed that this remains entirely in the plasma fraction, 1.2 ng of zinc introduced as a contaminant would not affect the determination of plasma zinc. In contrast, for chromium, the quantity introduced (0.2 ng) would be entirely unacceptable since it would be greater than that present in serum samples (1, 12). For chromium in urine, there has been a continuous decline in baseline estimates of urinary chromium output from 7.2 μg/day to 0.16 μg/day as contamination control procedures have improved with time (1). Other crucial factors in the effective control of contamination are the duration of storage before analysis, the use of sample containers and handling accessories made of materials (e.g. titanium) which do not interfere with the proposed analyses, and the control of humidity and dust. Practical methods of dealing with problems related to sampling, sample preparation and storage have been discussed elsewhere (13, 14).

21.1.4 Loss of trace elements before and during analysis

Except in non-destructive instrumental analytical procedures, the first sample treatment usually involves chemical dissolution or fusion. During this stage, loss of an analyte can occur by gaseous evolution, absorption, adsorption onto the surfaces of instruments and containers, sputtering, spraying, agitation or adsorption onto precipitated or undissolved solid particles With botanical samples, the problem of undissolved residues is particularly serious when contaminating soil or other siliceous minerals absorb trace elements from analyte solutions.

With biological materials, the most hazardous steps from the point of view of the loss of trace elements are ashing, drying and evaporation to dryness. The volatility of an element at these stages depends on its chemical form in the sample. Dry ashing of biological materials, especially of samples intended for multielement analysis (even at low temperatures), should generally be avoided (Table 21.1). Elements such as boron can be lost even during freeze-drying, e.g. if boron is present in the aqueous phase as boric acid, and is not stabilized by an appropriate base. Apart from the loss of intrinsically volatile compounds of the trace elements, several elements have been shown to be lost from a variety of matrices (15).

Table 21.1. Loss of trace elements during dry ashing of biological samples—investigational results[a]

Element	Matrix	Procedure, mode of incorporation into sample	Ashing temperature (°C)	Time (hours)	Loss (%)
Aluminium	Animal liver	Chemical analysis	450	?	16
	Animal kidney	Chemical analysis	450	?	12
Arsenic	Ox blood (dry)	Radioisotope, spiking	850	16	35
			550	16	29
			450	16	28
	Rat bone	Radioisotope,	450	16	44
	Rat blood	intravenous	450	16	86
	Rat kidney		450	16	82
Cobalt	Animal liver	Chemical analysis	450	?	14
	Mollusc	Radioisotope, metabolized	450	?	26
			800	?	22
Chromium	Brown sugar	Chemical analysis	450	?	13
	Unrefined sugar	Chemical analysis	450	?	47
	Molasses	Chemical analysis	450	?	52
	Rat blood	Chemical analysis	500	16	4
			700	16	51
	Rat liver	Chemical analysis	500	16	6
Lead	Human rib	Chemical analysis	600	16	< 5
			710	16	40
Mercury	Fish (whole)	—	110	24	81
Manganese	Mollusc	Radioisotope, metabolized	450	?	15
			800	?	21
Strontium	Ox blood	Radioisotope, spiking	450	16	9
	Rat blood	Radioisotope,	450	16	16
	Rat kidney	intravenous	450	16	5
Zinc	Mollusc	Radioisotope, metabolized	450	?	33
			800	?	44

[a] Information pooled from reference 16.

Wet ashing is relatively safe if the ashing mixture is used with discretion (and appropriate choices are made, firstly, of "open" or "closed" digestion systems, secondly, of the mixture of acids and, thirdly, of the oxidizing conditions maintained during ashing). However, chlorides of arsenic(III), antimony(III), tin(IV), selenium(IV), germanium(IV) and mercury(II) are volatile, and can be lost even when they are formed by reactions with other chlorides or with chloride-rich acids used for ashing. Similarly, boron can also be lost from acid media if fumes escape during dissolution.

Loss of non-volatile elements can occur as a result of failure to recover them from residues following wet ashing. Thus determinations of chromium in brewer's yeast in which a significant fraction of total chromium was present in the insoluble matrix have yielded conflicting results because of inconsistencies in the recoveries achieved by different analytical procedures (1). In a recent investigation involving apple and peach leaves, it was shown that significant fractions of chromium (6–25%), iron (up to 9%) and scandium (up to 59%) were associated with the insoluble fraction following wet digestion (15). Oven drying at temperatures exceeding 100 °C (Table 21.2) and even freeze-drying are unsuitable for certain elemental species, since they can be lost under these conditions (Table 21.3). In addition, sulfide-rich matrices can cause additional problems by inhibiting the release into solution of elements such as copper and mercury. Detailed information on the trace analysis of biological materials is available elsewhere (13, 17).

21.1.5 Storage and preservation

Since the stability of a chemical constituent during storage depends on matrix type, it may be important to preserve the sample in its natural state as far as possible. This is true of organic compounds (e.g. organometallic species, vitamins and enzymes) or when autolysis of the sample causes analytical problems (e.g. generation of sulfides). Conventional storage is then inadequate. Cryogenic preservation is one method of ensuring that specimens retain much of their biochemical identity. The storage of materials for trace-element analysis requires safe, clean, uncontaminated and non-degradable containers. Polyethylene vials and bottles are acceptable for use in storing dry powders for several years as very low temperatures are not required. If such temperatures are desired, polyethylene is not suitable and polytetrafluoroethylene bags or bottles are recommended. Even so, it is prudent to verify that the containers have not been treated with chemical agents (e.g. anticoagulants, antibacterial and antifungal agents, pigments or surface lubricants) which can introduce trace-element contaminants.

Many dry biological standard reference materials have been stored satis-factorily at reference laboratories for 10 or more years at room temperature (about 20 °C) without any special precautions. Similarly, the International Union of Pure and Applied Chemistry has demonstrated that freeze-dried blood serum prepared as a standard for selenium is stable for over 7 years at − 20 °C.

Table 21.2. Loss of trace elements during oven drying of biological samples[a]

Element	Matrix	Procedure, mode of incorporation into sample	Drying temperature (°C)	Time (hours)	Loss (%)
Cobalt	Mollusc	Radioisotope, metabolized	110	?	14
Iodine	Human urine	Radioisotope, metabolized	110	24	4
			120	24	7
	Rat blood		120	24	7
	Rat serum		120	24	8
	Rat red cells		120	24	10
Lead	Oyster	Radioisotope, metabolized	60	48	17
			100	48	20
Manganese	Mollusc	Radioisotope,	110	?	14
	Oyster	metabolized	50–120	48	No loss
Mercury	Human urine	Mercury-203, organic, intravenous	80	72	3
			110	24	15
			120	24	25
	Plankton	Chemical analysis	60	50	51–60
	Rat liver	Radioisotope, metabolized	80	72	5
			110	24	3–10
			120	24	5–15
	Rat brain		120	24	5–16
	Rat muscle		120	24	5–21
Selenium	Herbage	Chemical analysis	100	12	No loss
	Human urine	Selenium-75, organic, intravenous	80	72	12–30
			110	24	30–50
			120	24	50–65
	Oyster	Radioisotope, metabolized	100	24	< 5
			120	24	< 20
Zinc	Mollusc	Radioisotope, metabolized	110	?	9

[a] Information pooled from reference 16.

21.2 Foods

The problems encountered in determining trace elements in dietary materials are similar to those encountered with biomedical samples. The elements calcium, chlorine, magnesium, phosphorous, potassium, sodium and sulfur

Table 21.3. Loss of trace elements during freeze-drying of biological samples[a]

Element	Matrix	Procedure, mode of incorporation into sample	Pressure (Pa)	Time (hours)	Loss (%)
Iodine	Water	Chemical analysis	1.3–6.7	48–72	39
	Human urine	Radioisotope, metabolized	1.3–6.7	48–72	2
Manganese	Oyster	Radioisotope, metabolized	?	24	No loss
Mercury	Fish	Chemical analysis	?	?	20
	(homogenate)	Radioisotope, spiking	?	?	16–39
	Butterfish (gunnel)	Chemical analysis	?	?	50–64
	Human brain (pons)	Chemical analysis	?	?	18–57
	Sea cucumber	Chemical analysis	?	?	59
	Water	Chemical analysis	1.3–6.7	48–72	39
	Guinea-pig muscle	Mercury-203 (methylmercury)	6.7	24	3
	Guinea-pig muscle	Mercury-203 (phenylmercury)	6.7	24	No loss
	Human urine	Mercury-203, organic	6.7	48	2
Selenium	Human urine	Selenium-75, organic, intravenous	6.7	48	3

[a] Information pooled from reference *16*

occur in foods at rather high concentrations and their determination is not particularly difficult. However, with trace elements the situation is different; analytically, they can be divided into three subgroups: (1) those easy to determine routinely by several techniques (e.g. iron and zinc); (2) those not always easy to assay, particularly at low concentrations (e.g. arsenic, selenium and tin); and (3) those (e.g. cadmium, chromium, lead, manganese, mercury, molybdenum and nickel) which require a high level of analytical expertise because of the low concentrations present, detection limit problems, matrix interferences, incomplete recoveries and related methodological difficulties (*18–22*). The problem of representative sampling of foods is discussed in

Chapter 22 with respect to minor and trace elements in total diets (see also reference 23).

At low concentrations, the analysis of dietary material presents considerable difficulties, depending on whether the matrix is simple (e.g. drinking-water and beverages) or complex (dairy products). Meat and a few other food products contain some trace elements at very high concentrations and are generally easy to analyse. The implications of these various conditions are important when single foods are analysed, something that may present an array of problems. The moisture content of foods varies widely, ranging from 94% in leafy vegetables to 60% in meat, 20% in grains and cereals, and up to 10% in oils and fats (20). Elimination of this moisture is useful as a means of preconcentration of some foods (e.g. milk), but may not be adequate for others. The fat content of foods can cause difficulty, e.g. a high-fat product such as cheese will present a real challenge if dissolution steps are involved. (Oxidation of samples rich in fats and oils with perchloric acid should be avoided because of explosion risks.)

The concentrations of several trace elements vary considerably even in foods belonging to similar groups, and those of both minor and trace elements vary widely between foods belonging to different groups. The freeze-drying of mixed diets helps to reduce the problems of low trace-element content of specific foods since a sixfold enrichment of the components is achieved. Experience with the composite analysis of freeze-dried total diet demonstrates the possibility of extending analytical coverage to over 30 elements of biological significance (24).

21.3 Quality assurance

Quality assurance encompasses quality control, quality assessment and maintenance of a quality standard. Quality control covers the procedures established to control errors, while quality assessment is the process of verifying that the measurement system is operating within acceptable limits. Both internal and external quality-assurance programmes are of crucial importance in maintaining a satisfactory level of performance (as a measure of quality control and assessment) in any laboratory. Procedures for implementing the necessary steps are discussed elsewhere (25). Quality standard refers to the degree of desired overall quality of a given analytical investigation, as discussed below.

21.3.1 Quality standards

The standards set for the quality of an analytical result should depend on the end use of the results. Thus, if the aim is merely to scan different biological matrices in order to establish their elemental concentration profiles, a modest quality standard is sufficient. Similarly, for most biomedical trace-element research, results with a total uncertainty of 5–10% should suffice. In contrast, an exceptionally high quality standard (< 1% total uncertainty) is mandatory for legal purposes or the certification of reference materials. Although many aspects of quality assurance can, and should, be expressed in numerical terms, quality itself is a subjective concept. The first operational decisions therefore relate to the degree of quality (quality standard), or tolerance limits, required for the purpose of the investigation for which the analyses are being made. If the tolerance limits set are narrower than the investigation really requires, or are not practically attainable, this can cause unnecessary expense and loss of time.

21.3.2 Reference materials

Frequent analysis of reference standards is the key to eliminating procedural inconsistencies in establishing quality control. Such standards are invaluable aids in the exposure of systematic errors associated with analytical methods. Ideally, at least two reference standards should be available. These should be of matrix type similar to that of the samples being analysed and have analyte concentrations representative of the entire working range of interest (i.e. at least one at the low end and one at the high end) (5).

Analytical quality-assurance materials can be classified as *primary* and *secondary* reference materials. Primary reference materials are known either as certified reference materials or as standard reference materials. These are prepared and certified under the rigid conditions necessary for maintaining high analytical quality. They are thus very expensive to prepare and are usually produced by established institutions such as the IAEA in Vienna, the Bureau of Reference Materials of the European Economic Community in Brussels, the National Institute of Standards and Technology (formerly the National Bureau of Standards) in the USA and the National Institute of Environmental Sciences in Japan (1, 26, 27).

Primary reference materials are indispensable. Ideally, they should be used for validating new analytical methods, verifying performance when changes are made in an existing method, and for monitoring analytical proficiency in a laboratory by means of periodic external and internal quality-control programmes.

Secondary reference materials are defined as carefully prepared "in-house" control standards characterized by analytical methods that are evaluated by the use of an appropriate primary reference material. Well characterized secondary reference materials, as working control materials, are sufficient for a variety of purposes. For example, they satisfactorily meet the day-to-day requirements of quality assurance in an analytical laboratory and may provide an adequate source material for the development of quality-control charts.

241

Although many biological reference materials are currently available (1, 27, 28), the range does not meet all present analytical requirements: for the elements aluminium, antimony, fluorine, silica, tin and vanadium, few or no reference materials are available. A major problem is that trace-element determinations are generally subject to large errors, and it is essential to select a reference material whose matrix resembles that of the sample with respect not only to composition but also to the relationships between the analyte and the principal matrix constituents. Only then can the sources of systematic errors arising from matrix effects be identified. For example, using instrumental neutron activation analysis, it was possible to determine both mercury and selenium in human milk even in small samples, but not in cow's milk (29). The levels of these two elements were comparable in both, yet the matrix effects resulting from the 10-fold greater levels of phosphorus and calcium in cow's milk made analytical performance unsatisfactory.

In addition to the existing single-food reference materials such as milk powder, rice and wheat powder, considerable attention has been recently focused on the analysis of inorganic nutrients in mixed and total diets. These are prepared on the basis of food as eaten, either by a duplicate sampling technique or by preparing composites made up of individual foods so as to represent a typical meal. Concentrations of several trace elements in biological, dietary and environmental reference materials have been certified (1, 27, 28). In particular, for nutritionally important trace elements such as chromium, copper, iron, selenium and zinc, a wide range of reference matrices is available. A reasonably satisfactory situation also exists for arsenic, cadmium, cobalt, lead, manganese, mercury and nickel, but not for elements such as aluminium, iodine and molybdenum. For boron, fluorine, lithium, silicon, tin and vanadium, the situation is particularly unsatisfactory and must be improved. Demands for the development of speciated reference materials (e.g. of methylmercury, organotin species, and arsenic species) can be expected.

21.4 Analytical techniques

Analytical techniques such as atomic absorption spectrophotometry (AAS) (flame and flameless), atomic emission (direct-current and inductively coupled plasma), chemical and electroanalytical methods, gas and liquid chromatography, mass spectrometry in different modes, nuclear-activation techniques and X-ray fluorescence offer sufficiently low detection limits to make them suitable for investigating a variety of biomatrices.

Low detection limits alone are not sufficient, however, to remedy the situation described on p. 233 in which analytical data on trace elements are regarded with scepticism. Ignorance of various interferences, e.g. matrix-related problems (see below), flaws in sample and standard preparation (see section 21.1), and inadequate calibration procedures (see section 21.3.2) all contribute to this regrettable situation. The analyst is therefore by far the most important component of any analytical system (1).

21.4.1 Choice of type of assay

The analyst is faced with the choice between multielement and single-element assays, which is affected by a number of factors. Thus, even though sometimes only partly quantitative, multielement assays are useful in obtaining simultaneous elemental composition profiles of a given specimen. For example, the non-destructive procedures offer the possibility of generating data simultaneously (including repeated determinations on the same test portion) for several elements for purposes of comparison. They also offer the possibility of internal quality control so that unusual situations involving any specific element can be evaluated. Moreover, in a carefully designed study, multielement assays can provide very useful information at relatively low cost. However, some elements must be determined alone because of serious analytical problems. Clinical, environmental and nutritional laboratories dealing with specific elements frequently need single-element assays. In a laboratory performing a wide range of analyses, therefore, a combination of both single- and multielement capability may be essential for effective functioning.

21.4.2 Choice of analytical technique

The choice of an analytical technique depends on a number of factors, including: (1) susceptibility to matrix effects; (2) the range of elements covered; (3) the detection limits; and (4) suitability for the matrix of interest. The susceptibility of an analytical technique to matrix effects depends on the sample composition. With some matrices, these effects are of major importance, but others can be avoided by a modification of the technique. The susceptibility of various analytical techniques to matrix-related analytical problems is shown in Table 21.4.

Matrix effects and their influence on a range of analytical techniques are discussed elsewhere (1, 16, 30, 31).

The usefulness of an analytical method for trace-element analysis, also depends on the range of elements covered and the order of magnitude of its detection limits for the elements at the top and bottom of its sensitivity range. Detection limits will not be the same for all elements, so that simultaneous multielement determination will require compromises in experimental conditions that will affect the accuracy and precision of at least a few elements. Even when there is a method of choice for the analysis of a particular element, its

243

Table 21.4. Susceptibility of analytical techniques to matrix effects

Susceptibility to matrix effects	Technique
Very high	Fluorimetry
High	Atomic absorption spectrophotometry (AAS)-furnace, optical emission with direct-current plasma (DCP) and microwave-induced plasma (MIP), X-ray fluorescence and proton-induced X-ray fluorescence (PIXE), voltammetry, gas and high-pressure liquid chromatography (HPLC)
Medium	AAS-hydride generation, some types of mass spectrometry (MS) and optical emission spectrometry
Low	AAS-flame (at > 100 ng/g range for many elements), AAS (with Zeeman correction), atomic emission spectrometry with inductively coupled plasma (ICP-AES) and neutron activation analysis (NAA)

performance will depend on the concentration of the element in question and that of others in the matrix. Concentration ranges also vary widely between different types of biomaterials and foods. These changes in relationships between elements may necessitate modifications to the technique for specific applications in order to maintain optimum performance and prevent any decline in detection limits.

The most important criterion of the suitability of a method, however, is whether it is appropriate for the matrix of interest; useful guidance is available elsewhere (1, 16). Using a set of four representative biological matrices, namely bovine liver, porcine muscle, Bowen's kale and human serum, an advisory group designated by the International Atomic Energy Agency evaluated the performance of different analytical techniques (Table 21.5). For elements such as copper, iron and zinc, several methods were suitable. Thus, for zinc (Table 21.6), many methods can generate results with a 1% CV (16). On the other hand, for elements such as fluorine, iodine, tin and vanadium, the choice was limited (16). The analytical techniques studied nevertheless reached detection limits below the ng/g level for chromium, manganese and vanadium, i.e. the level at which these elements are expected to occur in some specimens. Detection capabilities are discussed elsewhere (30).

21.4.3 Special analytical problems

The bulk element composition of a biological matrix often influences both the risk of interferences during the measurement of analyte signals and the choice of

Table 21.5. Analytical methods applicable to four biological matrices (blood serum, animal muscle, bovine liver and a plant material, kale) with a better than 10% CV[a]

Element	A1	A2	A3	C1	C2	E	M	N1	N2	N3	X
Antimony		x					x		x	x	
Arsenic		x					x		x	x	
Cadmium		x					x		x		
Calcium	x	x		x		x	x	x	x	x	
Chlorine				x	x			x	x		
Chromium	x		x						x		
Cobalt		x							x	x	
Copper	x	x	x		x	x	x		x	x	x
Fluorine									x		
Iodine									x		
Iron	x	x	x	x	x	x	x	x	x	x	x
Lead		x	x		x						
Magnesium	x		x		x		x		x	x	
Manganese	x	x	x			x	x		x	x	
Mercury		x						x	x	x	
Molybdenum		x	x				x		x	x	
Nickel		x	x						x		
Phosphorus		x	x	x	x	x	x		x		
Potassium	x			x		x			x		
Selenium		x	x					x	x	x	
Silicon		x	x	x	x	x	x		x		
Sodium	x			x		x		x	x		
Thallium		x							x		
Tin		x							x		
Uranium									x		
Vanadium							x		x		
Zinc	x	x	x	x	x	x	x	x	x	x	x

[a] Source: reference 16.

[b] A1: atomic absorption spectrophotometry (AAS); A2: AAS–flame atomization using special sample techniques or after preconcentration and separation of the analyte; A3: AAS–electrothermal atomization in graphite furnace; C1: chemical methods; C2: electro-chemical methods; E: emission spectroscopy–inductively coupled plasma source; M: mass spectrometry—spark source; N1: neutron activation analysis (NAA)—instrumental methods; N2: NAA with single-element separation; N3: NAA with group separation (simple scheme involving removal of alkali metals, halogens and phosphorus); X: X-ray analysis—proton-induced X-ray fluorescence.)

Table 21.6. Applicability of different analytical methods to the determination of zinc in biological matrices[a]

Method	Blood serum	Bowen's kale	Animal muscle	Bovine liver
Atomic absorption — flame	+ + +	+ + +	+ + +	+ + +
Atomic emission — inductively coupled plasma	+ + +	+ + +	+ + +	+ + +
Neutron activation — instrumental	+ + +	+ + +	+ + +	+ + +
Neutron activation — radiochemical	+ + +	+ + +	+ + +	+ + +
X-ray — proton-induced emission	+ + +	+ + +	+ + +	+ + +
Atomic absorption — graphite furnace	+ +	+ +	+ +	+ +
Chemical	+ +	+ +	+ +	+ +
Electrochemical	+ +	+ +	+ +	+ +
Mass spectrometry — spark source	+ +	+ +	+ +	+ +

[a] + + + = determinable with high precision (1% CV); + + = determinable with low precision (10% CV).

analytical technique. Prior knowledge of the probable element composition profile of a matrix is of great help in formulating analytical strategies. Even among samples of the same type, matrix composition can vary significantly and pose unexpected analytical problems. As previously mentioned, cow's milk contains approximately ten times more calcium and phosphorus than human milk and, depending on the analytical technique used, this may cause difficulties in determining the concentrations of certain trace elements (29).

The analytical problems relating to certain "difficult to determine" trace elements (arsenic, cadmium, cobalt, copper, chromium, iodine, lead, manganese, mercury, molybdenum and nickel) in foods are best illustrated by an IAEA study. This involved the reinvestigation in 1987 of reference materials IAEA A-1 (milk powder) and IAEA H-4 (animal muscle), first analysed in 1980. The expertise of the analysts selected covered all the major analytical techniques (22) which were validated by analyses of other reference materials. The results are given in Table 21.7. The data reported in 1980 were obtained by a large number of participant laboratories, those for 1987 by a select group of analysts. This comparative study indicated in most instances that improvements in the analytical control of contamination and of matrix-related inter-

Table 21.7. Comparison of old and new data for selected elements in IAEA milk powder and animal muscle (ng/g dry weight, overall mean ± SD)

Element	Milk powder (IAEA A-11)		Animal muscle (IAEA H-4)	
	Specialist data[a] (1987)	Multicentre data[b] (1980)	Specialist data[a] (1987)	Multicentre data[b] (1980)
Arsenic	4.85 ± 0.2	48 ± 16	5.95 ± 0.35	5.7 ± 1.5
Cadmium	1.7 ± 0.2	526 ± 638	4.9 ± 1.0	44 ± 39
Cobalt	4.5 ± 0.8	5 ± 1	3.1 ± 1.0	2.7 ± 1
Chromium	17.7 ± 3.8	257 ± 262	9.1 ± 2.2	60 ± 40
Copper	378 ± 31	838 ± 450	3650 ± 345	3960 ± 960
Iodine	87 ± 6	1469 ± 1548	14.3 ± 1.7	11; 150[c]
Lead	54 ± 10	267 ± 255	< 25; 160; 260[d]	220 ± 190
Manganese	257 ± 6	377 ± 177	466 ± 42	520 ± 80
Mercury	3.2 ± 0.6	2.5 ± 0.7	6.8 ± 0.4	13.7 ± 5.4
Molybdenum	92 ± 9	1266 ± 1649	41 ± 2.8	50 ± 10
Nickel	54 ± 28	931 ± 920	64 ± 37	970; 1020[c]

[a] Results of 1987 reinvestigation (*22*).
[b] Results of 1980 IAEA intercomparison.
[c] Only two results reported.
[d] Only three results reported.

ference and in, particular, the effective use of primary reference materials to monitor performance, reduced both the absolute values and the variability of the estimates of the concentration of many analytes. Inconsistencies remained, such as embarrassing discrepancies in estimates of lead in animal tissue but, in general, the results showed unequivocally that improved monitoring of analytical procedures increases the reliability of the data produced.

21.4.4 Trace-element speciation and bioavailability

In conventional studies of dietary trace-element intakes, comparisons are often made and conclusions drawn in the context of recommended dietary allowances. However, it is being increasingly recognized that the proportion of element intake that is biologically available is often determined by its speciation chemistry, which can differ between foods. Ideally, the bioavailability of the various elements present in single or mixed foods should be determined before any attempt is made to interpret data on their contents in diets or foods. However, the characterization of element "species" in complex biological and dietary media is difficult, partly because of inadequate detection limits and the danger of causing changes in speciation states during analysis. Many biochemical methods for the isolation of metallocomplexes are in use, but introduce problems of loss and contamination of the element and its species. Radioactive labelling of organoarsenic compounds has been used in animal studies (32). A two-stage system designed to stimulate the gastric and intestinal digestion of food *in vitro* in combination with inductively coupled plasma mass spectrometry has been successfully used in recent investigations (30). Several techniques based on gas chromatography, high-pressure liquid chromatography and anodic stripping voltammetry have also been applied to speciation chemistry (33). Many analytical methods can be used for speciation studies provided that their limitations are recognized (30). The usefulness of stable isotopes in studying the influence of bioavailability phenomena in mineral metabolism has been stressed in recent reviews (34). There is no radiation risk, they are widely accepted for *in vivo* use and, when measured by either mass spectrometry or *in vitro* neutron activation techniques, have speeded up progress in research on mineral metabolism.

21.5 Establishment of trace-element analysis laboratories in developing countries

21.5.1 Analytical objectives

Analysts in many laboratories in developing countries wish to acquire the analytical competence to determine at least the limited range of analytes needed to support various bioenvironmental and nutritional research activities. These analytes can be divided into the following two categories: (1) minor elements (calcium, chlorine, magnesium, phosphorus, potassium, sodium and sulfur) and trace elements (cadmium, copper, iodine, iron, lead, mercury, selenium and zinc) for which analyses are frequently required; and (2) a number of trace elements (aluminium, arsenic, boron, chromium, fluorine, lithium, manganese, molybdenum, nickel, silicon, tin and vanadium) for which analytical data are needed less frequently. Although for elements such as calcium, phosphorus and sulfur classical analytical methods such as gravimetry and volumetry are applicable, the emphasis here is on trace-element determinations and on instrumental methods.

A basic fact to be taken into account in establishing any trace-element analytical laboratory is that as previously mentioned, the analyst is the most important component of any analytical system. Even the best instruments can yield poor data in the hands of an unskilled analyst; even modest equipment can generate meaningful results when used by a knowledgeable one.

If appropriately trained and experienced analysts are available, method selection becomes contingent on the potential and limitations of laboratory facilities and techniques. From the analytical point of view, biologically relevant trace elements can be divided into four classes. For Class 1 elements, among which are copper, iron and zinc, methods applicable to several types of matrices are available, and flame atomic absorption equipment will often suffice to meet most analytical requirements. Dedicated systems for specific analytes can be operated and maintained economically. For Class 2 elements, such as chromium, manganese, molybdenum, nickel and selenium, graphite furnace atomic absorption is often an appropriate technique provided that trained staff are available who are familiar with it and with its frequently unique matrix problems especially when analyte concentrations are low. The determination of Class 3 elements, which include aluminium, arsenic, cadmium, lead and mercury, presents particular difficulties for the non-specialist laboratory either because of the need for individual element-specific analytical techniques (e.g. for mercury) or, for some elements (e.g. aluminium and lead), because of the ubiquity of potential sources of contamination. For Class 4 elements, namely boron, cobalt, fluorine, lithium, silicon, tin and vanadium, the need for specific analytical techniques often requiring the allocation of considerable time and resources usually precludes analyses by non-specialist laboratories. Although elements such as boron and silicon (spectrophotometry), lithium (flame AAS) and fluorine and iodine (various forms of potentiometry) can be determined by simple and well established techniques, formidable problems are encountered in dealing with certain matrices, especially at low concentration levels. To some extent, special techniques are also needed for elements in Classes 2 and 3 (e.g. aluminium, cadmium, chromium, lead, manganese and mercury). Ultimately the analyst's ability to understand the overall impact of the analytical problem is the key to the successful application of a chosen technique.

21.5.2 Basic laboratory facilities

Of vital importance among the factors to be considered when establishing a trace-element analytical laboratory is the need to control contamination from the laboratory air, fixtures, equipment, reagents and personnel (especially the analyst). The impact on the quality of analysis of extraneous contamination from laboratory surroundings depends, for some elements (aluminium, lead and zinc), on the concentration of the analyte in question. For example, when the analytes to be determined are present at concentrations in the range 1–100 μg/g, laboratory design will be very different from that required when lower concentrations have to be determined. Environmental contamination is often the limiting factor. Guidance on the design of appropriate laboratory facilities to handle such concentration ranges is available elsewhere (1, 16, 31).

The stability of the electrical power supply to the laboratory is a matter of vital importance that must be addressed during the planning of the facility. The availability of clean working surfaces on which to handle samples during their preparation is a fundamental requirement for all trace-element laboratories. These should preferably be accompanied by a Class 100 clean-air hood equipped with high-efficiency particulate air filters with laminar flow. Areas protected from contamination should be large enough to permit preliminary sample handling, particle size reduction and sample homogenization. A separate work bench, preferably remote from areas where samples are handled, should be provided exclusively for the preparation of primary standards. Facilities for sample storage, usually consisting of a refrigerator of adequate size and a freezer, and a dependable microbalance are an integral part of any reasonably equipped laboratory. Dust-free ventilation and a liberal supply of purified water of specified purity are essential.

Walls should be covered with a non-flaking coating (e.g. latex paint) and floors should be covered with good-quality linoleum or with polyvinyl chloride or ceramic tiles. Commercially available "tacky" mats help to remove dust from footwear and should be placed at the entrance to laboratories. Such conditions will help to provide an environment suitable for the determination of many elements belonging to Classes 1 and 2. The working surfaces of laboratories engaged in routine food analysis for calcium, magnesium, phosphorus, silicon and sodium, and in some cases copper, iron, manganese and zinc, should be covered with clean polyethylene sheets. Disposable sheets of bleached filter paper are a suitable alternative.

From the experience gained during international studies (1, 35) and during the analysis and certification of biological reference materials (22, 24, 28), it is possible to identify suitable analytical methods for the determination of frequently assayed minor and trace elements in different matrices. Recommended methods are given in Table 21.8, methods that are relatively simple and inexpensive being listed in the first column, while methods for which expensive operational training is usually required and/or extensive financial support, either for the initial purchase of the equipment or its operation, are listed in the other two columns. The methods listed in the second column are of particular importance for laboratories dealing with a wide range of biological matrices and aiming to develop expertise and provide a service by determining biologically relevant trace elements.

Both inductively coupled plasma atomic emission spectrometry (ICP-AES) and neutron activation analysis (NAA) are established multielement techniques. The former has several practical advantages; however, if a neutron source (reactor) is available, the latter can offer attractive possibilities. Among other multielement techniques, inductively coupled mass spectrometry has great potential but involves expensive instrumentation and elaborate operational procedures; its use is only likely to be feasible in specialist centres. The methods listed in the third column are specialized ones or means of extending the applicability of a particular technique to include a specific assay.

Many colorimetric, fluorimetric or potentiometric methods that have been successfully used for the determination of a number of elements have been replaced by atomic absorption techniques which are usually quicker and sometimes more readily automated. However, laboratories located in remote areas where servicing of sophisticated equipment is difficult may still wish to rely on non-automated and less complex colorimetric or fluorimetric techniques. Although often more labour-intensive and comparatively slow, they can yield excellent data if meticulous attention is paid to detail during the procedures. Several excellent studies on problems related to iodine and selenium currently rely on such methods. For example, the catalytic technique for iodine determination is particularly suitable for certain specific purposes such as the assay of iodide in milk, and therefore continues to be of great practical significance.

21.5.3 Quality surveillance and control

Surveillance of the quality of trace-element analysis in a good laboratory typically accounts for up to 20% of its working time, something that should be allowed for in planning analytical programmes. In addition to analysing certified reference materials and participating in proficiency exercises, each laboratory should, as a matter of principle, be able to develop selective "in-house" reference materials for routine use. This calls for the use of at least two different analytical techniques for the verification of the data for a given analyte. However, if methods are validated by the analysis of primary reference materials (see section 21.3.2), use of a single method can be sufficient to demonstrate that the performance of a laboratory is satisfactory. If specialist centres assist by conducting the multielement analysis of such in-house standards by ICP-AES or NAA, the value of such materials can be maximized.

21.5.4 Recommendations

Those responsible for trace-element analysis laboratories in developing countries often complain that primary reference materials cannot be obtained either because of their expense or because of the scarcity of the hard currency needed to buy them. This situation has prejudiced laboratory development and performance in a number of countries even though those hoping to develop such facilities are aware of the need for analytical quality control. Since it is impossible, even for international agencies, to provide reference materials free

Table 21.8. Suitability of specific analytical techniques for laboratories in developing countries

Analyte assayed	Technique		
	Simple and practicable	Difficult but feasible: greater resources required	For limited use: can be expensive

Frequently determined minor elements

Calcium	F-AAS, AES	ICP-AES, INAA	PIXE, X-RAY
Chlorine	SP	IC, INAA	PGAA, PIXE, X-RAY
Magnesium	F-AAS, AES	ICP-AES	INAA
Phosphorus	SP	ICP-AES	PGAA, PIXE, X-RAY
Potassium	F-AAS, AES	ICP-AES, INAA	PGAA, PIXE, X-RAY
Sodium	F-AAS, AES	ICP-AES, INAA	PGAA, PIXE, X-RAY
Sulfur	SP	IC	PGAA, PIXE, X-RAY

Frequently determined trace elements

Cadmium	ASV	GF-AAS, RNAA	ICP-AES
Copper	F-AAS, ASV, SP	ICP-AES, RNAA	PIXE, X-RAY
Iodine	POT (CAT, ISE)	RNAA	EPNAA, PAA, X-RAY
Iron	F-AAS, ASV, SP	GF-AAS, INAA, ICP-AES	PIXE, X-RAY
Lead	ASV	GF-AAS, ICP-AES	IDMS, PIXE, X-RAY
Mercury		CV-AAS, INAA	GC
Selenium	SP (FLU)	HG-AAS, INAA	GC-MS
Zinc	F-AAS, ASV, SP	GF-AAS, ICP-AES, INAA	PIXE, X-RAY

Less frequently determined trace elements

Aluminium		GF-AAS, ICP-AES	INAA
Arsenic	SP	HG-AAS, RNAA	X-RAY
Barium	F-AAS, AES	INAA, ICP-AES	X-RAY
Boron	SP, AES	ICP-AES	NA-MS, PGAA
Bromine		INAA	X-RAY, PIXE
Caesium	F-AAS, AES	INAA, ICP-AES	
Chromium		GF-AAS, INAA/RNAA	GC-MS
Cobalt	SP	GF-AAS, INAA, ICP-AES	
Fluorine	POT (ISE), SP, IC		NAA
Lithium	AES	F-AAS/GF-AAS, ICP-AES	IDMS, NA-MS
Manganese	F-AAS	GF-AAS, ICP-AES, INAA	PIXE, X-RAY
Molybdenum	SP	GF-AAS, INAA/RNAA	ICP-AES
Nickel	ASV, SP	GF-AAS, ICP-AES	NAA, X-RAY
Rubidium	F-AAS, AES	GF-AAS, INAA, ICP-AES	X-RAY
Silicon	SP	ICP-AES	NAA, PIXE, X-RAY
Strontium	F-AAS, AES	GF-AAS, INAA, ICP-AES	X-RAY
Tin	—	HG-AAS, INAA/RNAA	ICP-AES
Vanadium	—	GF-AAS, RNAA	ICP-AES

Table 21.8 *(continued)*

AAS	atomic absorption spectrophotometry	
	CV-AAS	cold vapour AAS
	F-AAS	flame AAS
	GF-AAS	graphite-furnace AAS
	HG-AAS	hydride-generation AAS
AES	atomic emission spectrophotometry	
	ICP-AES	inductively coupled plasma AES
ASV	anodic stripping voltammetry	
GC	gas chromatography	
GC-MS	gas chromatography–mass spectrometry	
IC	ion chromatography	
IDMS	isotope-dilution mass spectrometry	
NAA	neutron activation analysis	
	EPNAA	epithermal NAA
	INAA	instrumental NAA
	RNAA	radiochemical NAA
NA-MS	neutron activation–mass spectrometry	
PAA	photon activation analysis	
PGAA	prompt gamma activation analysis	
POT	potentiometry	
	CAT	catalytic techniques
	ISE	ion-selective electrode
SP	spectrophotometry	
	FLU	fluorimetry for selenium
X-RAY	X-ray fluorescence	
	PIXE	proton-induced X-ray fluorescence

of charge over long periods of time, other approaches are needed. One possibility is to encourage at least one laboratory in a particular area to acquire the ability to prepare good-quality secondary reference materials linked to proper primary reference materials (see section 21.3.2) and to become the regional quality-control laboratory in that area. Such regional specialist laboratories should possess the facilities for, and the expertise in, several analyte-specific methodologies, supported by at least one of the multielement analytical techniques listed in Table 21.8.

Proper and sustained analytical quality control can be less costly but nevertheless effective if costs are shared, e.g. between developing countries in a particular region. In any case, its cost is trivial compared with the consequences of generating and acting on inaccurate results.

A programme to promote regional self-reliance in preparing secondary reference materials and to provide technical guidance and analytical help is being developed under the aegis of the Asian Society for Reference Materials

(ASREM) (36). Potential users in developing countries in Asia are encouraged to participate in ASREM's activities. Recognition by United Nations agencies of the activities of groups such as ASREM would be helpful in promoting analytical work in other areas.

Guidance from established laboratories must form an essential part of all efforts to improve the analytical resources of developing countries. Efforts to promote such guidance must play a greater role in future programmes of work.

It is also vitally important that courses be organized periodically in different regions to provide practical training in newer analytical techniques. Such training is indispensable and specially designed workshops on trace-element analysis are essential. For example, bench workers in some laboratories frequently lack the ability to prepare good and accurate primary and working standards suitable for a range of analytical applications. Many analysts need to be educated in the proper use of reference materials through participation in proficiency courses offered by external organizers. It is difficult, if not impossible, to conduct an effective quality-assurance programme without such outside support. The IAEA has made a good beginning in promoting such activities through its regional training programmes and its efforts should be supported by other United Nations agencies so that the scope of such programmes can be extended.

21.6 Biomonitoring

21.6.1 Choice of specimens

The context in which information is required on the composition of a biological specimen must be clearly defined. The criteria governing the acceptability of samples for the clinical diagnosis of deficiency or toxicity, for the biological monitoring of environmental pollution, for nutritional surveillance and monitoring, and for forensic investigations differ markedly and have been discussed elsewhere (1). An indication of the suitability of various human tissues and body fluids for use in the biomonitoring of a number of trace elements and in assessing exposure to toxic elements is given in Tables 21.9 and 21.10, respectively. The feasibility of the selective monitoring of essential and other trace elements through the analysis of whole blood and its components or of hair, urine, faeces or milk is assessed below and has also been discussed elsewhere (1).

21.6.2 Examples

Blood (including serum, plasma and erythrocytes) and saliva

Because of the effectiveness of homoeostatic control mechanisms, the levels of essential elements in blood are not always good indicators of the adequacy or

Table 21.9. **Suitability of human clinical specimens for biological monitoring programmes**[a]

Metal	Specimen	Exposure assessment	Risk assessment
Antimony	B	+	?
Aluminium	U	+ +	?
Aluminium	B	+ + +	+ + +
Arsenic (inorganic)	U	+ +	+
Arsenic (organic)	U	+ +	?
Cadmium	B, U	+ + +	
Chromium	U	+ +	+
Cobalt	U	+	?
Lead (inorganic)	B	+ + +	+ + +
Lead (organic)	U	+	+
Manganese (inorganic)	B, U	?	?
Manganese (organic)	U	+ +	?
Mercury (inorganic)	B, U	+ +	+ +
Mercury (organic)	B, H	+ + +	+ + +
Nickel	B, U	+	?
Selenium	B, U	+ +	+ +
Tin	B, U	?	?
Vanadium	B, U	+	?

[a] Pooled information from reference *1*. B = whole blood, plasma or serum; U = urine; H = hair; + = weak, + + = moderate; + + + = well established association; ? = not known.

Table 21.10. **Human clinical specimens suitable for assessing exposure to toxic elements**[a]

Tissues	Arsenic	Cadmium	Lead	Inorganic mercury	Methylmercury
Blood	x	x	x	x	x
Bone			x		
Brain				x	x
Faeces		x	x		
Hair	x		x[b]		x
Kidney		x	x	x	
Liver		x	x		x
Placenta		x	x		
Teeth			x		
Urine	x	x	x	x	x

[a] Pooled information from reference *1*.
[b] Sampling and preparatory steps critical.

255

inadequacy of the nutrient status of the body. The presence of "abnormal" levels of copper, iron, selenium and zinc in certain populations has led to speculations as to nutritional inadequacies and subacute disease states, as following the discovery of high levels of copper in the blood of aboriginals in some settlements in Australia and in the inhabitants of Tokelau, signs of probable low zinc status among sections of the population of western Asia, and abnormally high or low values of selenium in various other parts of the world (37). Of these four elements, selenium is the most sensitive to variations in dietary supply. While the monitoring of blood for copper, iron, selenium and zinc does not present serious problems, the interpretation of the analytical data requires careful consideration of their physiological relevance and limitations.

For elements such as arsenic, chromium, lead, mercury, nickel and thallium, the levels in blood rise following exposure. Lead can be monitored using whole blood or erythrocytes (about 95% of lead is bound to erythrocytes). The level of lead in blood is a good indicator of current exposure, and reflects a dynamic equilibrium between exposure, absorption, distribution and elimination under conditions of moderately high exposure. For cadmium and mercury, because of their low concentrations in blood, a high level of analytical skill is essential. The results of several studies indicate that the cadmium levels in the blood of smokers are significantly higher than those in non-smokers (1–3 ng/g vs. 0.1 ng/g) (1, 38), and that frequent eaters of fish have elevated levels of mercury in their blood (39).

A combination of blood serum analysis with that of saliva, milk and urine can be more reliable than single-specimen analysis. The fluorine status of the body has been assessed from such multiple analyses (40); analyses of saliva have proved useful for monitoring lithium levels (41).

Hair

External contamination is a major source of some trace elements in hair and caution is therefore necessary in data interpretation. Contamination with selenium from hair rinses is a common problem and even preanalytical washing may contribute to "inaccurate" results (42).

The biological relevance of levels of essential elements in hair is doubtful, since fluctuations in the homoeostatic control of the pool which supplies it may mean that they do not properly reflect a nutritional deficiency. An evaluation of the results obtained for a number of trace elements in hair in several countries (37) has shown that, despite appreciable differences in living habits, it is difficult to detect definite differences in the composition of hair samples procured from different population groups within the same country (43). However, these data do usefully reflect gross tendencies for a few elements in a group of countries. Thus, compared with zinc levels in European samples (220–250 $\mu g/g$), marginal to low (100–140 $\mu g/g$) values have been observed in several countries such as Bangladesh, Egypt, South Africa (Bantu subjects) and Turkey. Relatively low concentrations of copper in hair have been reported in samples from Bangladesh, Nigeria, Pakistan and Turkey (7–11 $\mu g/g$) as compared with the commonly reported 15–25 $\mu g/g$ in most European countries and in American subjects (37).

In contrast, hair is a good indicator specimen for mercury (44, 45), and especially for methylmercury (46), as well as for arsenic (47) and possibly also for lead (48) and thallium (49). Both mercury (especially methylmercury) and zinc have a higher rate of transfer to hair (46). After ingestion of organic mercury compounds has terminated, the level of mercury in hair decreases in parallel to that in blood (39). At present, mercury in hair is considered a meaningful parameter for assessing the intake of methylmercury.

It is generally difficult to relate the concentration levels of trace elements found in hair to specific metabolic events in the body, especially when dealing with nutritional mineral-deficiency problems.

Urine

Because the daily water output in urine is so variable, the analysis of 24-hour samples is essential.

For elements such as copper, selenium and zinc, subnormal levels are found in urine when dietary intake is deficient. Because of difficulties in interpreting the results of analyses of urinary samples, however, such data should only be used to supplement information obtained from analyses of blood, serum, erythrocytes and hair from the same subjects. If consistently lower values are found in all the specimens, this may point to some form of deficiency. However, paradoxical findings, such as the increased levels of zinc in urine in cases of alcoholism, stress or tissue injury, or increased urinary chromium output following strenuous exercise or high intakes of sugar, can complicate interpretation.

Urine composition can provide a useful index of occupational exposure, particularly for elements such as arsenic, chromium, lead, mercury, nickel and thallium (50–54). Thus urine concentrations provide an adequate indication of exposure to metallic mercury or more rarely to inorganic mercury salts. On the other hand, to detect exposure to alkyl mercury salts, blood will also have to be analysed because urinary excretion does not reflect exposure to this particular source of mercury (55).

Table 21.11. *Reference concentrations for 25 trace elements in adult human clinical specimens*[a]

Element	Liver (µg/kg)	Whole blood (µg/l)	Blood serum (µg/l)	Urine (µg/day)	Milk (µg/l)	Hair (µg/kg)
Aluminium	0.3–2	2–8	1–5	10–100	< 1?	3–10[b]
Arsenic	5–15	2–20	< 1–5	10–30	0.25–3	100–300
Barium	10?	0.5–2.5	?	2–4	?	400–2000
Boron	< 100	20–50	15–45	500–3000	< 50?	1000–2000
Bromine	1000–2000	3000–6000	3000–6000	2–10[b]	1000–2000	2–10[b]
Cadmium	500–2000	0.3–1.2[c] 1–4[d]	0.1–0.3	1–5	< 1	250–1000
Cobalt	30–150	5–10	0.1–0.3	0.5–2	0.2–0.7	50–300
Chromium	5–50	< 5?	0.1–0.2	0.2–2	< 1.0–2.0	300–1200
Caesium	5–20	1.5–4.5	1–2	5–20	1–5	100–1000
Copper	5000–7000	800–1100[e] 1000–1400[f]	800–1100[e] 1100–1400[f]	30–60	200–400	15–25[b]
Fluorine	100–300	200–500	20–50	500–1500	10–25	?
Iodine	100–200	40–60	60–70	100–200	40–80	400–1000

Iron	150–25C[b]	425–500	800–1200	100–200	300–600	30–60[b]
Lead	300–600	50–150	<1	10–20	1–5	2–20[b]
Lithium	<?	0 4–1	0.2–0.8	25–100	<1?	10–100
Manganese	1000–20C0	8–12	0.5–1	0.5–2	3–10	500–1500
Mercury	30–15C	2–20	<1	5–20	1–3	500–2000
Molybdenum	400–800	1–3	<0.1–0.5	20–30	1–4	50–200?
Nickel	10–50	1–5?	<1–2	2–8	10–20	20–200?
Rubidium	400–6000	2000–4000	0.1–0.3	1000–4000	300–1200	1000–2000
Selenium	250–400	90–130	75–120	25–50	10–25	500–1000
Silicon	25–100[f]	?	300?	3–12[b]	?	4–10[b]
Tin	100–1000	<1	<1	1–2	<1–2	800?
Vanadium	5–20	0.1–0.5	0.1–1.0	0.2–1	0.1–0.3	50–150
Zinc	40–60[b]	6000–7000	800–1100	400–600	1000–2000	150–250[b]

[a] Pooled data from references 1, 8, 35, 37, 38, 43, 56–59. ? = uncertain.
[b] In mg/kg or mg/l.
[c] Non-smokers.
[d] Smokers.
[e] Males.
[f] Females.

Faeces

For elements such as aluminium, cadmium, chromium, manganese, nickel, tin and vanadium, which are poorly absorbed by the gut, analysis of faecal samples can give very useful information after suspected dietary exposure or in routine screening. For evaluating the intake and intestinal resorption of cadmium, faecal analysis is simple and probably more meaningful than analysis of the diet wherever a normal rate of absorption can be assumed, and provides useful data even on individuals. However, the data from faecal analyses reflect only intakes shortly before sampling (i.e. current exposure levels), and do not provide information on accumulation with time.

Milk

Milk is comparable to blood in its trace-element profile. One advantage of using milk (of which samples are often readily available) for the assessment of chromium and manganese is that metal instruments, such as the needles used for venepuncture, are not required for specimen collection. Marked geographical differences in the elemental composition of milk have been found in recent studies (35).

21.6.3 Reference ranges

The interpretation of data on the elemental composition of human tissues and body fluids has often to be based on the use of "references ranges" of values that take into account factors such as differing dietary habits and geochemical and other environmental influences that may result in anomalies in the trace-element content of samples. For biologically essential elements subject to homoeostatic control, such ranges are likely to be narrow in populations of healthy subjects. For non-essential elements, the ranges can be broad, depending on the level of exposure of the subjects. Thus aluminium, which is not an essential element, is therefore not subject to homoeostatic control. The amounts entering human systems are highly variable, intakes fluctuating from low to very high, depending on the type of food consumed and other factors. Indeed, it is questionable whether a "normal" value exists for this element in blood serum. The same is also true for some other non-essential elements. Table 21.11 shows a set of recommended reference concentrations for several trace elements derived from a global literature survey conducted between 1982 and 1988 (56) and revised during the preparation of this report.

21.7 Conclusions

Obtaining analytically meaningful and biologically interpretable data on trace elements in biomedical investigations is a tedious task and requires the dedicated efforts and multidisciplinary skills of analytical chemists and medical scientists. The problems described in this chapter re-emphasize the fact that good analytical measurements are not only essential for success in trace-element research but mandatory when the results are to be used for diagnostic and related purposes.

References

1. Iyengar GV. *Elemental analysis of biological systems*, Vol. 1. Boca Raton, FL, CRC Press, 1989.
2. ACS Committee on Environmental Improvement. Guidelines for data acquisition and data quality evaluation in environmental chemistry. *Analytical chemistry*, 1980, **52**: 2242–2246.
3. Currie L, Parr RM. Detection in analytical chemistry. In: *Proceedings American Chemical Society Symposium Series 361*. Washington, DC, American Chemical Society, 1988: 171–193.
4. Dybczynski R, Veglia A, Suschny O. *Report on the intercomparison run IAEA-A-11 for the determination of inorganic constituents of milk powder*. Vienna, International Atomic Energy Agency, 1988 (Report RL/68).
5. Parr RM. Quality assurance of trace element analysis. *Nutrition research*, Suppl. 1: 5–11.
6. Cornelis R, Versieck J. Critical evaluation of the literature values of 18 trace elements in human serum or plasma. In: Brätter P, Schramel P, eds. *Trace element analytical chemistry in medicine and biology*. Berlin, de Gruyter, 1980: 587–600.
7. Heydorn K et al. Sources of variability of trace element concentrations in human serum. In: *Proceedings of the IAEA Symposium on Nuclear Activation Techniques in the Life Sciences*. Vienna, International Atomic Energy Agency, 1978: 129–142.
8. Versieck J, Cornelis R. *Trace elements in human plasma or serum*. Boca Raton, FL, CRC Press, 1979.
9. Iyengar GV et al. Elemental composition of platelets, part I: sampling and sample preparation of platelets for trace element analysis. *Clinical chemistry*, 1979, **25**: 699–704.
10. Iyengar GV. Presampling factors in the elemental composition of biological systems. *Analytical chemistry*, 1982, **54**: 554A–558A.
11. Iyengar GV. Autopsy sampling and elemental analysis: errors arising from post mortem changes. *Journal of pathology*, 1981, **134**: 173–180.
12. Behne D, Iyengar GV. Spurenelementanalyse in biologischen Proben. [Trace element analysis in biological specimens.] In: *Analytiker Taschenbuch*, Band 6. [*Analysts' handbook*, Vol. 6] Heidelberg, 1986: 237–280.
13. Pritchard MW, Lee J. Agricultural samples. In: McKenzie HA, Smythe LE, eds. *Quantitative trace analysis of biological materials*. Amsterdam, Elsevier, 1988: 367–1387.
14. Iyengar GV, Iyengar V. Clinical samples. In: McKenzie HA, Smythe LE, eds.

Quantitative trace anlaysis of biological materials. Amsterdam, Elsevier, 1988: 401–417.

15. Greenberg RR et al. Dissolution problems with botanical reference materials. *Fresenius Zeitschrift für analytische Chemie*, 1990, **338**: 394–398.

16. *Elemental analysis of biological materials.* Vienna, International Atomic Energy Agency, 1980 (Technical Report No. 197).

17. Bock R. *Decomposition methods in analytical chemistry.* New York, Halsted Press, 1979.

18. Horwitz W, Kamps LR, Boyer KW. Quality assurance in the analysis of foods for trace constituents. *Journal of the Association of Official Analytical Chemists*, 1980, **63**: 1344–1354.

19. Kumpulainen J. Chromium. In: McKenzie HA, Smythe LE, eds. *Quantitative trace analysis of biological materials.* Amsterdam, Elsevier, 1980: 451–462.

20. Cunningham WC, Stroube WB. Application of an instrumental activation analysis procedure to analysis of food. *Science of the total environment*, 1987, **63**: 29–43.

21. Jones JW. Food samples. In: McKenzie HA, Smythe LE, eds. *Quantitative trace analysis of biological materials.* Amsterdam, Elsevier, 1988: 331–352.

22. Byrne AR et al. Results of a co-ordinated research programme to improve certification of IAEA milk powder A-11 and animal muscle H-4 for eleven "difficult" trace elements. *Fresenius Zeitschrift für analytische Chemie*, 1987, **326**: 696–698.

23. *Guidelines for the study of dietary intakes of chemical contaminants.* Geneva, World Health Organization, 1983 (unpublished document WHO EFP/83.53; available on request from Nutrition, World Health Organization, 1211 Geneva 27, Switzerland).

24. Iyengar GV et al. Preparation of a mixed human diet material for the analysis of nutrient elements, selected toxic elements and organic nutrients: a preliminary report. *Science of the total environment*, 1987, **61**: 235–252.

25. Taylor JK. *Quality assurance in chemical measurements*, Chelsea, MI, Lewis, 1987.

26. Wolf WR, ed. *Biological reference materials*, New York, John Wiley, 1985.

27. Ihnat M. Biological reference materials for quality control. In: McKenzie HA, Smythe LE, eds. *Quantitative trace analysis of biological materials.* Amsterdam, Elsevier, 1988: 331–352.

28. Cortes Toro E, Parr RM, Clements SA. *Biological and environmental reference materials for trace elements, nuclides and organic microcontaminants*, Vienna, International Atomic Energy Agency, 1990 [IAEA/RL/128 (Rev. 1)].

29. Iyengar GV et al. Determination of cobalt, copper, iron, mercury, manganese, antimony, selenium and zinc in milk samples. *Science of the total environment*, 1982, **24**: 267–274.

30. Toelg G. Where is analysis of trace elements in biotic matrices going to? In: Brätter P, Schramel P, eds. *Trace element analytical chemistry in medicine and biology.* Berlin, de Gruyter, 1988: 1–24.

31. McKenzie HA, Smythe LE. Design of laboratories for trace and ultra-trace analysis. In: McKenzie HA, Smythe LE, eds. *Quantitative trace analysis of biological materials.* Amsterdam, Elsevier, 1988: 39–47.

32. Sabbioni E, Edel J, Goetz L. Trace metal speciation research in environmental toxiciology research. *Nutrition research*, 1985, Suppl. 1: 32–43.

33. Batley GE. *Trace element speciation: analytical methods and problems.* Boca Raton, FL, CRC Press, 1989.

34. Janghorbani M, Ting BTG. Stable isotope methods for studies of mineral/trace element metabolism. *Journal of nutritional biochemistry*, 1990, 1: 4–19.

35. *Minor and trace elements in breast milk. Report of a Joint WHO/IAEA Collaborative Study.* Geneva, World Health Organization, 1989.

36. Iyengar GV. Analytical quality control materials for developing countries: a new initiative. *Food laboratory news*, 1990, 6-1: 20–22.

37. Iyengar GV. Reference values for the concentrations of As, Cd, Co, Cr, Cu, Fe, I, Hg, Mn, Mo, Ni, Pb, Se and Zn in selected human tissues and body fluids. *Biological trace element research*, 1987, 12: 263–295.

38. Friberg L, Vahter M. Assessment of human exposure to Pb and Cd through biological monitoring: results of a UNEP/WHO global study. *Environmental research*, 1983, 30: 95–128.

39. Kershaw TG, Dhahir PH, Clarkson TW. The relationship between blood levels and the dose of methylmercury in man. *Archives of environmental health*, 1980, 35: 28–32.

40. Paez D, Dapas O. Biochemistry of fluorosis — comparative study of the fluoride levels in biological fluids. *Fluoride*, 1982, 15: 87–92.

41. Preskorn SH, Darrel RA, McKnelly WM. Use of saliva lithium determinations for monitoring lithium therapy. *Journal of clinical psychology*, 1978, 39: 756–761.

42. Bos AJJ et al. Incorporation routes of elements into human hair: implications for hair analysis used for monitoring. *Science of the total environment*, 1985, 42: 157–169.

43. Skypeck HH, Joseph BJ. The use and misuse of human hair in trace metal analysis. In: Brown SS, Savory J, eds. *Chemical toxicology and clinical chemistry of metals.* London, Academic Press, 1983: 159–163.

44. Airey D. Total mercury concentrations in human hair from 13 countries in relation to fish consumption and location. *Science of the total environment*, 1983, 32: 157–180.

45. Goyar RA, Mehlman MA. *Toxicity of trace elements.* New York, John Wiley, 1977.

46. Al-Shahristani H, Shihab KM. Variations of biological half life of methyl mercury in man. *Archives of environmental health*, 1974, 28: 342–345.

47. Houtman JPW et al. Arsenic levels of human hair as an indicator for environmental exposure. In: *Symposium on Nuclear Activation Techniques in the Life Sciences.* Vienna, International Atomic Energy Agency, 1979: 599–614.

48. Chattopadhyay A, Roberts TM, Jervis RE. Scalp hair as a monitor of community exposure to lead. *Archives of environmental health*, 1977, 32: 226–236.

49. Brockhaus A et al. Intake and health effects of thallium among a population living in the vicinity of a cement plant emitting thallium containing dust. *International archives of environmental health*, 1981, 48: 375–380.

50. Lauwerys RR, Buchet JP, Roels H. The relationship between cadmium exposure or body burden and the concentration of cadmium in blood and urine in man. *International archives of occupational and environmental health*, 1976, 36: 275–285.

51. Roels H et al. Comparison of renal function and psychomotor performance in

workers exposed to elemental mercury. *International archives of occupational and environmental health*, 1982, **50**: 77–93.

52. Buchet JP, Lauwerys R, Roels H. Comparison of several methods for the determination of arsenic compounds in water and in urine. Their application for the study of arsenic metabolism and for the monitoring of workers exposed to arsenic. *International archives of occupational and environmental health*, 1980, **46**: 11–29.

53. Brune D et al. Accumulation of heavy metals in tissue of industrially exposed workers. In: *Symposium on Nuclear Activation Techniques in the Life Sciences.* Vienna, International Atomic Energy Agency, 1978: 643–655.

54. Grandjean P. Monitoring of environmental exposures to toxic metals. In: Brown SS, Savory J, eds. *Chemical toxicology and clinical chemistry of metals.* London, Academic Press, 1983: 99–112.

55. Lundgren KD, Swensson A, Ulfvarson U. Studies in humans on the distribution of mercury in the blood and the excretion in urine after exposure to different mercury compounds. *Scandinavian journal of clinical and laboratory investigation*, 1967, **20**: 164–166.

56. Iyengar GV, Woittiez JRW. Trace elements in human clinical specimens: evaluation of literature data to identify reference values. *Clinical chemistry*, 1988, **34**: 474–481.

57. Hamilton EI. *Chemical elements and man*, Springfield, IL, Charles C. Thomas, 1979.

58. Heydorn K. *Neutron activation analysis in clinical trace element analysis.* Boca Raton, FL, CRC Press, 1984.

59. Minoia C et al. Trace element reference values in tissues from inhabitants of the European Community. *Science of the total environment*, 1990, **95**: 89–105.

22.

Assessment of dietary intakes of trace elements

22.1 Introduction

Observations of usual (or "habitual") dietary intakes of trace elements in different population groups are generally not directly useful for estimating requirements or safe ranges of population intakes. However, when the range of intakes occurring *naturally* is sufficiently wide for recognizable symptoms of deficiency or excess to be observed in at least some of the groups examined, useful information can be obtained from which the safe ranges of population intakes can be estimated. This has been the case, historically, for deficiencies of iodine, iron, selenium and zinc, and for excesses of arsenic, selenium and several other toxic elements.

Such considerations motivated the WHO Expert Committee in 1973 (*1*) to recommend further studies on dietary intakes of trace elements, and their relationships to the development of pathological changes. Since then, many such studies have been reported. The main purpose of the present chapter is to survey some of these reports of dietary intakes in different population groups, and to comment on their relationship to the safe ranges of population intakes now proposed.

During the preparation of this report, particular attention was paid to any obvious anomalies that emerged between reported intakes and the proposed lower and upper limits of the safe ranges of trace-element intakes under discussion. The details of this exercise are not presented here since only its outcome is of interest. Suffice it to say that there were important consequences for zinc. For example, surveys of dietary intake prompted the decision to set the CV of zinc intake at 25% (rather than 20%) for most age groups, a step which led on to a reappraisal of the evidence on dose/response relationships from studies of dietary differences in the bioavailability of zinc (see Chapter 5). Furthermore, the initial factorial estimates of the zinc requirements of females led to the obviously incorrect conclusion that lactating women consuming virtually any of the diets for which compositional and intake data were available would develop zinc deficiency. This anomaly, by prompting a reappraisal of the factors used to estimate requirements, suggested, for the first time, that postnatal reutilization of zinc from the resorbing maternal uterus and skeleton may reduce the need for zinc of dietary origin.

Before the data on actual dietary intakes in different population groups are reviewed, a brief description is given of some of the main methodologies employed. This will clarify understanding of the potential sources of uncertainty in estimates of dietary intake. Since it is hoped that this report may stimulate readers to conduct their own dietary surveys, this brief review may help to draw their attention to some of the factors to be taken into account in designing new studies.

22.2 Methods of assessing dietary intakes of trace elements

The protocol of every study should describe its objectives and how the population of individuals should be defined, their representatives selected and their food intakes sampled (e.g. by duplicate diets or market basket samples). Such important details are often ignored. For general guidance on this subject, the reader is referred to any of a number of standard texts (2–7).

Information on dietary intakes of trace elements by individuals or groups can be obtained either by direct methods based on the actual analysis of foods consumed or by indirect methods involving computation from standard food tables. This section reviews briefly some of the practical advantages and disadvantages of these methods; further details are given in references 2–7.

22.2.1 Direct methods based on food analyses

The direct analysis of food samples, identical to those consumed by individuals or groups over a period of time, can accurately predict the actual dietary intake of trace elements over that period. Two basic methodologies are currently used.

Duplicate portion or duplicate diet studies

Theoretically, the most accurate method for estimating trace element intakes is by the collection and careful analysis of an exact copy of the foods eaten, preferably weighed, to replicate the diet consumed by an individual. The duplicate portions are generally precisely weighed over a 24-hour period and this procedure is repeated over several such periods to allow an estimate of typical food intake to be made. Identical studies on several individuals are used to estimate group mean or population mean intakes.

Exact and repetitive weighing of a duplicate portion of diet by an active individual is arduous and may greatly change that individual's normal daily eating routine. Fewer foods may be consumed and individuals may change their usual eating pattern for ease of collection. They may choose more prepackaged items of known weight, eat more monotonously or restrict eating outside the home. Financial incentives result in individuals choosing more expensive items than usual or decreasing their normal intake for profit. How representative the portion collected will be depends on the motivation and interest of the subject and the careful explanation and monitoring of the study by the researcher. The technique is both time-consuming and expensive.

Since a duplicate diet study requires an invasive and detailed survey technique it is usually only possible for researchers to collect data on small samples. However, for the comparison of the average diets of particular population groups from particular areas, sample sizes of 20 or more individuals are preferable to facilitate statistical analyses of the data. For epidemiological studies it is always useful to collect at least three 24-hour duplicate portions to reflect daily variations in food choice. The population sample chosen should be a representative cross-section of individuals in that population, and be randomly selected where possible. Duplicate portions should always be weighed rather than estimated, and thought should be given to the effect that the collection of an extra food portion may have on the dietary practices of the individual studied.

Although literature describing the intrinsic validity of duplicate diet studies is scarce, it has been suggested that some underestimation (up to 20%) of the true intake may occur (8). However, when the study population is well defined and properly supervised, underestimation may be reduced to as little as 5–10%. It becomes more significant when the collection period exceeds 24 hours.

This technique is the method of choice for a number of trace elements for which food-table or past analytical data for individual foods are sometimes unreliable (e.g. arsenic, chromium, fluorine, mercury and lead) or usually unavailable (e.g. most minor and trace elements except calcium, chlorine, copper, iron, magnesium, manganese, phosphorus, potassium, selenium, sodium and zinc).

Total diet or market basket studies

In this technique a diet typical of a particular country, area or population group is constructed, and the foods are purchased and prepared for consumption before analysis. Methodology varies, but the construction of the diet is often based on reports on household food purchases or disappearance data for the population. To be of value, such reports should clearly indicate the number of individuals whose dietary patterns have been studied and must also account for meals consumed out of the household. Food is collected in a number of regions or areas as appropriate, and preparation and sampling are often centrally coordinated; the diets are prepared by standard methods. This method does not assess the variability of intakes by individuals or reveal extreme intakes, but provides a useful basis for the comparison of individual studies. If continued over an appreciable time it can expose trends in trace-element intake.

22.2.2 Indirect methods involving computation from food tables

For the study of nutrient intakes in large population groups, computation from an account of the food type and quantity consumed, using standard food tables, remains the most practical and cost-effective method. However, the nutrient-intake data estimated from dietary surveys will always be dependent on the quality and completeness of the food tables available. Tabulated data are often based on the analysis of pooled samples of foods intended to represent an average for a country or area, so that those prepared in one country are usually not appropriate for use in another. This is a particular problem for trace elements since their concentrations in some foods may be highly dependent on the geochemical environment, soil conditions and cultural practices in the regions in which they are grown.

Raw foods are often analysed as such and cooked food values then calculated; this can cause errors depending on whether cooking leads to trace-element contamination from utensils or the environment or, alternatively, to losses in cooking water; with selenium, losses may occur by thermal volatilization. The composition of manufactured foods may vary over time depending on the availability and cost of raw ingredients to manufacturers. Trace-element analysis of foods is rarely seen as a priority, and data may therefore often be unavailable. Values described as "not detectable" in food tables are often taken as zero, leading to a negative bias. Methods of sampling and food analysis can differ between reports.

Despite these problems, reasonable agreement on some average trace-element intakes can be reached, based on analysed and calculated nutrient intakes, particularly when the population size is large.

Methods of recording the type and quantity of foods consumed in a population include food balance sheets for recording the per capita food intake of large groups, and "recall" studies involving retrospective collection of data on foods consumed by individuals. Food frequency questionnaires compiled by experienced survey workers and self-conducted recording of personal consumption, weighed or unweighed, over periods typically between 3 and 7 days are other possible approaches. The advantages and disadvantages of the various methods have been described elsewhere (see, for example, reference 7).

The validity of dietary-intake studies can be monitored either by comparing the 24-hour excretion of urinary nitrogen or of electrolytes before and during the survey collection period or by comparing estimated energy intake with estimates of basal metabolic rate (*9*). Authors are strongly encouraged to report energy intake, and heights and weights of subjects when recording trace-element intakes, to facilitate appraisal of the validity of survey data.

22.2.3 Intakes from non-dietary sources

Water

In any properly designed study, intakes of trace elements in drinking-water are included as part of the assessment of total intake, and this is indeed true of most of the studies summarized in this section. Nevertheless, there may sometimes be reasons for wishing to make a separate assessment of intakes from drinking-water, e.g. when drinking-water composition is influenced strongly by local variables such as the geochemical characteristics of the rocks surrounding an aquifer, or by the "hardness" of the water supply and the type of water piping used locally. In such circumstances it may be much more difficult to obtain a representative sample of drinking-water than a representative total diet.

Very occasionally, trace elements in drinking-water can account for a major proportion of total element intake (see Table 22.1) (*10, 11*). More usually, they account for between 2% and 20% of intake (Table 22.1). Typically, water makes a significant contribution to the intakes of chromium, fluorine and lead. In some localities it may also provide a large additional contribution to the intakes of arsenic, cadmium, copper, mercury, selenium and zinc.

Air

For the majority of trace elements only negligible quantities are absorbed by breathing normal air. Higher concentrations of some toxic trace elements may be inhaled as a result of industrial exposure, although the amount inhaled may not correlate with the amount absorbed. Lead is the best documented trace element found in air; intakes of between 1.5 and 30 μg/day by inhalation have been estimated in rural and urban areas in the United Kingdom (*12*).

Soil

This can be ingested accidentally on unwashed fruit and vegetables or, in some parts of the world, deliberately, in the common habit known as geophagia. As considered in greater detail in Chapters 3 and 23, soil ingestion can inhibit the absorption of some trace elements (e.g. iron, zinc (*13*) and copper). In other circumstances, geophagia can make a significant contribution to trace-element nutrition, e.g. for copper, iron, manganese and zinc (*14*).

Table 22.1. Contribution of drinking-water to dietary intake of selected elements

Constituent	Concentration in water			Unit	Contribution to dietary intake (%)[d]		
	Typical[a]	Maximum[b]	Guideline value[c]		Typical	Maximum	Guideline value
Aluminium	0.1		0.2	mg/l	4		9
Arsenic	2	50	10 (P)	μg/l	10	238	48
Cadmium	1		3	μg/l	14		43
Chloride	20	179	250	mg/l	1	6	9
Chromium	5	112	50 (P)	μg/l	20	448	200
Copper	0.1	0.45	2 (P)	mg/l	13	60	267
Fluoride	0.3	7	1.5	mg/l	40	933	200
Iodine	5	18		μg/l	5	19	
Iron	0.3	2.2	0.3	mg/l	5	34	5
Lead	5		10	μg/l	19		37
Manganese	0.02	1.32	0.5 (P)	mg/l	1	85	32
Mercury	0.05		1	μg/l	2		43
Molybdenum	3	68	70	μg/l	5	113	117
Nickel	5	75	20	μg/l	7	100	27
Selenium	3	6.6	10	μg/l	10	22	33
Sodium	20	220	200	mg/l	1	13	11
Zinc	0.1	1.5	3	mg/l	2	30	60

[a] Typical concentrations of elements in drinking-water, as surmised from references reviewed in the WHO *Guidelines for drinking-water quality* (*10*).

[b] Maximum concentrations occurring in water supplies in the United States, as reported by the National Research Council (*11*).

[c] From the WHO *Guidelines for drinking-water quality* (*10*). Values for arsenic, cadmium, chromium, copper, fluoride, lead, manganese, mercury, molybdenum, nickel and selenium are guideline values representing upper limits of concentration based on *health criteria*. Values for aluminium, chloride, iron, sodium and zinc represent upper limits of concentration based on parameters that may give rise to *complaints from consumers*. Values marked "P" are provisional.

[d] Contribution to dietary intake assuming a consumption of water of 2 l/day. Values are expressed as a percentage of the median adult dietary intakes quoted in Table 22.2.

22.3 Interpretation of data on dietary trace-element intakes

Two main sources of uncertainty limit the value of dietary survey data as criteria for identifying pathologically relevant anomalies in trace-element supply, namely uncertainties in: (i) the estimates of usual (or "habitual") dietary intake; and (ii) the estimates of population requirements. Such doubts provide the principal justification for the view that observed relationships between trace-element supply and estimated requirement should never be used as the *sole* criteria by which the need for intervention is assessed. Such action should always be backed by additional evidence from biochemical, anthropometric or other indicators of pathological change.

The collection of accurate data on the usual trace-element intake of a population or group is not a simple task. In practice, many sources of variability affect the estimation of a mean population intake, including sampling errors and analytical errors of the kind discussed in Chapter 21, all of which may include systematic biases and random errors. Depending on the study design, there may also be components of variability reflecting the inter- and intrapersonal differences in food consumption during the study period. In practice, these different sources of variability have seldom been studied in detail for trace elements and are therefore commonly of unknown magnitude. However, even in the best of circumstances (when the investigator has studied all sources of variability exhaustively, and has minimized the most important), the uncertainty of the final estimate of a mean population intake derived from studies with an adequate sample size is rarely better than about $\pm 5\%$; it is often safer to assume $\pm 20\%$ (CV).

22.4 Observed dietary intakes of trace elements

22.4.1 Sources of information

The main source of information used here is a global literature survey and database prepared by IAEA (*15*) which focuses on dietary intake data reported during the last 20 years. Each value in the database is the mean value (or sometimes the median, if thus reported) of dietary intake for a particular element in a particular study group. The reports sometimes present data for "children" or "adults" without discriminating between the sexes; in others, the numbers of individual samples are not reported.

Preliminary results from an ongoing IAEA research programme (*16*) are included and reported separately since this was the only study known to the Expert Consultation in which all the samples, from a variety of different countries, have been collected and analysed by strictly comparable procedures and with careful attention to analytical quality control.

Irrespective of the above limitations, the raw data from those of the above-mentioned studies in which it is believed that reasonable standards of analytical quality control were met are summarized in Table 22.2, but this covers the intakes of adults only, irrespective of sex. Additional information on the intakes of copper, selenium and zinc for specific age groups and sexes is given in

Table 22.2. *Statistical summary of literature data[a] and IAEA data[b] on daily dietary intakes per adult person per day*

Element	No. of studies[c]	Percentile of intake[a]					IAEA study[b]		Unit
		0 (min.)	10	50 (median)	90	100 (max.)	Range	No. of studies[d]	
Aluminium	26	2.2	2.8	4.5	15	17	3.0–17	11	mg
Antimony	10	0.20	0.28	2.6	22	23			µg
Arsenic	28	3.0	7.6	42	170	330	3–160	11	µg
Barium	4	0.18		0.30		0.72			mg
Boron	8	1.3		1.6		3.7			mg
Bromine	10	2.3		4.0		7.8			mg
Cadmium	50	8.0	8.6	14	49	200	8–25	11	µg
Caesium	15	4.4	4.7	8.8	74	75			µg
Calcium	110	210	450	760	1200	1650	320–920	10	mg
Chlorine	10	3000		5670		13000	5340–13000	3	mg
Chromium	38	20	25	50	105	285	59–106	6	µg
Cobalt	22	6.2	6.6	15	39	43			µg
Copper	136	0.6	1.0	1.5	2.8	5.8	1.1–2.0	10	mg
Fluorine	15	0.4	0.5	1.5	3.4	3.5			mg
Iodine	37	0.05	0.08	0.19	0.34	1.05	0.05–0.26	10	mg
Iron	141	5.1	8.6	13	21	47	8.1–30	9	mg
Lead	54	7	25	54	175	510	21–160	11	µg
Lithium	6	22		38		107		10	µg
Magnesium	71	120	195	300	430	680	190–420		mg
Manganese	77	1.6	2.2	3.1	6.8	8.8	2.2–8.6	10	mg
Mercury	30	0.7	2.0	4.6	42	76	3–76	7	µg

Table 22.2 *(continued)*

Element	No. of studies[c]	Percentile of intake[a]					IAEA study[b]		Unit
		0 (min.)	10	50 (median)	90	100 (max.)	Range	No. of studies[d]	
Molybdenum	31	0.06	0.07	0.12	0.26	0.52	0.08–0.25	4	mg
Nickel	33	0.08	0.10	0.15	0.36	0.60	0.1–0.4	11	mg
Phosphorus	61	470	930	1300	1640	2010	630–1600	10	mg
Potassium	53	500	1930	2670	3780	4500	2300–3900	6	mg
Rubidium	21	1.2	1.4	2.2	6.0	7.0			mg
Scandium	11	0.11	0.12	0.38	2.0	2.2			μg
Selenium	85	8	23	60	130	1340	34–133	9	μg
Silver	3	4.5				7.1			μg
Sodium	42	1570	2020	3510	5630	6900	3500–6900	6	mg
Strontium	10	1.0		1.5		3.9			mg
Tin	7	0.10		0.65		2.4	0.1–1.6	4	mg
Vanadium	15	6.2	7.3	16	47	63	10–63	10	μg
Zinc	171	4.2	7.0	10	14	19	8.3–14	9	mg

[a] From IAEA (*15*); statistical summary of data for adults only (each data point being the mean or median of a study reported in the literature).

[b] From Parr et al. (*16*); range of country-median intakes normalized to 10 MJ of energy per day.

[c] No. of studies (n) in the IAEA literature survey (*15*); if $2 \leq n \leq 4$ then only the minimum and maximum values are quoted; if $5 \leq n \leq 10$ then only the minimum, median and maximum values are quoted; otherwise the minimum, 10th percentile, median, 90th percentile and maximum values are quoted.

[d] Each survey in the IAEA study is from a different country.

Table 22.3. Both tables incorporate data from the survey now being conducted by IAEA (*16*) and both summarize data from the entire IAEA database (*15*) irrespective of the sample sizes of the surveys for which the mean or median is reported. The data given represent *total* trace-element intakes and, while not making allowances for differences in trace-element bioavailability, they illustrate the following interesting features.

Of 38 studies in which chromium intake was monitored by carefully controlled analytical procedures, at least three indicated that the diets analysed were unlikely to supply enough of the element to meet probable requirements. Among elements for which very tentative estimates of basal requirements were offered, principally on the basis of studies with non-human species, intakes of nickel appeared lower than might be desirable in five of 40 dietary regimens. In addition, tentative estimates of a requirement for arsenic (page 218) suggest, implausibly, that 11 of 37 groups for which diets were sampled might not have received enough of this element, for which reasonable evidence of essentiality now exists from studies with experimental animals. The present estimates of

Table 22.3. Statistical summary, for selected elements and study groups, of daily dietary intakes per person per day

Element and group[b]	No. of studies[c]	0 (min.)	10	50 (median)	90	100 (max.)
		Percentile of intake[a]				
Zinc (mg)						
Children	39	4.1	4.9	7.9	13.0	22.3
Adults (unspecified)	62	4.2	6.8	10.0	15.0	16.4
Females	46	4.7	5.7	8.5	10.9	13.8
Pregnancy and lactation	17	7.9	8.1	9.6	12.9	13.4
Males	36	6.6	9.1	12.0	15.4	18.5
Vegetarians	10	7.6		9.5	14.9	15.0
All adults	171	4.2	7.0	10.0	14.3	18.5
IAEA study[d]	*9*	*8.3*		*10.0*		*14.0*
Selenium (μg)						
Children	12	19	19	54	120	130
Adults (unspecified)	54	8	25	60	145	1340
Females	14	22	23	58	105	130
Pregnancy and lactation	4	38		79		97
Males	10	36		71		215
Vegetarians	3	10				65
All adults	85	8	23	60	132	1340
IAEA study[d]	*9*	*34*		*61*		*133*

Table 22.3 (continued)

Element and group[b]	No. of studies[c]	Percentile of intake[a]				
		0 (min.)	10	50 (median)	90	100 (max.)
Copper (mg)						
Children	25	0.5	0.6	1.3	3.9	4.1
Adults (unspecified)	50	0.7	1.1	1.4	2.2	5.8
Females	35	0.6	0.8	1.3	2.0	3.6
Pregnancy and lactation	11	1.4	1.4	1.6	2.9	3.0
Males	30	0.8	1.0	1.7	2.7	4.8
Vegetarians	10	1.4		2.9		3.7
All adults	136	0.6	1.0	1.5	2.8	5.8
IAEA study[d]	*10*	*1.1*		*1.4*		*2.0*

[a] From IAEA (*15*); statistical summary of data for various population groups ranging in size from 2 to 6925 individuals (each data point being the mean or median of a study reported in the literature).

[b] "Adults (unspecified)" refers to adults in general but excludes studies in which adults were identified specifically as males, females, pregnant or lactating females, or vegetarian; data for children cover a wide age range and are therefore not strictly comparable.

[c] No. of studies (*n*) included in the literature survey (*15*); if $2 \leq n \leq 4$ then only the minimum and maximum values are quoted; if $5 \leq n \leq 10$ then only the minimum, median and maximum values are quoted; otherwise the minimum, 10th percentile, median, 90th percentile and maximum values are quoted.

[d] From Parr et al. (*16*), each data point being a country-median intake normalized to 10 MJ of energy intake per day; the number of countries reported is the number for which data are available from this IAEA study.

requirements for arsenic may well require revision in the light of future studies. Estimates of arsenic tolerance suggest that three of the 37 diets analysed contained undesirably high concentrations of arsenic, but the validity of this conclusion must be questioned in the absence of evidence as to the forms of the element present; certain organic derivatives of arsenic in food are relatively innocuous.

Among other elements usually noted for their potential toxicity, the IAEA database includes 24 estimates of fluoride intake, two of which significantly exceeded provisional estimates of tolerable intakes from water and diet. Corresponding relationships between the number of surveys in which the contents of lead, cadmium or mercury were found to be in excess of proposed upper tolerable limits are, for lead, 1/63; for cadmium, 1/60; and for mercury, 2/43.

Iron supply and the worldwide significance of its relationship to iron-deficiency anaemia have been considered in a separate report (*17*).

22.4.2 Relationships of observed dietary supply to proposed safe ranges of population mean intakes

Estimates of the safe ranges of population mean intakes have been derived for the specific purpose of interpreting data derived from carefully conducted surveys of dietary trace-element content. Use of the estimates for this purpose presupposes that the fractions of the populations sampled are truly representative with respect to age and sex distribution and, where relevant, to characteristic dietary habits and other social or ethnic parameters. Even when such criteria are met, it is prudent to set a lower limit of sample size when interpreting data for any specific group or population. It is suggested here, arbitrarily but not inflexibly, that such surveys should be based on data from at least 20 individuals if it is intended to compare the results with the estimates of acceptable population intakes described in this report. The relatively small number of studies that meet all these criteria for dietary intakes of zinc, copper or selenium in the comprehensive IAEA database are presented in Figures 22.1, 22.2 and 22.3, respectively, in which the mean values reported are shown as a percentage of the estimates of minimum mean population intakes likely to meet *normative* requirements for these elements. Data for each WHO region are plotted together.

These three diagrams show how few studies meet the criteria needed to assess population intakes of trace elements and their relationship to population requirements and tolerance, as well as the very uneven distribution of such studies between the different regions. There is a particular lack of relevant studies in regions where food preferences exist for diets from which zinc availability is liable to be low (Table 22.4 and Figure 22.1). The uneven geographical distribution of studies of copper and selenium intakes is equally regrettable. However, this is probably of less significance than in the assessment of the adequacy of zinc nutrition in that geographical differences in food preferences are less closely associated with the selection of foods differing in the bioavailability of copper and selenium than is true for zinc. Nevertheless, for virtually all the elements there is an urgent need for more precise information on the trace-element intakes of populations in developing countries and socially disadvantaged communities.

22.4.3 Trace-element supply and basal requirements of specific age groups

A summary of the medians and distributions of data for age-related intakes of zinc, copper and selenium in the entire IAEA database is presented in Table 22.3. Although statistically heterogeneous because of the wide range of sample sizes or the frequent absence of information on this factor, these data

Figure 22.1. Mean or median dietary intakes of zinc reported from surveys based on 20 or more individuals (from reference 15) and their relationships to estimates of population minimum intakes needed to meet normative requirements for zinc ($Zn_{Plmin}^{normative}$)

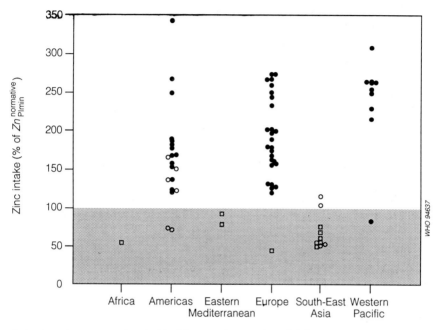

Estimates take account of probable differences in zinc bioavailability according to the dietary compositional criteria given in Table 5.5; availability categories: ● = high; ○ = moderate; □ = low. Data are for all ages and are grouped according to the WHO regions in which the studies were conducted.

have been examined with respect to the relationships between actual intakes and the estimates of population minimum acceptable mean intakes of specific age groups. Data for both sexes at different stages of development are presented as "box plots" (*18*) (for interpretation, see Figure 22.4); these summarize the range and distribution of median intakes from individual studies expressed as a percentage of the recommended minimum population mean intake needed to meet *basal* requirements of zinc, copper and selenium, as shown in Figures 22.5, 22.6 and 22.7 respectively.

Despite their statistical limitations, these diagrams show that, for zinc and copper, population intakes unlikely to meet basal requirements have been reported for most age groups considered in the IAEA database. The selenium intake of some ill-defined groups of adults also appears to be unsatisfactory but,

Figure 22.2. Mean or median dietary intakes of copper reported from surveys based on 20 or more individuals (from reference 15) and their relationships to estimates of population minimum mean intakes needed to meet normative requirements for copper (Cu$_{Plmin}^{normative}$)

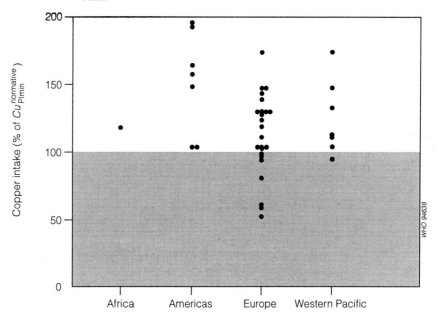

Data are for all ages and are grouped according to the WHO regions in which the studies were conducted. Data meeting the criteria for inclusion were not available for the Eastern Mediterranean or South-East Asia Regions.

regrettably, at the time of writing there were no data from areas where the selenium-responsive disorder, Keshan disease, exists in children (see Chapter 6).

22.5 Population intakes and normative minima

The limited evidence available from surveys defining population dietary intakes of zinc, copper and selenium and the estimates of the safe ranges of *normative* intakes of these elements are considered below. For the reasons indicated above, the discussion is confined to studies in the IAEA database in which the sex of subjects is defined (unless it is deemed irrelevant in the estimates of the tolerable range of intakes) and to the groups or "populations" surveyed that include 20 or more individuals.

Figure 22.3. Mean or median dietary intakes of selenium reported from surveys based on 20 or more individuals (from reference 15) and their relationships to estimates of population minimum mean intakes needed to meet normative requirements for selenium (Se$_{\text{PImin}}^{\text{normative}}$)

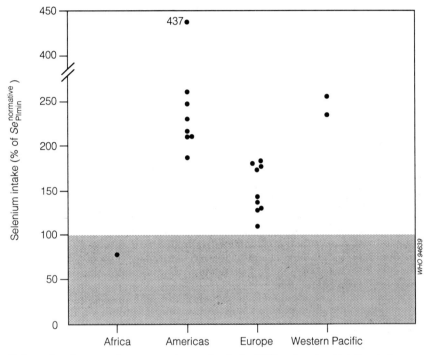

Data are for all ages and are grouped according to the WHO regions in which the studies were conducted. Data meeting the criteria for inclusion were not available for Eastern Mediterranean or South-East Asia Regions.

22.5.1 Zinc

The data for zinc presented in Figure 22.1 indicate that, of the studies in which mean population intakes fall below estimates of the minimum needed to meet normative requirements ($Zn_{\text{PImin}}^{\text{normative}}$), 14 out of 15 are associated with communities consuming diets from which dietary zinc was judged to be only moderately or poorly available according to the criteria outlined in Table 5.5, page 92. All were studies conducted either on subjects in developing countries or on immigrant communities originating from such countries. This finding adds urgency to the need already emphasized for additional surveys on an adequate scale and subject to proper analytical control in developing countries.

Table 22.4. Influence of assumed bioavailability of dietary zinc on the interpretation of zinc survey data[a]

Parameter	Assumed bioavailability of zinc[b]		
	High[c]	Moderate[d]	Low[e]
No. of surveys in category	148	47	15
Percentage with mean/median below Zn^{basal}_{PImin}	0	11	60
Percentage with mean/median below $Zn^{normative}_{PImin}$	1	40	100

[a] Derived from reference *15*; all available data are included irrespective of the number of individuals in the study.

[b] For the criteria used to categorize zinc bioavailability from the diet, see Table 5.5.

[c] Studies in this group were performed in the following countries (no. of studies in parentheses): Australia (2), Belgium (1), Brazil (1), Canada (9), Denmark (6), Finland (5), France (11), Germany (4), Italy (9), Netherlands (2), New Zealand (14), Poland (1), Spain (2), Sweden (11), Switzerland (2), United Kingdom (26), USA (40), former USSR (1) and former area of Yugoslavia (1).

[d] Studies in this group were performed in the following countries (no. of studies in parentheses): Brazil (2), Canada (4), China (4), India (8), Islamic Republic of Iran (1), Japan (10), Myanmar (2), Philippines (1), Sudan (1), Sweden (2), Thailand (3), Turkey (1), United Kingdom (3) and USA (5).

[e] Studies in this group were performed in the following countries (no. of studies in parentheses): India (2), Islamic Republic of Iran (2), Malawi (1), Morocco (1), Nigeria (2), Thailand (2) and Turkey (5).

Most mean or median intakes in the IAEA database refer to study groups in the developed regions of the world (mainly North America, Europe and Australasia), for which it is reasonable to assume that most diets contain zinc in highly available forms. These study groups appear to be at negligible risk of failing to meet their basal or normative requirements.

The important influence of the estimate of bioavailability assigned to dietary zinc on the interpretation of data from the full IAEA database is illustrated in Table 22.4. Thus, of the 148 diets predicted to contain zinc in a highly available form, only one would have failed to meet normative requirements. In contrast, diets with zinc in forms of moderate or low availability would have failed to meet basal requirements in 11% or 60% of cases, respectively. Despite the uncertainties mentioned earlier as to the precise geographical origins of the individuals under study, there are strong indications that suspected relationships between the geographical or ethnic origins of communities and their apparent propensity to consume diets from which the availability of zinc is either moderate or low warrant much closer study.

Figure 22.4. "Box and whisker" plot illustrating the relationship of the median and range of medians of all studies of population iodine intake reported in reference 15 to estimates of desirable minimum population mean intakes (see Table 6.5)

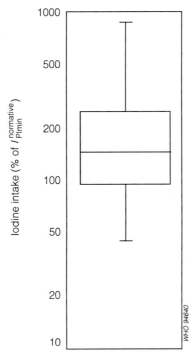

A "box and whisker" plot is a convenient graphical illustration of some of the main parameters of a set of data (18). It is particularly useful for representing data for which the nature of the underlying statistical distribution is unknown (as in Table 22.2, which deals with a mixture of means and medians, and the medians thereof). The values indicated in the figure are the maximum (875), upper quartile (252), median (158), lower quartile (90) and minimum (42) of the 43 values of the daily iodine intake (reported in reference 15) expressed as a proportion (%) of the minimum mean intake likely to meet normative requirements for iodine. The width of the box is proportional to $\sqrt{n}$ (where n is the number of mean or median values in each data set). The most "robust" value in a box plot is the median (i.e. this is the value in which the user can have the highest degree of confidence). A lesser degree of confidence applies to the 25th and 75th percentiles, particularly if these are not distributed symmetrically around the median. The lowest degree of confidence applies to the maximum and minimum values (since these could be statistical outliers caused by some unidentified problem in the design or execution of the project).

As with most other mammalian species, it is clear that differences in the availability of zinc from human diets are likely to have as important an influence on the adequacy of zinc nutrition as will changes in the total intake of zinc. It is not yet possible to define in quantitative terms how the risks of development of

Figure 22.5. Ranges of mean/median dietary intakes of zinc reported for all surveys recorded in the IAEA database (15) and their relation to minimum mean intakes needed to meet basal requirements (Zn_{Plmin}^{basal}) of specific age groups (for interpretation, see Figure 22.4)

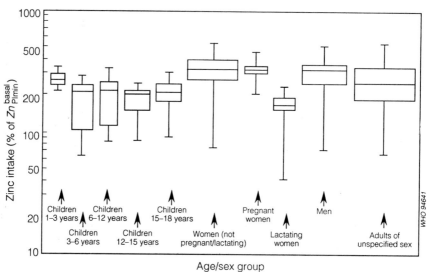

Figure 22.6. Ranges of mean/median dietary intakes of copper reported for all surveys recorded in the IAEA database (15) and their relation to minimum mean intakes needed to meet basal requirements (Cu_{Plmin}^{basal}) of specific age groups (for interpretation, see Figure 22.4)

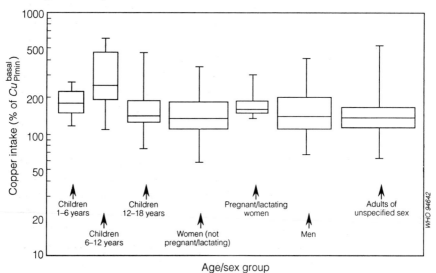

Figure 22.7. Ranges of mean/median dietary intakes of selenium reported for all surveys recorded in the IAEA database (15) and their relation to minimum mean intakes needed to meet basal requirements (Se$_{Plmin}^{basal}$) of specific age groups (for interpretation, see Figure 22.4)

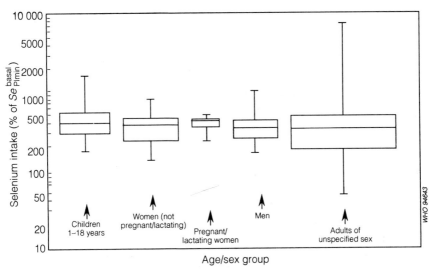

zinc deficiency are influenced by dietary composition. However, low zinc absorption is to be expected when the phytate/zinc molar ratio exceeds 15 (other studies quoted in Chapter 3 suggest that adverse effects might develop if the ratio exceeds 5) or if the ratio Ca × phytate/Zn is greater than 150 mmol/1000 kcal. In the current IAEA study (15), values for all three analytes are available for population groups in 10 countries. In three (China, the Islamic Republic of Iran and Sudan) the phytate/zinc molar ratios are approximately 10, and the Ca × phytate/Zn ratios are of the order of 60–70 mmol/1000 kcal. While such values are not conclusive evidence of a nutritional problem, they indicate a need for care in avoiding further dietary increases in potential antagonists of zinc utilization (see Chapter 3).

Although requirements are greatly increased during growth and may increase in women during lactation, there does not generally seem to be an increased risk of failing to meet the relevant basal requirements in the segments of the population concerned (Figure 22.5). However, most studies show mean intakes of available zinc below the proposed minimum basal mean values in developing countries and, in such situations, children and lactating women are probably at greatest risk of failing to meet their basal requirements.

It is emphasized that no account has been taken of differences in body weight between populations in different countries. Indian "standard man", for example, has a body weight of only 50 kg (*19*) compared with the 65 kg assumed throughout this report. However, even if this factor is taken into account, it is unlikely to affect the conclusion that zinc nutrition in developing countries should be a priority area for future research. In such countries there is obviously a dearth of reliable information, not only on zinc intakes and bioavailability (including the distribution of usual intakes), but also on the dietary concentrations of potential antagonists or promoters of absorption, such as protein, phytate and calcium.

22.5.2 Copper

Relationships between survey data for dietary intakes of copper and estimates of $Cu_{\text{PImin}}^{\text{normative}}$ are illustrated in Figure 22.2, in which again the only evidence from the IAEA database that is included is derived from studies containing more than 20 individuals of defined sex. The scarcity of adequately planned studies is again evident, with insufficient data from Africa, the Eastern Mediterranean and South-East Asia. The apparently higher proportion of European studies suggesting undesirably low population mean intakes of copper needs to be investigated more closely to determine whether it is a truly characteristic feature of diets of the eastern German communities from which these particular samples were drawn. Before it is concluded that intakes of copper are likely to be reasonably adequate in the Americas, the western Pacific fringe and the remainder of Europe, it must be strongly emphasized that none of the surveys covered in Figure 22.2 were representative of those socially and nutritionally disadvantaged communities in which food preferences lead to the consumption of diets providing as little copper as those reported to induce clinical signs of deficiency elsewhere (see Chapter 7). More extensive sampling of such communities is desirable.

When all the IAEA data are considered, approximately 10% of reported mean intakes are below the proposed minimum basal mean $(Cu_{\text{PImin}}^{\text{basal}})$ and approximately 25% are below the corresponding minimum normative mean population intake $(Cu_{\text{PImin}}^{\text{normative}})$. Intakes five times higher than the basal minimum mean are observed in some population groups, but these are still well below the upper limit of the safe range of mean population intake $(Cu_{\text{PImax}}^{\text{tox}})$ (12 mg/day for men) and there is no evidence from the IAEA database that the copper intake from diets for young children is sufficiently high to cause concern in the communities studied.

Vegetarian mean intakes of copper appear to be twice as high as those of omnivores (Table 22.3), or even higher. In view of the uncertainties that exist in estimating dietary intakes and requirements for copper (Chapter 7), it cannot yet be concluded that copper deficiency is a significant nutritional problem in any specific region of the world or segment of the population. However, many of the reported mean intakes are sufficiently close to Cu_{PImin}^{basal} to justify further studies of this issue (see Chapters 7 and 23).

22.5.3 Selenium

The geographical coverage of surveys of selenium intake is even less complete than those for the other elements considered. For example, if, as recommended, consideration of the population mean is restricted to samples containing not less than 20 individuals, the IAEA database includes no reference to population mean intakes of selenium in areas where the selenium-responsive cardiomyopathy of Keshan disease is endemic. The failure to investigate selenium intakes over substantial regions of the world is regrettable. However, the picture emerging from Figure 22.3 strongly supports other evidence that, for geochemical reasons, the contents of selenium in staple crops (e.g. of cereals) in North America is often significantly higher than in those in Europe. Thus, it is particularly unfortunate that representative analyses of selenium intakes are not available for many of the developing countries in Africa, South-East Asia, and the Eastern Mediterranean, in many of which the geochemical characteristics do not favour selenium accumulation.

Despite the absence of reports from major surveys, it is known that selenium intakes can be highly variable from one region to another, particularly in China, which contains regions where the intakes from indigenous crops can be either very high or very low. Data from Finland are also variable, and include results from studies conducted before and after the introduction of a policy to increase selenium intake by measures which have included the importation of selenium-rich North American cereal grains and the fortification of fertilizers with selenium. Fewer than 5% of the studies included in the full IAEA database report mean values below the estimate of the basal population minimum (Se_{PImin}^{basal}) and only 20% mean values below the proposed minimum normative population mean ($Se_{PImin}^{normative}$). No particular age group or sex appears to be especially at risk (Table 22.3). Most of the low intakes reported were from countries already known to have soils of low selenium content or availability (e.g. New Zealand, Sweden and some regions of China). Only one sample had a selenium content exceeding the proposed Se_{PImax}^{tox} (400 μg/day) for adults, namely a composite sample of diets taken from an area in China where human selenosis was known to be endemic (20).

For most developing countries, reliable data on selenium nutrition are still not available. Additional dietary surveys in these countries would be useful to help to identify population groups at risk of deficient or excessive intake. It would be prudent to include the measurements of iodine intake in such surveys in view of growing evidence of the role of selenium in iodine utilization (see Chapter 3).

22.5.4 Iodine

In the light of the geographically widespread clinical evidence of the significance of iodine-related diseases, it is remarkable that relatively few studies of population intakes of iodine have been conducted. The entire set of survey data in the IAEA database is represented diagrammatically in Figure 22.4. In even fewer studies has an attempt been made to relate population intakes to the incidence and severity of pathological manifestations of iodine deficiency or excess.

Without doubt, this situation reflects the frequently unequivocal clinical manifestations of at least one form of iodine deficiency (thyroid hyperplasia) and the fact that iodine status is so readily assessed by means of measurements of urinary iodine output and the plasma activity of thyroid-stimulating hormone. Furthermore, all these criteria are of value for the monitoring of responses to the administration of iodine supplements (e.g. of iodized salt) or injections (e.g. iodized poppyseed oil) (see Chapter 4).

The success of these approaches has reduced the priority given to quantitative investigation of the factors governing the absorption, utilization and excretion of iodine. The scarcity of such data has made it impossible to obtain estimates of the minimum tolerable population basal intakes of iodine, nor has it proved feasible to quantify the influence of characterized dietary goitrogens on iodine requirements. While these limitations have been relatively insignificant from the point of view of attempting to detect and eliminate overt manifestations of severe deficiency, they are assuming greater importance in efforts to clarify the significance of the wider range of covert pathological manifestations of deficiencies that are now being identified and to define the distribution of marginal deficiencies, particularly those associated with intakes of goitrogens and with concurrent depletion of selenium reserves (see Chapters 4 and 6).

22.6 Conclusions

Measurements of dietary intake are not in themselves sufficient to provide a reliable assessment of nutritional health with respect to trace elements; however, they do give some guidance as to whether or not existing intakes are adequate to maintain health in already healthy individuals. Data of this kind can also help to identify regions, or segments of a population, in which dietary intakes of trace elements are excessively high or low.

For nearly all of the elements discussed in detail here, data on dietary intakes provide evidence of unacceptably low trace-element intakes in at least some population groups. Previously, only a handful of trace elements (namely fluorine, iodine, iron and selenium) have been recognized as being of wide-spread public health significance from a nutritional standpoint. Now, genuine concern arises as to the necessity of adding zinc to this list, especially for population groups in developing countries consuming diets from which zinc is of low bioavailability.

Since there is an almost complete lack of reliable data on trace-element intakes in most developing countries, large gaps exist in the knowledge of this important aspect of nutrition in much of the world's population. Obviously, this important issue needs to be addressed in future research. However, it is not only in the developing countries that new data are needed. Nutritional habits and lifestyles are changing practically everywhere. In developed countries, the trend is towards reduced energy intake, leading possibly to changes in trace-element status (21). Obviously, it would be wise to keep this situation under review.

Priority topics for future research include: (i) studies of the relationships between biochemical, functional and immunological indices of trace-element status on the one hand and dietary trace-element intake on the other; (ii) further analyses of trace elements in individual foods, and in water supplies, to improve the reliability of assessments of trace-element intake by indirect methods; (iii) studies of the effects of meal composition and nutrient–nutrient interaction on trace-element absorption and utilization; (iv) further investigation of trace-element intakes in regions, or segments of the population, in which intakes of essential elements appear to be below normative requirements; and (v) similar investigation in regions, or segments of the population, in which intakes have so far not been assessed—particularly in developing countries.

References

1. *Trace elements in human nutrition. Report of a WHO Expert Committee.* Geneva, World Health Organization, 1973 (WHO Technical Report Series, No. 532).
2. Marr JW. Individual dietary surveys: purposes and methods. *World review of nutrition and diet*, 1971, 13: 105–114.
3. Bingham S. The dietary assessment of individuals. Methods, accuracy, new techniques and recommendations. *Nutrition abstracts and reviews, Series A*, 1987, 57: 705–742.
4. Macdonald I, ed. *Monitoring dietary intakes.* Berlin, Springer-Verlag, 1991.
5. Basiotis PP et al. Number of days of food intake records required to estimate

individual and group nutrient intakes with defined confidence. *Journal of nutrition*, 1987, **117**: 1638–1641.

6. National Research Council. Nutrient adequacy: assessment using food consumption surveys. Washington, DC, National Academy Press, 1986.

7. Gibson RS. *Principles of nutritional assessment.* New York, Oxford University Press, 1990.

8. Errors in reporting habitual energy intake. *Nutrition reviews*, 1991, **49**: 215–217.

9. Goldberg GR et al. Critical evaluation of energy intake data using fundamental principles of energy physiology. I. Derivation of cut-off limits to identify under-recording. *European journal of clinical nutrition*, 1991, **45**: 569–581.

10. *Guidelines for drinking-water quality*, 2nd ed. *Volume 1. Recommendations. Volume 2. Health criteria and other supporting information.* Geneva, World Health Organization, Vol. 1 1993; Vol. 2 in press.

11. National Research Council, Safe Drinking Water Committee. The contribution of drinking water to mineral nutrition in humans. In: *Drinking water and health*, Vol. 3. Washington, DC, National Academy Press, 1980, Chapter 5.

12. Ministry of Agriculture, Fisheries and Food. *Survey of lead in food.* London, HMSO, 1982 (Food Surveillance Paper No. 10).

13. Cardar AO et al. Geophagia in Turkey: iron and zinc deficiency, iron and zinc absorption studies in response to treatment with zinc in geophagia cases. In: Prasad A et al., eds. *Zinc deficiency in human subjects.* New York, Alan R. Liss, 1983: 71–97.

14. Johns T, Duquette M. Detoxification and mineral supplementation as functions of geophagy. *American journal of clinical nutrition*, 1991, **53**: 448–456.

15. Parr RM et al. *Human dietary intakes of trace elements: a global literature survey mainly for the period 1970–1991: data listings and references.* Vienna, International Atomic Energy Agency, 1992 (Report IAEA-NAHRES-12).

16. Parr RM et al. Dietary intakes of trace elements and related nutrients in eleven countries: preliminary results from an IAEA co-ordinated research programme. In: Momcilovic B, ed. *Trace elements in man and animals—TEMA 7.* Zagreb, University of Zagreb, 1991: 13-3–13-5.

17. *Requirements of vitamin A, iron, folate and vitamin B_{12}.* Rome, Food and Agriculture Organization of the United Nations, 1988 (Food and Nutrition Series No. 23).

18. McGill R, Tukey JW, Larsen WA. Variations of boxplots. *American statistician*, 1978, **32**: 12–16.

19. *Compilation of anatomical, physiological and metabolic characteristics for a reference Asian man.* Vienna, International Atomic Energy Agency, 1991 (Report IAEA-JR-RC-451).

20. Yang G et al. Studies of safe maximal daily dietary selenium intakes in a seleniferous area in China. *Journal of trace elements and electrolytes in health and disease*, 1989, **3**: 77–86.

21. Pietrzik K, ed. *Modern lifestyles: lower energy intake and micronutrient status.* London, Springer-Verlag, 1991.

23.

Detection and anticipation of the risks of development of trace-element-related disorders

Trace-element-related disorders can be detected by a comparison of dietary analyses with estimates of the tolerable ranges of trace-element intakes, but only when this approach is supported by an adequate understanding of the other variables that influence risk. In this chapter, the principal factors that modify susceptibility to such disorders are briefly considered and the influence of environmental conditions on trace-element supply outlined. The limitations of existing diagnostic criteria are reviewed and the importance emphasized of drawing on evidence derived from a wide variety of lines of enquiry if nutritional disorders are to be identified more effectively.

Relationships between abnormalities in trace-element supply and suboptimal human health are often difficult to recognize. None the less they should always be considered when seeking the causes of disorders which may have nutritional origins. Although exposures to substantial excesses of the anionic trace elements fluorine, iodine and selenium are readily identified from characteristic clinical features, the clinical signs of marginal deficiencies or excesses of other trace elements are usually non-specific and less obvious.

As shown in summary in Table 23.1, deficiencies of a number of trace elements share many pathological features. As with the effects of other nutrient deficiencies and imbalances on health, the tissues with the most rapid turnover and highest metabolic activities are those most susceptible to anomalies in trace-element supply. Linear growth, cellular and humoral immunity, haematopoiesis, reproduction, and the turnover of the gastrointestinal mucosa and skin are therefore particularly affected. The fact that they are also susceptible to deficiencies of most other nutrients and many disease processes complicates the unequivocal identification of the trace-element-related components of nutritional diseases that are the consequence of a multiplicity of deficiencies. Clinical features alone may be insufficient to identify the nutrients involved in such situations. It is emphasized here that consideration of the circumstances known to modify the risks of development of trace-element-related effects on health can contribute to their identification under these conditions.

Table 23.1. Pathological effects of essential-trace-element deficiencies in human subjects and animal models [a]

Pathological effect	Iodine	Zinc	Copper	Selenium	Chromium	Molybdenum
Growth retardation	+	+	+	±	±	−
Anaemia	±	±	+	±	−	−
Integumental lesions	+	+	+	±	−	−
Impaired immunity	+	+	+	+	−	−
Intestinal/ pancreatic "atrophy"	?	+	+	±	−	−
Hepatic necrosis	−	−	±	+	−	−
Cardiac functional changes	+	−	+	+	−	−
Reproductive disturbance	+	+	+	±	?	?
Neurological defects	+	+	+	−	−	+
Skeletal lesions	−	+	+	−	−	−

[a] + = prominent effect; ± = marginal or needing confirmation; − = not reported.

23.1 Predisposing factors

The risks of development of trace-element-related health defects are aggravated by factors that increase susceptibility to many other nutritional problems (see Table 23.2). Although each pathogenic category listed in Table 23.1 is important, their relative significance as causes of disease not only differs between elements but reflects the influence of social and ethnic differences in dietary composition on trace-element bioavailability.

The task assigned to the Expert Consultation was to define the trace-element requirements and tolerances of normal (i.e. healthy) populations. However, this must not be allowed to obscure the probability that the complex interaction of factors involved in the etiology of undernutrition syndromes is frequently responsible for the development of trace-element deficiencies (1).

Clinical signs of concurrent trace-element deficiency may not be obvious in untreated cases of undernutrition. Since the individuals concerned are in a catabolic state, appreciable amounts of trace elements may be mobilized from

Table 23.2. Factors increasing susceptibility to development of trace-element-responsive disease

Factor	Elements depleted
Inadequate dietary intake/low absorbability of element	
Some vegetable-based diets	Zinc
Incorrectly formulated therapeutic and synthetic diets (e.g. for enteral and parenteral nutrition, diets for management of inborn errors of metabolism)	Copper, chromium, molybdenum, selenium, zinc
Intestinal infections (bacteria, protozoa, helminths)	Zinc
Nutrient interactions with dietary components and drugs	Copper, iodine, zinc
Systemic defects in element absorption and utilization	
Selective inborn errors of metabolism (including copper excess in Wilson disease, Indian childhood cirrhosis)	Copper, molybdenum, zinc
Maldigestion:	
After surgery: gastric and intestinal resection	Zinc
Gastric atrophy	Zinc
Inflammatory bowel disease	Zinc
Exocrine pancreatic insufficiency ⎫ Enteropathies ⎭	Copper, zinc
Increased loss	
Catabolic states, protein-losing enteropathies	Copper, zinc
Renal failure, renal dialysis, and diuretic therapy	Chromium, zinc
Chronic blood loss and haemolysis	Zinc
Chelating agents (specific and non-specific)	Copper, zinc
Exfoliative dermatoses	Zinc
High physical activity	Chromium
Increased demand	
Preterm neonates; infancy; childhood; adolescence	Copper, zinc
Pregnancy and lactation; rapid tissue synthesis; postcatabolic convalescence	Copper, chromium, selenium, zinc

the breakdown of body tissues (e.g. muscle) and from the loss of bone mass. Reutilization of these adventitiously released elements, which are otherwise lost from the body, may preserve trace-element-dependent functions in other tissues during "adaptation" to undernutrition. However, once the causes of catabolism (e.g. infections) have been removed and the supply of energy and other major nutrients becomes sufficient to initiate recovery (2), the need for many trace elements and other micronutrients for the synthesis of new tissue increases. Breakdown of 1 g (wet weight) of muscle releases about 50 μg of zinc, 1 μg of copper, 0.1 μg of manganese and 0.1 μg of selenium. During rehabilitation, this catabolic release of trace elements from tissues ceases, and the patient, usually a child, must then depend on adequate exogenous supplies of these elements both to restore tissue reserves and to meet additional requirements for the synthesis of new tissue. Thus, as with the intracellular cations magnesium and potassium, it is during the anabolic phase of recovery that the undernourished child is most vulnerable to specific trace-element deficiencies.

This has been well demonstrated in Jamaica, where undernourished, oedematous children have been shown to absorb zinc poorly (3). However, in convalescent undernourished children, zinc supplements have reduced the energy cost of weight gain (4, 5), improved the healing of cutaneous ulcers (6), reversed thymic atrophy (7), and restored sodium transport across the cell membranes of leukocytes *in vitro* (8). Other reports indicate that zinc supplements have improved weight gain in similar convalescent children in Bangladesh (9) and Chile (10).

While these situations develop because of the increased demand for zinc during rehabilitation, other deficiencies reflect inadvertent therapeutic use either of foods intrinsically low in specific trace elements or of foods from which they have been removed during the refining process. Thus, copper deficiency has developed during the nutritional rehabilitation of malnourished children in Chile (11) and Peru (12); in the former, those who received copper supplements maintained their plasma copper concentrations, had fewer respiratory tract infections and gained weight more rapidly (11, 13). Problems resulting from selenium (14) and chromium (15) deficiency may also arise in such children, but have been less extensively described.

Impaired immunity secondary to trace-element deficiencies (e.g. of copper, selenium and zinc) possibly contributes to the detrimental synergism between infection and undernutrition (16–18). In particular, infective diarrhoea increases the loss of endogenous copper and zinc (19), and it has been reported that oral zinc supplements shorten the duration of infective diarrhoea in young children (20).

23.2 Detection

23.2.1 Health surveillance

Surveillance of the health and nutrient status of the population (21) can reveal problems which reflect the impact of trace-element supply on health. Such studies tend to focus on particularly vulnerable groups such as neonates, infants, other growing children and adolescents, and pregnant and lactating women.

The strategy of nutritional surveillance depends on the monitoring of statistics on infant and child mortality, the height of children at school entry, maternal mortality, the prevalence of low birth weight, life expectancy, and, where possible, psychomotor development and nutritional status (21). Any problem thus identified needs to be further analysed by characterizing the types of malnutrition, the groups affected and the potential causes, such as socio-economic factors and the nature of the food consumed. As indicated in Table 23.1, abnormalities in the supply of several elements can have one or more pathological effects. An outstanding example is provided by the multiplicity of effects of iodine deficiency. The public health implications of deficiencies or excesses of many other trace elements have not yet been adequately explored.

23.2.2 Surveys of reproductive efficiency

Surveys of reproductive efficiency tend to focus on birth weight. However, the range of reproductive failures that result from abnormalities of nutrient supply also includes sexual dysfunction, chromosomal abnormalities of germ cells, sperm abnormalities, subfecundity, maternal illness during pregnancy, early and late fetal death, intrapartum and neonatal death, intrauterine growth retardation, altered sex ratios, multiple births, congenital structural or func-tional abnormalities (e.g. psychomotor retardation), infant death, infant morbidity, and possibly childhood malignancy (22). The importance of appreci-ating the variety of these potential outcomes is emphasized by the occurrence of nearly all of them in at least one human trace-element deficiency, namely iodine-deficiency disorders (see Chapter 4). Comparative studies of a range of element deficiencies and toxicities in domestic livestock and experimental animal models (23, 24) point to their importance in many species.

Thus, the incidence of congenital anomalies and neonatal deaths in pigs and poultry is high in the endemic selenium toxicosis area of Enshi Province, China (25). However, it is not clear whether human reproduction is similarly affected either in this area or in the seleniferous zones of the USA (26) and Venezuela (27). Similarly, little has been reported on possible reproductive anomalies in women living in regions where selenium deficiency is endemic in other species.

Excessive exposure to aluminium, arsenic, cadmium, lead, lithium, man-ganese, mercury, selenium or zinc can cause fetal death and congenital abnor-malities in animal models (24). However, the exposure required to produce such effects is seldom achieved in human experience except in industrial environments, or when bioconcentration of a toxic element occurs. The latter is typified by the occurrence of mercury poisoning around Minamata Bay,

Japan, where methylmercury generated by pollution of the marine food chain was ingested by humans and their livestock. This and other problems associated with environmental contamination with mining or industrial effluents (28, 29) or the consumption of seed grain treated with a mercurial pesticide (29) are reviewed in Chapter 16. The potential risks associated with agricultural practices leading to the entry of toxic elements into the food chain can be minimized by legislation regulating the disposal of such metal-rich wastes on soil and by suggesting limits on the consumption of liver, kidneys and other offal derived from animals grazing on contaminated areas (29).

The results of experiments on animal models suggest that the trace-element deficiencies most likely to affect human reproduction are those of copper, iodine, selenium and zinc. Geographical regions where these deficiencies are endemic in livestock are therefore appropriate areas in which to seek analogous effects on human reproduction. Such considerations justify the speculation, for example, that in western Asia and Turkey the occurrence of anencephaly together with an endemic undernutrition syndrome involving zinc deprivation may indicate a causal relationship with maternal zinc deficiency (24).

23.2.3 Monitoring of infant and child health and growth

Infants might be suspected to be particularly susceptible to deficiencies of most trace elements. However, with the exception of some cases of zinc deficiency in breast-fed infants aged about 3 months (30), and of copper deficiency in 6–9-month-old infants fed inappropriately on unmodified cow's milk, in some instances supplemented with honey (31, 32), trace-element deficiencies have not been unequivocally recognized in otherwise healthy, full-term infants. Although the absolute concentrations of copper, manganese and zinc in human milk decline with increasing duration of lactation (33), this does not seem to cause nutritional problems, and human breast milk is clearly the most appropriate food for full-term infants (34). In contrast, preterm low-birth-weight infants are at risk of copper (31) and zinc (30) deficiency. The many problems involved in feeding the low-birth-weight and/or preterm infant have been recently reviewed elsewhere (34).

Although the bioavailability of trace elements from soya-based infant formulae is less than that from formulae based on cow's milk or from human breast milk, no trace-element-related clinical problems have yet been attributed to the consumption of appropriately fortified formulae (35). Despite this, there are no published systematic data from which to estimate the quantitative or qualitative consequences of modifying the trace-element supply to infants by replacing maternal milk by milk or milk products derived from other species.

The importance of trace-element deprivation in the complex etiology of growth faltering encountered in weanlings and preschool children merits closer investigation. Growth retardation was a feature of the earliest reports of zinc deficiency in association with less severe undernutrition syndromes (36), and the potential contribution of this and other trace-element deprivations to "stunting" syndromes has recently been reviewed (37). As indicated in Chapter 5, this problem is not restricted to developing countries, as demonstrated by the beneficial effects of zinc supplements on the linear growth and weight gain of some short-statured children in Denver, USA (38) and Guelph, Canada (39).

It has been assumed that the reduced stature of children and adults at high altitudes represents a genetic trait or an adaptational response secondary to low ambient temperatures and oxygen pressure. However, leaching of soils in these areas exposed to heavy rainfall would reduce the content, in particular, of copper, iodine, selenium and zinc. Thus, for example, endemic iodine-deficiency diseases and selenium deficiency are more prevalent in mountainous areas, and it seems possible that, in such areas, other trace elements may be limiting (40).

23.2.4 Use of diagnostic criteria of deficiency and toxicity

Ideal clinical and biochemical criteria from which to assess whether the intake of specific trace elements is sufficient to influence the risks of deficiency or toxicity have yet to be developed. In their absence, it is generally assumed, or hoped, that the composition of physically and ethically accessible body fluids and tissues faithfully reflects trace-element "status". Blood or plasma is frequently selected for trace-element analysis but with equally frequent disregard of the difficulty of assessing the physiological relevance of the results.

Ease of access to a tissue for purposes of sampling and precise analysis is no guarantee of the metabolic and pathological relevance of the results. Furthermore, since tissues respond differently to deficiency or excess of specific elements, the detection of pathologically significant anomalies may well require the use of tissues other than blood or liver (41).

Single measurements of plasma trace-metal (e.g. copper, zinc) concentrations are of limited value as criteria of trace-element "status" because of their susceptibility to a wide variety of pathophysiological changes. Typical examples are the marked increase in plasma copper and the decrease in plasma iron and zinc during the acute phase of responses to infection or stress. The use of hair as the sole indicator of copper and zinc intakes or deficiencies is not technically difficult but, because of frequent failure to characterize the variables influencing the growth patterns of hair and because of the risks of adventitious contamination, such data are difficult to interpret for individual subjects (42, 43). Carefully controlled, the technique may, however, be useful in population studies of chronic exposure.

The invasive character of muscle or liver tissue sampling for the study of their trace-element content clearly limits their suitability for population studies. Furthermore, their trace-element contents may merely reflect changes secondary to disturbances in the tissue content of other nutrients (44). Analyses of leukocyte pellets as functional and compositional criteria of trace-element status offer an approach that frequently cannot be exploited because of failure to take into account the variation in the elemental content of white cell subsets, each differing in age and half-life and thus in their historical experience of changes in trace-element status. The proportions of such subsets also change in response to disease or physiological development. Compositional analyses of leukocytes and discrete leukocyte subsets were found to be of particular value in at least one clinical situation (undernutrition) where elemental supplementation was beneficial (9).

23.2.5 Dietary surveys

The value of dietary surveys and food composition tables is limited (45) because few provide complete data for the trace elements of particular interest (copper, iodine, selenium, zinc and possibly chromium fluoride, manganese and molybdenum). Many composition tables do not cover an adequate range of representative foodstuffs for populations with a diversified diet. Data for the staple foods of many developing countries are scarce, and little or no account is taken of the variable influence of environmental and cultural conditions on the trace-element content of foods.

It may appear commendable to establish more comprehensive databases of dietary trace-element intake for populations likely to be at risk — in, for example, socially disadvantaged communities or populations in developed countries subsisting on a restricted range of foods. However, the value and purpose of such an exercise should be critically assessed before it is undertaken. Success is contingent not only on the availability of expensive analytical equipment and expertise but also on the feasibility of interpreting the data obtained. This applies particularly to the cationic elements (e.g. iron and zinc), for which assessments of element intake alone say nothing about the bioavailability of the particular mineral. To gauge this, even approximately, additional information on the dietary content and biological effects of constituents antagonizing or facilitating trace-element utilization is essential.

The interpretation of comparisons of intake data with estimates of requirements should take into account the quality of the data from which the requirements were estimated, and the precise physiological and statistical limitations governing their applicability. These matters are considered in the sections of this report dealing with individual elements.

For all these reasons, single analyses of diets, like single assays of the functional activity of metabolic systems, are inappropriate indices of possible trace-element deprivation. While repeated analyses indicating compositional or functional anomalies add certainty to the diagnosis, an unequivocal diagnosis is rarely achieved without careful monitoring of metabolic, functional or clinical responses to supplementation.

23.3 Soil and geochemical factors

Variables modifying the trace-element content of foods or of drinking-water can profoundly influence the risk that anomalies in trace-element intake may be sufficient to cause diseases attributable to deficiency or excess. In general, urban communities, which usually obtain their foods and sometimes their water supplies from a variety of geographical sources, are less likely to be exposed to such risks than rural communities relying heavily on locally grown crops as constituents of diets consisting of a limited number of food items. Such limitations on the range and geographical origins of staple foods and water markedly increase the effect of the composition of the rocks and soils in an area on the entry of trace elements into food chains or into drinking-water collected from surface sources or artesian wells.

Examples of geochemical and soil variables likely to influence significantly the trace-element intake of rural populations are given in Table 23.3. The examples given are not exhaustive, but they do illustrate the following points:

- The geochemical composition of rocks from which some soils are derived can influence, directly or indirectly, both the balance of elements within those soils and the trace-element content of food crops. Regional deficiencies of chromium, copper, iodine, iron, selenium and zinc and excesses of arsenic, cadmium, fluoride, lead and selenium arise from such causes.
- Differences in soil moisture and acidity or alkalinity arising either from natural causes or from cultivational and irrigation practices, industriali- zation or urbanization can markedly affect the uptake of specific elements. Irrigation with alkaline groundwaters, especially of certain types of shales and of some mineralized granites, greatly increases molybdenum and selenium uptake. Iron-rich irrigation waters restrict the uptake of selenium into the food-chain. Extensive water leaching of some acid arenaceous soils low in organic matter increases the magnitude of iodine losses, and reduces the intrinsic availability of soil selenium and zinc. High soil acidity strongly potentiates crop uptake of aluminium, iron and manganese.

297

Table 23.3. Soil and geochemical features associated with typical trace-element anomalies in human food-chains

Nature of anomaly	Environmental origins
Deficiencies	
Low iodine	Excessive leaching of iodine from acid soils low in organic matter and clay mineral fractions, and especially from soils derived from glaciation
Low selenium	Soils intrinsically low in selenium such as extensively leached acid arenaceous soils Soils rich in iron and manganese with low pH, capable of "fixing" selenium in immobile forms; many lateritic soils
Low zinc	Calcareous soils from which zinc uptake is poor; leached arenaceous soils
Toxicities	
High arsenic	Waters from hydrothermal sources; soils derived from detritus of mineral ore (especially gold) workings
High fluoride	Water from aquifers including drainage from certain rhyolite-rich rocks, black shales or coals; soils derived from fluoride-containing residues of mineral deposits
High selenium	Groundwater of high pH derived from a wide variety of soil/rock types
High zinc	Soils incorporating products of weathering of zinc-rich mineralized deposits (e.g. sphalerite) or black shales

- The impact of such geochemical and soil variables on human trace-element intake depends markedly on the types of crops that are dietary staples. In general, the trace-element composition of leguminous crops, pulses and cruciferous crops fluctuates widely as such variables change. In contrast, the trace-element content of cereal grains, although frequently lower, is less readily affected (46). It should be noted, however, that the selenium content and to a lesser extent the zinc content of cereal grains are markedly influenced by soil conditions and type.

The influence of geochemical and soil conditions on trace-element supply is considered in greater detail elsewhere (46). FAO reports (47, 48) on a wide range of studies in different countries demonstrate the importance of considering the intrinsic properties of indigenous soils as trace-element sources. Disappointingly little is known about the geographical distribution of abnormalities influencing iodine and selenium uptake, but apart from this, extensive information banks have been developed for many countries which define the mineral characteristics of rocks and soils in the context of surveys either of potential mineral resources or of the cropping potential of soils. Such information should be fully exploited in investigations of the causes of deficiencies of copper, iodine, selenium, zinc and possibly of boron, chromium and fluorine and of toxicoses due to fluoride, iron, molybdenum and selenium.

Those responsible for large-scale irrigation schemes or the introduction of modified soil-cultural practices should see it as their duty to request information from such sources on the possible effects of these developments on trace-element flux from parent rocks through soils to edible crops before they are imposed on rural communities. Failure to take this precaution has already caused extensive problems resulting from excesses of fluoride and selenium in some communities. It has also caused crop failures and decreased animal productivity from the inadvertent potentiation of trace-element-related disorders caused by deficiencies of cobalt, copper, manganese, selenium and zinc or by excesses of fluorine, iron and selenium and, in animals, of molybdenum.

The FAO Soil Resources, Management and Conservation Service has published two relevant reports, the first containing trace-element information at the country level and including details of crop responses to trace elements in 15 developing countries (47). The second provides global information on the trace-element status of soils in a wider range of developing countries (48). More detailed information for specific countries can often be obtained from their ministries of agriculture or national soils institutes, as applicable.

Information on the availability of relevant geochemical survey data can be obtained from:

The Secretariat,
International Geochemical Correlation Programme,
Department of Environmental Sciences,
UNESCO/IUGS,
Place de Fontenoy,
75700 Paris, France

or:

International Division,
British Geological Survey,
Keyworth,
Nottingham,
NG12 4GG, England.

Plants have a wide tolerance of many trace elements, and show marked species variability in the extent to which they are accumulated. The feasibility of cropping different species or cultivars in order deliberately to modify dietary mineral supply has not been extensively examined but there is sufficient evidence to indicate that this approach may be of value. The variability of the trace-element content of specific crops differs markedly for the different elements; copper has been found to vary four-fold, zinc, seven-fold, boron 21-fold and molybdenum up to 46-fold depending on soil and crop management (47). Maize concentrates selenium better than rice; when, in the Enshi Province of China, it was grown as an alternative crop because droughts had caused the failure of the usual rice crop, recycling of maize ash as a fertilizer contributed to an accumulation of selenium in an already selenium-rich soil thereby causing selenium toxicosis in the local livestock and human population (25). Fluorosis may be more frequent in populations subsisting on sorghum rather than maize, because the former retains more fluoride from cooking water (49). Changes in dietary sources and an increasing intake of processed foods can reduce trace-element intake. Separation procedures, e.g. peeling, milling and refining, increase the loss of elements such as chromium, iron and zinc from flours and sugars (50).

23.4 Geophagia

Geophagia, the involuntary or sometimes deliberate eating of earth, usually clays, is a widespread practice in the animal kingdom and in many human communities (51). It is a form of pica likely to have pathological implications when it impairs the intestinal uptake of trace elements such as iron and zinc. However, it is also suggested, though not proved, that geophagia is sometimes an evolved adaptive attempt to compensate for mineral deficits or imbalances. The differing properties of various clays clearly affect their ability to meet this need. Eating of clays with high cation-exchange capacities that release many elements under acid conditions can significantly supplement the intakes of copper, iron, manganese and zinc of some subsistence communities (e.g. in the United Republic of Tanzania and in Central America). They may also release macrominerals, the need for which may be the underlying cause of geophagia. In contrast, eating of other clay types may cause elemental deficiencies. In parts of Turkey, geophagia is believed to impair the utilization of iron and zinc, giving rise to a distinctive geophagic or clay-eating syndrome associated with growth retardation, anaemia and delayed puberty (52).

Quantitative data on the extent of the mineral imbalances created by geophagia are scarce. However, it appears highly probable that geophagia or the deliberate or adventitious contamination of foods with calcareous soils can increase the intake of calcium sufficiently to potentiate inhibition of zinc absorption from vegetable-based diets high in phytate (see Chapter 5). Such causal relationships have been invoked to account for the development of zinc deficiency in some rural communities in Western Asia. The consumption of iron-rich lateritic soils or of iron-rich waters draining from them must be expected to influence adversely the utilization of copper, zinc and probably selenium in other regions.

23.5 Water

The risks of the appearance of trace-element-related effects on health can be influenced substantially by changes in the source of drinking-water or ground-water. The effects of irrigation, soil water economy and solar evaporation on the entry of elements into the food-chains of rural populations are most clearly evident in communities where food choice, particularly for the young, is largely restricted to a few locally grown staples and water is drawn from a single source.

High soil moisture induced by irrigation or impeded drainage, especially if accompanied by a high pH and reducing conditions, favours the uptake of molybdenum by legume crops and of selenium by brassicas. In contrast, the aluminium, iron and manganese contents of many staple crops are increased markedly by acid soil conditions with a high water table. It has been claimed that copper and zinc toxicoses have resulted from the consumption of extremely acidic water contaminated by copper from conduits (53) or with zinc from galvanized tanks (54). An increased incidence of a Parkinsonian neurological syndrome in mining areas of Greece has been associated with an abnormally high content of manganese in drinking-water (55).

Aquifers in fluoride-bearing rocks or the irrigation of fluoride-rich soils can increase the intake of this element through drinking-water or food crops sufficiently to induce major problems of community health arising from severe fluoride intoxication (see Chapter 15). The increased consumption of water in arid environments may be sufficient to increase the risks of fluorosis (56).

The leaching of iodine from acid, mineralized soils is an important determinant of the geographical distribution of iodine deficiency. The distribution of selenium deficiency may be influenced similarly by the leaching of mineralized soils by rainwater.

23.6 Overall assessment

Uncertainty whether a health disorder, not attributable to infection alone, may be trace-element-related can often be removed by consideration of the potentiating variables considered above. The significance of individual factors will differ markedly in different situations (57–61). However, evidence of geochemical and soil anomalies, or of the adoption of high-risk agricultural practices or abnormal dietary preferences can often make it easier to decide whether to adopt more direct lines of enquiry into the possible existence of significant abnormalities of trace-element intake. Additional corroborative evidence may be available from the observation of related trace-element-responsive diseases in livestock (59), the regional distribution and identity of which can usually be ascertained from veterinarians or animal nutrition advisers. Such links between trace-element problems in livestock and humans are known for deficiencies of iodine, selenium and zinc and for chronic toxicities of mercury, molybdenum and selenium.

The investigative potential of such approaches for the detection of trace-element-related problems in the populations of developing countries has been considered in detail by Golden et al. (62), who have also discussed the importance of generalized malnutrition and infection in the etiology and control of such problems.

Appropriate priorities for the analysis of tissues or diets, or preferably both, are frequently suggested by evidence that one or more of the above factors influencing susceptibility may be operating. The subsequent measurement of tissue trace-element content, or of metabolic markers which reflect the physiological adequacy of trace-element status, can be useful both in the diagnostic investigation of individuals and in epidemiological investigations. In contrast, the comparison of the results of dietary trace-element surveys with estimates of the safe range of average population intakes provides information applicable principally to the communities or specific populations from which the dietary samples were drawn and the parameters of acceptability derived. Thus the primary value of the dietary survey is the indication that it may provide that more detailed investigation is justified of the possible relevance for health of the particular anomalies of trace-element supply that it reveals.

The decision whether to undertake such additional studies must often be influenced more by considerations of cost and feasibility than by their scientific value or limitations. Their value will increase once better techniques for assessing pathologically relevant changes in trace-element status become available. Until then, there is a need for wider agreement on "action criteria" appropriate for use in diagnostic work with the techniques currently available but for which the quantitative significance or pathological relevance is at present debatable.

In the face of such uncertainties, it may be decided to undertake a direct investigation of the effects of modifying trace-element supply by dietary intervention or supplement administration. The success of such intervention trials depends greatly on the care with which they are planned. Except where immunocompetence is the criterion whereby the value of modifying dietary trace-element intake is to be assessed, communities or individuals used for such trials should be treated to remove confounding variables such as parasitic and other infections. Account must also be taken in intervention trials of the possibility that the supply of more than one nutrient may be limiting. If so, responses to fortification with a single element may be transient or absent. Appropriate study designs could include the comparison of responses either to single and specific nutrients (including energy) or to the spectrum of nutrients whose adequacy is in question. Ethical considerations will influence experimental design and decisions whether briefly to withhold supplements of specific trace nutrients while attempting the rehabilitation of those suffering from disorders of complex nutritional origin.

The biological criteria used to monitor response should preferably reflect changes in the severity of a clearly established pathological condition (e.g. growth retardation in malnourished or socially deprived children) previously identified by the surveillance of community health or welfare. Before trials commence, the precision with which anthropometric and other data can be obtained must be realistically estimated; subtle effects escape detection if precision is poor. Wherever feasible, treatment should be randomly allocated and coded, and all procedures subjected to random scrutiny by supervisory staff ignorant of treatment codes.

Finally, ethical considerations may often preclude experimental investigations on the subjects at greatest risk. It is rarely acceptable to deliberately manipulate the composition of the diets of infants or pregnant women if there is pathological evidence that nutritionally related disorders exist in a community. Only two options are then open. First, the likely relevance of clinical or covert manifestations of trace-element deficiency or excess in other species of animal must be considered carefully in relation to those of the human communities believed to be at risk. Second, biochemical indications of metabolic anomalies must be sought and, despite their current limitations, assessed in relation to agreed criteria of element deficiency or excess. Guidelines on appropriate action criteria must be accompanied by advice as to feasible dietary or cultivational intervention policies likely to rectify detected anomalies in trace-element status.

Success in the detection and control of most trace-element-related aspects of ill-health will remain contingent on acceptance of the fact that their pathological signs are rarely specific and on an awareness of the need for multidisciplinary expertise in identifying risks and suggesting means for their elimination. It is now recognized that trace elements are important because of their direct influence on health. The possibility that they may also influence susceptibility to a large number of diseases, as suggested by an increasing number of studies (63–69), requires careful appraisal as techniques for monitoring the effects of changes in trace-element status improve. Such investigations should be accorded the highest priority in those developing countries where the children of socially disadvantaged communities subsist on monotonous diets based on a very limited number of locally produced foods.

23.7 Recommendations for future work

- The importance of multidisciplinary approaches to the assessment of the risks that trace-element-related problems will influence community health has been emphasized here. It is therefore recommended that international agencies should play a much more positive role in encouraging such multidisciplinary activity by supporting the organization of workshops and training courses specifically to consider the etiology, control and health significance of trace-element-related diseases. Their significance in the developing countries should be given particular attention, as should the impact of concurrent infectious disease on risk. Iron should be considered together with the metallic trace elements because of their frequent functional and metabolic interdependence.

- Field investigators and nutritional consultants have frequently been made aware of the diagnostic and predictive limitations of many possible indicators of trace-element status. The significance of the limitations of individual parameters is reduced if, in their interpretation, other relevant indices are considered. It would therefore be useful as an interim measure if advice on "action criteria" could be summarized in the form of guidelines that specifically emphasize the importance of considering all relevant physiological and environmental data when assessing the significance of anomalies in the composition of diets, blood and tissues.

References

1. Aggett PJ. Malnutrition and trace element metabolism. In: Suskind RM, Lewinter-Suskind L, eds. *The malnourished child.* New York, Raven Press, 1990: 155–176.
2. *The treatment and management of severe protein-energy malnutrition.* Geneva, World Health Organization, 1981.
3. Golden BE, Golden MHN. Zinc absorption in malnourished children. In: Momcilović B, ed. *Trace elements in man and animals — TEMA 7.* Zagreb, University of Zagreb, 1991: 14.10–14.11.
4. Golden BE, Golden MHN. Plasma zinc, rate of weight gain, and the energy cost of tissue deposition in children recovering from severe malnutrition on a cow's milk or soya protein based diet. *American journal of clinical nutrition,* 1981, 34: 892–899.

5. Golden MHN, Golden BE. Effect of zinc supplementaion on the dietary intake, rate of weight gain and energy cost of tissue deposition in children recovering from severe malnutrition. *American journal of clinical nutrition*, 1981, **34**: 900–908.

6. Golden MHN, Golden BE, Jackson AA. Skin breakdown in Kwashiorkor responds to zinc. *Lancet*, 1980, i: 1256.

7. Golden MHN, Jackson AA, Golden BE. Effect of zinc on thymus of recently malnourished children. *Lancet*, 1976, ii: 1057–1059.

8. Patrick J, Golden BE, Golden MHN. Leucocyte sodium transport and dietary zinc in protein energy malnutrition. *American journal of clinical nutrition*, 1980, **33**: 617–620.

9. Simmer K et al. Nutritional rehabilitation in Bangladesh — the importance of zinc. *American journal of clinical nutrition*, 1988, **47**: 1036–1040.

10. Castillo-Duran C et al. Controlled trial of zinc supplementation during recovery from malnutrition: effects on growth and immune function. *American journal of clinical nutrition*, 1987, **45**: 602–608.

11. Castillo-Duran C et al. Controlled trial of copper supplementation during the recovery from marasmus. *American journal of clinical nutrition*, 1983, **37**: 898–903.

12. Cordano A, Graham GG. Copper deficiency complicating severe chronic intestinal malabsorption. *Pediatrics*, 1966, **32**: 596–604.

13. Castillo-Duran C, Uauy R. Copper deficiency impairs growth of infants recovering from malnutrition. *American journal of clinical nutrition*, 1988, **47**: 710–714.

14. Mathias TM, Jackson AA. Selenium deficiency in kwashiorkor. *Lancet*, 1982, i: 1312–1313.

15. Gurson CT, Saner G. Effects of chromium on glucose utilisation in marasmic protein calorie malnutrition. *American journal of clinical nutrition*, 1971, **24**: 1313–1319.

16. Tomkins A, Watson F. *Malnutrition and infection*, Geneva, United Nations, 1989.

17. Fenwick PK et al. The effect of zinc deficiency and zinc repletion on the response of rats to infection with *Trichinella spiralis*. *American journal of clinical nutrition*, 1990, **52**: 166–172.

18. Fenwick P et al. The effect of zinc deficiency and repletion on the susceptibility of rats to infection with *Strongyloides ratti*. *American journal of clinical nutrition*, 1990, **52**: 173–177.

19. Castillo-Duran C, Vial P, Uauy R. Trace mineral balance during acute diarrhea in infants. *Journal of pediatrics*, 1988, **113**: 452–457.

20. Sachdev HP et al. A controlled trial on utility of oral zinc supplementation in acute dehydration diarrhoea in infants. *Journal of pediatric gastroenterology and nutrition*, 1988, **7**: 877–881.

21. Mason JB et al. *Nutritional surveillance*. Geneva, World Health Organization, 1984.

22. Edmonds L et al. Guidelines for reproductive studies in exposed human populations. In: *Guidelines for studies of human populations exposed to mutagenic and reproductive hazards*. New York, AD Bloom, 1981: 37–100.

23. Mertz W, ed. *Trace elements in human and animal nutrition*, 5th ed., Vols 1&2. Orlando, FL, & San Diego, Academic Press, 1986 & 1987.

24. Aggett PJ, Rose S. Soil and congenital malformations. *Experientia*, 1987, **43**: 104–108.

25. Yang G et al. Endemic selenium intoxication of humans in China. *American journal of clinical nutrition*, 1983, **37**: 872–881.

26. Cowgill UM. Selenium and neonatal death. *Lancet*, 1976, **ii**: 816–817.

27. Jaffe EG, Velez B. Selenium intake and congenital malformations in humans. *Archivos latinoamericanos de nutrición*, 1973, **23**: 515–517.

28. Harad M. Congenital Minamata disease: intrauterine methylmercury poisoning. *Teratology*, 1978, **18**: 285–288.

29. Oehme FW, ed. *Toxicity of heavy metals in the environment*. New York, Marcel Dekker, 1978.

30. Aggett PJ. Severe zinc deficiency. In: Mills CF, ed. *Zinc in human biology*. London, Springer, 1989: 259–279.

31. Shaw JCL. Copper deficiency and non-accidental injury. *Archives of disease in childhood*, 1988, **63**: 448–455.

32. Levy Y et al. Copper deficiency in infants fed cow milk. *Journal of pediatrics*, 1985, **106**: 786–788.

33. Casey CE, Neville MC, Hambidge KM. Studies in human lactation in secretion of zinc, copper and manganese in human milk. *American journal of clinical nutrition*, 1989, **49**: 773–785.

34. Akre J, ed. Infant feeding: the physiological basis. *Bulletin of the World Health Organization*, 1990, **67** (Suppl.).

35. Lönnerdal B. Dietary factors affecting trace element absorption in infants. *Acta paediatrica scandinavica*, 1989, Suppl. 351: 109–113.

36. Prasad AS et al. Zinc metabolism in patients with the syndrome of iron deficiency anemia, hypogonadism and dwarfism. *Journal of laboratory and clinical medicine*, 1963, **61**: 537–539.

37. Golden MHN. The role of individual nutrient deficiencies in growth retardation of children as exemplified by zinc and protein in linear growth retardation in less developed countries. In: Waterlow JC, ed. *Linear growth retardation in less developed countries*. New York, Raven Press, 1988: 143–163.

38. Walravens PA, Hambidge KM, Koepfer DM. Zinc supplementation in infants with a nutritional pattern of failure to thrive: a double blind controlled study. *Pediatrics*, 1989, **83**: 532–538.

39. Gibson RS et al. A growth-limiting, mild zinc deficiency syndrome in some Southern Ontario boys with low height percentiles. *American journal of clinical nutrition*, 1989, **49**: 1266–1273.

40. Iyengar GV, Gopal-Ayengar AR. Human health and trace elements; effects on high altitude populations. *Ambio*, 1988, **17**: 31–35.

41. Aggett PJ. The assessment of zinc status: a personal view. *Proceedings of the Nutrition Society*, 1991, **50**: 9–17.

42. Bradfield RB et al. Hair copper in copper deficiency. *Lancet*, 1980, **i**: 343–344.

43. Hambidge KM. Hair analysis: worthless for vitamins, limited for minerals. *American journal of clinical nutrition*, 1982, **36**: 943–949.

44. Golden MHN, Golden BE. Trace elements: potential importance in human nutrition with particular reference to zinc and vanadium. *British medical bulletin*, 1981, **37**: 31–36.

45. Southgate DAT. Trace element databases and food composition compilations. *Food chemistry*, 1992, **43**: 289–294.

46. Bowie SHU, Thornton I, eds. *Environmental geochemistry and health*. Dordrecht, Reidel, 1984.

47. Sillanpää M, ed. *Micronutrient assessment at the country level*. Rome, Food and Agriculture Organization of the United Nations, 1990 (FAO Soils Bulletin 63).

48. Sillanpää M, ed. *Micronutrients and the nutrient states of soils; a global study*. Rome, Food and Agriculture Organization of the United Nations, 1982 (FAO Soils Bulletin 48).

49. Krishnamachari KAVR. Skeletal fluorosis in humans: a review of recent progress in the understanding of the disease. *Progress in food and nutrition science*, 1986, **10**: 279–314.

50. Schroeder HA. Losses of vitamins and trace minerals resulting from processing and preservation of foods. *American journal of clinical nutrition*, 1971, **24**: 562–573.

51. Johns T, Duquette M. Detoxification and mineral supplementation as functions of geophagy. *American journal of clinical nutrition*, 1991, **53**: 448–456.

52. Minnich V et al. Pica in Turkey II. Effect of clay on iron absorption. *American journal of clinical nutrition*, 1968, **21**: 78–86.

53. Spitalny KC et al. Drinking water induced copper intoxication in a Vermont family. *Pediatrics*, 1984, **74**: 1103–1106.

54. Fox MRS. Zinc excess. In: Mills CF, ed. *Zinc in human biology*. London, Springer, 1989: 365–370.

55. Kondakis XG et al. Possible health effects of high manganese concentration in drinking water. *Archives of environmental health*, 1989, **44**: 175–178.

56. Brouwer ID et al. Unsuitability of World Health Organization guidelines for fluoride concentrations in drinking water in Senegal. *Lancet*, 1988, **1**: 223–225.

57. Beeson KC, Matrone G. *The soil factor in nutrition: animal and human*. New York, Marcel Dekker, 1976.

58. Allaway WH. Soil plant-animal and human inter-relationships in trace element nutrition. In Mertz W, ed. *Trace elements in human and animal nutrition*, Vol. 2. San Diego, Academic Press, 1986: 465–488.

59. Horvath DJ, Reid RL. Indirect effects of soil and water on animal health. *Science of the total environment*, 1984, **34**: 143–156.

60. Fan AM et al. Selenium and human health implications in California's San Joaquin Valley. *Journal of toxicology and environmental health*, 1988, **23**: 539–559.

61. Suliman HB et al. Zinc deficiency in sheep: field cases. *Tropical animal health and production*, 1988, **20**: 47–51.

62. Golden BE, Golden MHN. The detection of trace element deficiencies in the Third World. In: Momcilović B, ed. *Trace elements in man and animals — TEMA 7*. Zagreb, University of Zagreb, 1991: 14.5–14.6.

63. Jackson ML et al. The geochemical availability of soil zinc and molybdenum in relation to stomach and oesophageal cancer in the people's Republic of China and USA. *Applied geochemistry*, 1986, **1**: 487–492.

64. Jackson ML. Geochemical characteristics of land and its effect on human heart and

cancer death rates in the United States and China. *Applied geochemistry*, 1986, **1**: 175–180.

65. Kibblewhite ME et al. Evidence for an intimate geochemical factor in the etiology of oesophageal cancer. *Environmental research*, 1984, **33**: 370–378.

66. Salonen JT et al. Serum fatty acids, apolipoproteins, selenium and vitamin anti-oxidants and the risk of death from coronary artery disease. *American journal of cardiology*, 1985, **56**: 226–231.

67. Jackson ML, Zhang JZ, Li CS. Land characteristics affect heart and cancer death rates among Wisconsin counties. *Transactions of the Wisconsin Academy of Science, Arts and Letters*, 1985, **75**: 35–41.

68. Kinnunen E et al. The epidemiology of multiple sclerosis in Finland. *Acta neurologica scandinavica*, 1983, **67**: 255–262.

69. Sokoloff L. Kashin-Beck disease: current status. *Nutrition reviews*, 1988, **46**: 113–119.

24.

Conclusions and recommendations

In this report, trace elements have been divided into three groups from the point of view of their nutritional significance in humans, as follows: (1) essential elements; (2) elements which are probably essential; and (3) potentially toxic elements, some of which may nevertheless have some essential functions at low levels. For reasons related to recent improvements in analytical procedures and more rigorous criteria for the definition of deficiencies and toxicities, the estimates of requirements and tolerance given here tend to be lower than many of those suggested previously.

Comparisons of the data in Chapters 4–7 with recent estimates of population mean intakes suggest that a significant number of communities have intakes of copper, iodine, selenium or zinc lower than the estimates of normative requirements. While this situation does not automatically indicate that widespread pathological manifestations of deficiency exist, it does emphasize the need for closer scrutiny of dietary and other circumstances which may provoke covert pathological manifestations of ill-health.

The concepts underlying the determination of nutritional requirements, of recommended intakes to safeguard nutritional adequacy, and of the means of identifying population groups at risk have been outlined in Chapters 2 and 23. The application of these concepts to trace-element nutrition, however, is hampered by the scarcity of data that can be subjected to adequate statistical scrutiny. The collective judgement of the Expert Consultation has in some instances been called upon to complement the available data. This was particularly true during the estimation of normative requirements, in which subjective decisions were frequently necessary as to desirable levels of protection against possible future deficits or excesses in trace-element supply.

As in the 1973 report of the WHO Expert Committee on Trace Elements in Human Nutrition, the preparation of estimates of tolerable intakes of trace elements has frequently been hindered by a scarcity of data. This situation continues to reflect the relatively low priority previously accorded to investigations of trace-element-related effects on health that often take the form of ill-defined clinical manifestations lacking diagnostic specificity. With some trace elements, notably copper, iodine, molybdenum and selenium, the difficulties thus created have been minimized by exploiting relatively new evidence of their functional roles, together with the corresponding physiologically relevant biochemical indicators of deficiency or excess, to define tolerable levels of intake. However, for zinc and many of the "newer" essential trace elements, agreement has yet to be reached as to the most appropriate indicators of a satisfactory element status.

For all these reasons, the estimates of the safe ranges of element intakes have had to be derived by a variety of techniques. Thus data for iodine are based principally on the results of a substantial series of investigations of the prophylactic effectiveness of graded doses of iodine in areas of endemic deficiency. Increasingly, these data are being supported by evidence derived from the use of biochemical markers of iodine status. Estimates of requirements for copper and selenium rely substantially on biochemical criteria of adequacy or excess; for selenium, additional data from large-scale epidemiological studies are also available. Estimates of requirements for zinc have been based primarily on the factorial component analysis of probable demands for specific physiological processes. Supportive data have been obtained from zinc supplementation trials in socially deprived communities, and a substantial number of investigations are currently pointing to the value of zinc during the rehabilitation of malnourished children in developing countries. Estimates for the remaining elements have been derived mostly by extrapolation from evidence of essentiality or toxicity in non-human species. Any future attempts to confirm the essentiality of the "newer" trace elements lead, nickel, tin and vanadium are awaited with interest.

The Expert Consultation made the following recommendations:

● For virtually all trace-element-related disorders, except the obvious goitres of iodine deficiency and the dental discoloration of fluoride excess, pathological manifestations will remain difficult to detect until more specific pathologically relevant indicators of deficiency or excess become available. Greater priority should therefore be accorded to studies of the early pathological consequences of deficiency or excess and to the development of improved biochemical techniques for their detection. Such indicators are needed urgently not only for epidemiological studies but also to facilitate the quantitative assessment of requirements and, as indicated later, to permit more realistic assessment of the influence of diet on trace-element bioavailability.

Data from dietary surveys in 27 countries considered in Chapter 22 suggest that a usually small but nevertheless significant proportion of communities may have mean daily intakes of essential trace elements that are lower than the provisional estimates of the minimum mean intake considered to be safe.

310

- Whenever feasible, the estimates given here should be verified by means of statistically controlled intervention trials. Such action should be taken if mean dietary intakes of specific element are below or above estimates of the safe range of mean intakes and when other circumstances (see Chapter 23) increase the probable risks of pathological responses to element deficiency or excess. Such investigations should focus on the monitoring of pathophysiological responses to intervention rather than being confined to measurements of changes in trace-element status. Priority should be given to verification of the recommendations for iodine and zinc.

Social deprivation and extremes of climate and environment in the developing countries create the greatest risks that anomalies in trace-element supply may adversely influence health. Few data exist on the content and bioavailability of the essential and toxic trace elements of indigenous staple foods in such countries.

- Urgent action should be taken to acquire more information not only on the content of essential and potentially toxic elements in a wide range of staple foods of developing countries but also to determine the effect of cultural, climatic and environmental changes on the contents of these elements in diets derived from such foods.
- Such data must be accompanied by information on the dietary contents of factors known to influence trace-element bioavailability. Future studies could well be modelled on the existing IAEA International Dietary Surveys but with the proviso that compositional variables modifying trace-element utilization should also be considered analytically. There is also an urgent need to define more precisely the effects of such dietary antagonists and synergists so that their influence on the tolerable range of trace-element intakes can be more reliably predicted. Their influence is probably a major determinant of susceptibility to iodine and zinc deficiencies; it is also likely to influence susceptibility to fluorosis and the toxicity of heavy metals.
- While it is appreciated that the small number of internationally recognized centres of trace-element expertise established in response to the proposals in the 1973 WHO report have contributed significantly to world health, the number and scope of such centres should be increased. Collaboratively exploiting the expertise and costly technical facilities of the centres already established, they should serve the specific needs of the developing countries. The training and investigational facilities that they offer should place particular emphasis on the needs of regions with known marginal or inadequate food intakes and the special implications

311

for trace-element nutrition of concurrent infection, parasitism and general malnutrition. They should offer training courses demonstrating the value of multidisciplinary approaches to the detection of social, agricultural and environmental circumstances that increase susceptibility to trace-element-related effects on human health. Such centres should be given the funding necessary to provide adequate technical and analytical support and should be able to participate in internationally coordinated programmes in trace-element nutrition, modelled on the projects currently sponsored by the International Atomic Energy Agency.

- Finally, when new food standards are developed or food-manufacturing processes are modified, due consideration should be given to meeting the needs for essential trace elements. This applies especially to formulated foods designed for infants and young children, to food destined for disadvantaged communities, and whenever new sources of protein or unconventional staple foods are introduced into the diet.

Contributors

Principal authors and coordinators

Dr P.J. Aggett, Agricultural and Food Research Council, Institute of Food Research, Norwich, England (*Chapter 23*)

Dr G.H. Beaton, Department of Nutrition, University of Toronto, Canada, (*Chapter 2*)

Dr I. Dreosti, Division of Human Nutrition, Commonwealth Scientific and Industrial Research Organisation, Adelaide, Australia (*Chapter 7*)

Professor R.A. Goyer, Department of Pathology, University of Western Ontario, Canada (*Chapter 16*)

Dr B.S. Hetzel, International Council for the Control of Iodine Deficiency Disorders, Adelaide, Australia (*Chapter 4*)

Dr G.V. Iyengar, National Institute of Standards and Technology, Gaithersburg, MD, USA (*Chapter 21*)

Dr K. Kostial, Institute for Medical Research and Occupational Health, Zagreb, Croatia (*Chapter 16*)

Dr K.A.V.R. Krishnamachari, Regional Medical Research Centre, Indian Council for Medical Research, Chandrasekharpur, Bhubaneswar, India (*Chapter 15*)

Dr O.A. Levander, Vitamin and Mineral Nutrition Laboratory, United States Department of Agriculture/Agricultural Research Service, Beltsville Human Nutrition Research Center, MD, USA (*Chapter 6*)

Dr W. Mertz, United States Department of Agriculture/Agricultural Research Service, Beltsville Human Nutrition Research Center, MD, USA, (*Chapters 1, 11, 17, 18, 19*)

Professor C.F. Mills, Rowett Research Institute, Aberdeen, Scotland (*Chapters 3, 8, 23*)

Dr W.H. Nielsen, United States Department of Agriculture/Agricultural Research Service, Grand Forks Human Nutrition Research Center, ND, USA (*Chapters 9, 10, 12, 13, 14, 20*)

Dr R.M. Parr, Division of Human Health, International Atomic Energy Agency, Vienna, Austria (*Chapter 22*)

Professor M.A. Rish, Institute of Physiology and Biochemistry, State University of Samarkand, Uzbekistan, (*Chapter 8*)

Professor A.B. Sandström, Research Department, Human Nutrition, Royal Veterinary and Agricultural University, Frederiksberg C, Denmark (*Chapter 5*)

Joint FAO/IAEA/WHO Expert Consultation (Geneva, 18–22 June 1990)[1]

Members

Dr M. Abdulla, Department of Medical Elementology and Toxicology, Hamdard University, Hamdard Nagar, New Delhi, India

Dr P.J. Aggett, Agricultural and Food Research Council, Institute of Food Research, Norwich, England

Professor M. Anke, Faculty of Biology, Friedrich Schiller University, Jena, Germany

Dr G.H. Beaton, Department of Nutrition, University of Toronto, Canada

Dr I. Dreosti, Division of Human Nutrition, Commonwealth Scientific and Industrial Research Organisation, Adelaide, Australia

Dr B.S. Hetzel, International Council for the Control of Iodine Deficiency Disorders, Adelaide, Australia

Professor U.P. Isichei, Department of Chemical Pathology, Faculty of Medical Sciences, University of Jos, Jos, Nigeria

Dr G.V. Iyengar, National Institute of Standards and Technology, Gaithersburg, MD, USA

Dr K.A.V.R. Krishnamachari, Regional Medical Research Centre, Indian Council for Medical Research, Chandrasekharpur, Bhubaneswar, India

Dr O.A. Levander, Vitamin and Mineral Nutrition Laboratory, United States Department of Agriculture/Agricultural Research Service, Beltsville Human Nutrition Research Center, MD, USA

Dr W. Mertz, United States Department of Agriculture/Agricultural Research Service, Beltsville Human Nutrition Research Center, MD, USA (*Chairman*)

Professor C.F. Mills, Rowett Research Institute, Aberdeen, Scotland (*Rapporteur/ Technical Editor*)

---

[1] Addresses given are those valid at the time of the meeting.

Dr W.H. Nielsen, United States Department of Agriculture/Agricultural Research Service, Grand Forks Human Nutrition Research Center, ND, USA

Dr J. Parizek, Institute of Physiology, Academy of Sciences, Prague, Czechoslovakia

Professor M.A. Rish, Institute of Physiology and Biochemistry, State University of Samarkand, Uzbek Soviet Socialist Republic, USSR

Professor A.B. Sandström, Research Department, Human Nutrition, Royal Veterinary and Agricultural University, Frederiksberg C, Denmark

Dr P. Valeix, Centre for Research on Nutritional Anaemia (CRAN), Conservatoire national des Arts et Métiers, Paris, France

Professor Wu Bai Ling, Institute of Information Research, Academy of Military Medical Science, Beijing, China

Professor K. Yasumoto, Research Institute for Food Science, Kyoto University, Gokasho, Uji, Kyoto, Japan

Secretariat

Dr G.A. Clugston, Nutrition, World Health Organization, Geneva, Switzerland

Dr Keyou Ge, Institute of Nutrition and Food Hygiene, Beijing, China (formerly Food Policy and Nutrition Division, Food and Agriculture Organization of the United Nations, Rome, Italy)

Dr A. Pradilla, Nutrition, World Health Organization, Geneva, Switzerland

Dr R.C. Weisell, Food Policy and Nutrition Division, Food and Agriculture Organization of the United Nations, Rome, Italy

Additional contributors[1]

Dr M. Abdulla, Department of Medical Elementology and Toxicology, Hamdard University, Hamdard Nagar, New Delhi, India (*Chapters 2, 6, 22*)

Professor M. Anke, Faculty of Biology, Friedrich Schiller University, Jena, Germany (*Chapters 11, 17, 18, 19*)

Dr J.R. Arthur, Rowett Research Institute, Aberdeen, Scotland (*Chapter 6*)

Dr G.H. Beaton, Department of Nutrition, University of Toronto, Canada (*Chapter 6*)

Professor K.E. Bergmann, Institute of Social Medicine and Epidemiology, Berlin, Germany (*Chapter 15*)

---

[1] For the principal authors of individual chapters, see pages 313–314.

Dr I. Bremner, Rowett Research Institute, Aberdeen, Scotland (*Chapter 3*)

Dr R.F. Burk, Department of Medicine, Vanderbilt University, Nashville, TN, USA (*Chapter 6*)

Professor R.K. Chandra, Department of Pediatric Medicine and Immunology, University of Newfoundland, St John's Canada (*Chapter 5*)

Professor M.G. Cherian, Department of Pathology, Pharmacology and Toxicology, University of Western Ontario, Canada (*Chapter 3*)

Dr H. Crawley, Department of Nutrition, University of North London, England (*Chapter 22*)

Dr M. Fields, United States Department of Agriculture/Agricultural Research Service, Beltsville Human Nutrition Research Centre, MD, USA (*Chapter 7*)

Dr P.R. Flanagan, Department of Medicine, University of Western Ontario, Canada (*Chapter 3*)

Dr M. Franklin, Rowett Research Institute, Aberdeen, Scotland (*Chapters 3, 5*)

Professor R.S. Gibson, Department of Family Studies, University of Guelph, Ontario, Canada (*Chapter 7*)

Drs B.E. & M.H.N. Golden, Aberdeen University Medical School, Scotland (*Chapter 5*)

Professor K.M. Hambidge, Department of Pediatrics, University of Colorado Health Science Center, Denver, CO, USA (*Chapter 5*)

Dr G.V. Iyengar, National Institute of Standards and Technology, Gaithersburg, MD, USA (*Chapter 22*)

Dr M. Janghorbani, Department of Medicine, University of Chicago, IL, USA (*Chapter 21*)

Dr J. Kumpulainen, Central Laboratory, Agricultural Research Centre, Jokioinen, Finland (*Chapter 21*)

Professor J.C. King, Department of Nutritional Science, University of California, Berkeley, CA, USA (*Chapter 5*)

Dr L.M. Klevay, United States Department of Agriculture/Agricultural Research Service, Grand Forks Human Nutrition Research Center, ND, USA (*Chapter 7*)

Dr. N.F. Krebs, Department of Pediatrics, University of Colorado Health Science Center, Denver, Co, USA (*Chapter 5*)

Dr O.A. Levander, Vitamin and Mineral Nutrition Laboratory, United States Department of Agriculture/Agricultural Research Service, Beltsville Human Nutrition Research Center, MD, USA (*Chapter 2*)

Professor I. Lombeck, Institute of Toxicology and Children's Hospital, Düsseldorf, Germany (*Chapter 6*)

Dr W. Mertz, United States Department of Agriculture/Agricultural Research Service, Beltsville Human Nutrition Research Center, MD, USA (*Chapters 2, 5, 6, 7*)

Professor C.F. Mills, Rowett Research Institute, Aberdeen, Scotland (*Chapters 5, 7, 8, 16*)

Dr J. Parizek, Institute of Physiology, Academy of Sciences, Prague, Czech Republic (*Chapter 16*)

Professor A.S. Prasad, Department of Internal Medicine, Wayne State University School of Medicine, Detroit, MI, USA (*Chapter 5*)

Professor M.F. Robinson, Department of Nutrition, University of Otago, Dunedin, New Zealand (*Chapter 6*)

Dr E. Sabbioni, Life Sciences Unit, Environment Institute, Joint Research Centre, Ispra, Varese, Italy (*Chapter 21*)

Professor H.H. Sandstead, Department of Preventive Medicine and Community Health, University of Texas Medical Branch, Galveston, TX, USA (*Chapter 5*)

Professor A.B. Sandström, Research Department, Human Nutrition, Royal Veterinary and Agricultural University, Frederiksberg C, Denmark (*Chapters 3, 23*)

Dr R. Schelenz, International Atomic Energy Agency, Vienna, Austria (*Chapter 21*)

Dr J.R. Turnlund, United States Department of Agriculture/Agricultural Research Service, Western Human Nutrition Research Center, San Fransisco, CA, USA, (*Chapter 7*)

Dr W. Wolf, United States Department of Agriculture/Agricultural Research Service, Beltsville Human Nutrition Research Center, MD, USA (*Chapter 21*)

Professor G.Y. Yang, Institute of Nutrition and Food Hygiene, Beijing, China (*Chapter 6*)

Derivation and application of requirement estimates

1. Relationship of requirement estimates to the "recommended intake" or "safe level of intake" of earlier reports

Earlier joint FAO/WHO reports provided estimates of the *requirements of individuals* that lay in the upper tail of the distribution of such requirements, such that the published estimates were sufficient to meet the needs of almost all individuals in the class concerned (e.g. young adult men). For someone consuming a diet supplying this amount of the nutrient, there would be only a very low probability that individual's (unknown) requirement would not be met. Thus, that level of intake was deemed "safe" and could be recommended for the individual.

When the average *individual requirements* and the variability of the distribution are known, a "safe level of intake" can be estimated (see Fig. 2.1, p. 9) from:

$$\text{Safe level of intake} = \text{Mean}_{\text{Requirements}} + 2\,\text{SD}_{\text{Requirements}} \tag{1}$$

Such an estimate is explicitly related to individual intakes and indicates the level of intake at which a randomly selected individual is at low risk of inadequate intake *(1)*.

The present report is concerned with population (group) mean intakes and the distribution of such intakes rather than the intakes of particular individuals. Here the lowest acceptable limit of the population (group) mean intake is estimated in such a way that the following condition is satisfied:

$$\text{Group mean}_{\text{Intakes}} - 2\,\text{SD}_{\text{Intakes}} = \text{Mean}_{\text{Requirements}}$$

If this condition is met, very few individuals in the population group would be expected to have intakes below their own requirements. It follows that:

$$\text{Lower limit of population mean intakes} = \text{Mean}_{\text{Requirements}} + 2\,\text{SD}_{\text{Intakes}} \tag{2}$$

so that:

$$E_{\text{PImin}}^{\text{normative}} = E_{\text{R}}^{\text{normative}} + 2\,\text{SD}_{\text{Intakes}}$$

and:

$$E_{Plmin}^{basal} = E_R^{basal} + 2\ SD_{Intakes}$$

Equation (2) can be rearranged to give:

Lower limit of
population mean intakes $= Mean_{Requirements} \times \dfrac{100}{100 - 2\ CV_{Intake}}$ $\qquad$ (3)

where CV_{Intake} is the coefficient of variation $\left(\dfrac{SD}{mean} \times 100\right)$ of the usual intake.

Thus, for zinc, where CV_{Intake} has been estimated to be 25%:

$$Zn_{Plmin}^{basal} = Zn_R^{basal} \times 2$$

For copper, where CV_{Intake} was estimated to be 20%, the corresponding equation is:

$$Cu_{Plmin}^{basal} = Cu_R^{basal} \times 1.67$$

The mathematical distinction between the estimates obtained from Equations 1 and 2 lies in the nature of the variability involved—variability of *requirements* as opposed to variability of *intakes*. The conceptual distinction lies in the use to which the estimate is to be put—whether it is to be applied to the usual intake of an individual or to the average intake of a group or population.

A Subcommittee of the United States National Research Council (2) provided the empirical demonstration that the prevalence of inadequate intakes, estimated by means of an examination of the joint distribution of *intakes* and *requirements*, is relatively insensitive to the variability of *requirements* as long as the *requirement* distribution is symmetrical (but not necessarily normal) and the *intake* and *requirement* distributions are essentially independent of one another (low correlation). Further empirical testing showed that this insensitivity to the variability of requirements is also contingent upon the absolute variability of the *intake* distribution being greater than that of the *requirement* distribution. For the nutrients under consideration in the present report, all these conditions are believed to be satisfied provided that relatively homogeneous groups of people (e.g. adult men) are considered. While the term "populations" is used, this really refers to large groups or population subgroups that have been classified by age, sex and physiological characteristics (see also the discussion of "population" on p. 324). The approach to the estimation of the lower limit of safe population mean intakes is based on the empirical relationship between the variabilities of intake and requirement. What *is* required is an explicit estimate of the variability of usual intakes and, in this report, it has been assumed that in most instances the *intake* distribution approximates normality. In fact, actual intake distributions are often somewhat skewed. The approach adopted in the estimation of a suitable normal distribution is discussed below. In most circumstances, fitting the normal distribution will result in a reasonable estimate of the lower limit of the safe range of population mean intakes (E_{SRl}) but some underestimation of the upper limit of the safe range.

Table A1 provides a comparison of what might have been the old *recommended intake* or *safe level of intake* with the new *lower limit of safe population mean intakes*. Since the present report does not provide estimates of the variability of requirement, two different requirement variabilities, namely CV = 12.5% and CV = 15%, are used in the table. The variabilities of intake are as assumed earlier (for adults, 25% for zinc and 20% for copper).

2. Estimation of CV$_{Intake}$

While the derivation of the lower limit of the population intake is insensitive to the variability of requirement, it is fully sensitive to the estimate of variability of

Table A1. Comparison of possible individual and group safe levels of intake (mg/day)[a]

Element and age/sex group	CV$_{Requirement}$ = 12.5%		CV$_{Requirement}$ = 15%	
	"Safe level of intake" (individual)	E_{Plmin}^{basal} (group)	"Safe level of intake" (individual)	E_{Plmin}^{basal} (group)
Zinc				
Male (adult)	3.5[b]	5.7[c]	3.6[d]	5.7[c]
Female (adult)	2.5	4.0	2.6	4.0
Copper				
Male (adult)	0.89[b]	1.19[e]	0.93[d]	1.19[e]
Female (adult)	0.76	1.01	0.79	1.01

[a] For illustrative purposes only; zinc is assumed to be moderately bioavailable (see Table 5.6, page 95).
[b] $E_R^{basal} \times 1.25$.
[c] $E_R^{basal} \times 2.0$.
[d] $E_R^{basal} \times 1.3$.
[e] $E_R^{basal} \times 1.67$.

usual intake. This can be estimated from observed intakes of large groups of individuals although, at the time of preparation of this report, few published estimates were available for the elements of interest.

2.1 Problem of small group size

Some cautionary statements about the estimation of this variability are in order. First, although SD and CV are easy to compute, a reliable estimate of SD or CV is one of the more difficult parameters to obtain. Sampling exercises, discussed later (see Table A3 on p. 325 for example), readily show that quite substantial sample sizes are required for the reproducible estimation of SD from a very large population. Repeated sampling with small population sizes (25–50) reveals wide variation in the estimated SD. The impact of the number of days on which data are collected is also discussed later (see Table A4 on p. 328 for example). Together, these factors (small samples, small number of days) undoubtedly explain a substantial part of the wide range of reported CVs for zinc and copper intakes. Recognizing this, the Expert Consultation sought out recent large survey databases (3, 4) for which it could be confidently assumed that intakes of the elements were estimated with reasonable accuracy and where sample sizes suggested that variability of intake could be reliably estimated.

2.2 Dealing with skew

However, it was noted that, in these studies in the United Kingdom (3) and Australia (4), there was statistically significant skewing of the intake distributions. Data for zinc from the United Kingdom study are shown in Fig. A1. Since the Expert Consultation was primarily interested in the lower tail of the intake distribution, an expedient approach to describing variation was taken. Reported intakes below the median level were fitted to the lower half of a normal distribution from which the SD was then estimated. This procedure actually yielded a CV of 25.5% for adult males (as compared with the estimate of 25% adopted by the Expert Consultation after examination of data for several ages in both the Australian and United Kingdom surveys). The CV_{Intake} estimates presented in this report must be seen as based on actual data but tempered by the judgement of the Expert Consultation. It would certainly be desirable to accumulate and carefully examine more SD estimates for intake data, based on large data sets with apparently reliable intake estimates.

2.3 Need to examine usual intakes

Another critical factor in the estimation of CV_{Intake} is that it refers to the variability of *usual* intakes. This is discussed again later (see p. 326). There is

Figure A1. Distribution of zinc intakes in adult males in the United Kingdom (3)

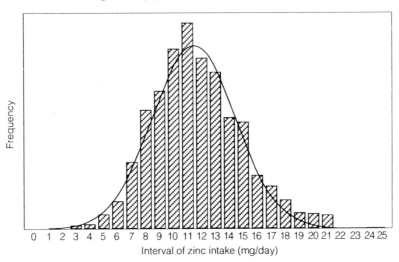

Interval of zinc intake (mg/day)

WHO 94660

The histogram represents reported data based on 7-day mean intakes of 1087 individuals. The curve represents the distribution of usual intakes assumed by the Expert Consultation (CV of 25% around the observed median intake). The normal distribution actually fitted to the lower half of the United Kingdom distribution has a CV of 25.5% (not shown). The intervals end at the levels shown (0.1–1.0 = 1, etc.). The curve is plotted for the mid-points.

now a substantial volume of literature demonstrating that nutrient intakes vary markedly from day to day for the same individual (within-person variation). When data are collected on a number of days and averaged for each individual, the within-person variance is reduced. The observed variance of dietary data then represents a summation of the remaining within-person variance and the between-person variance in usual intake. The latter has to be estimated, which implies either that data sets based on information collected on a number of days (at least 3 and preferably more) must be selected or that statistical adjustments of the observed variance must be made before the derived SD can be accepted as an estimate of the SD of usual intakes. The Expert Consultation undertook such statistical adjustments of some of the available data sets and noted greater consistency of derived estimates of the *between-person* SD, but still found substantial ranges of values, probably attributable to small sample sizes and to differing dietary sampling methodologies.

It is conceivable that the variability of usual intake differs with cultural group (patterns of the usual diets consumed). This also warrants examination in the future.

Table A2 exemplifies the effects that differing true variabilities of usual intake would have on Zn_{PImin}^{basal} and Cu_{PImin}^{basal} for adult males. It is emphasized that these examples are intended to serve as a warning to users of this report. In the judgement of the Expert Consultation, the estimates adopted in this report are reasonable and the best estimates that could be made with the information available.

As noted in Chapter 2 (pages 7–21), if appropriate data are available for examination, rather than re-estimating the SD and CV of intakes for the particular group, a more direct approach to assessment of intakes can be adopted. In this approach, no assumption is made about the variability of intakes except that the distribution under examination does represent the distribution of *usual* intakes. However, in planning (defining desirable goals for group mean intakes), some assumption about the distribution of intakes between individuals in the group is unavoidable.

3. Estimation of availability for utilization

With some elements, the proportion that can be utilized depends on the nature of the diet consumed when the element is ingested. This is particularly true for zinc. In the chapters dealing with individual elements, the evidence relating to the estimates adopted in this report has been reviewed. It should be obvious that, if the availability estimate is changed, the corresponding changes in the estimates of minimum population mean intake will be similar in magnitude to those shown in Table A2 for the effect of changes in the estimates of variability of usual intake. The Expert Consultation emphasized the need for improved

Table A2. Impact of different estimates of the variability of usual intake on the lower limit of population mean intakes for adult males

Assumed CV of usual intake	Derived Zn_{PImin}^{basal}	Derived Cu_{PImin}^{basal}
15%	4 1	I.U
20%	4.8	1.2[a]
25%	5.7[a]	˙ 1.4
30%	7.2	1.8
35%[b]	9.5	2.4

[a] Estimate adopted in this report.
[b] Variabilities as high as this (or higher) have been reported for some unadjusted 1-day data sets (including the inflationary effect of within-person variance).

estimates of zinc utilizability and for better ways of predicting the extent of utilization that should be expected with particular diets.

With regard to the question of the variability of element availability for diets within the group of individuals under examination, it has already been suggested (Chapter 2) that, where there is reason to believe that this might be significant in, for example, different cultural groups within the larger population group, the population group should be stratified and appropriate element availability estimates applied before any assessment of zinc intake is made. Even when this is done, it must be assumed that some variation in the element availability of the diets consumed by individuals will remain. It has been shown empirically that, if this variation is randomly distributed through the population, use of an average availability estimate does not seriously bias the assessment of intakes (2, 5).

4. The meaning of "population" in this report

Throughout this report the term "population mean intake" has been used to describe the requirement estimates presented. It has been repeatedly emphasized that the actual meaning of this term is *group* mean intake. The immediate question that arises is "when does a group become a population?" or "what is the minimum group size to which the estimates are applicable?" This can be seen as a question of sampling. If the aim is to assess a population defined, for example, by national or regional boundaries, then it is necessary that: (a) the population should be sampled in a random manner or at least that sampling weights should be known for each stratum that has been randomly sampled; and (b) the sample size should be sufficient to provide reliable estimates of the true population intake parameters. Discussion of the design of surveys is beyond the scope of this report. However, the impact of sample size on the estimation of the two parameters of interest in this report, the mean intake and the SD (or CV) of intake, can be illustrated very simply by the example presented in Table A3.

For the purpose of this exercise, a population of 10 000 individuals was taken which had a sample mean of 99.965 and an SD of 25.1595 (CV = 25.2%). From this "population", random samples of 25, 50, 100, 250 or 1000 individuals were drawn without replacement. For each sample, the mean and SD were computed. Table A3 shows the ranges of values obtained for the samples drawn. It should be readily apparent that, with small samples, the sample means and standard deviations are relatively unreliable estimates of the true population mean, even though they are correct descriptions of the individual samples themselves. It follows that, if the purpose of the examination is to assess the true population, group sizes must be very large for reliable results to be obtained.

Table A3. Simulation of effect of sample size in representation of a "population"

Sample size	No. of samples[a]	Sample mean		Sample SD value	
		Minimum	Maximum	Minimum	Maximum
10 000[b]	1	99.96		25.16	
25	400	85.89	116.40	13.95	34.78
50	200	91.51	107.70	16.67	31.30
100	100	91.85	105.15	21.29	30.01
250	40	96.98	102.57	22.68	26.82
1 000	10	98.72	101.10	24.60	25.47

[a] Samples drawn at random without replacement from a generated normal distribution of 10 000 simulated observations (mean and SD shown in table).
[b] Original data set.

This does not imply that the estimates given in this report are inapplicable to smaller groups. However, the estimate of the group variation (the CV of intake) is a serious limitation. The estimates used in this report have been based, as far as possible, on large sample survey data. Table A3 shows that, if a small sample is extracted from the population surveyed, the actual SD could be quite different from the true population SD and, by inference, quite different from the variability estimates used in the report in the derivation of $E_{\text{PImin}}^{\text{normative}}$ and $E_{\text{PImin}}^{\text{tox}}$. This would generate errors in the assessment of such a small group. Conversely, as has been noted earlier (Chapter 2), if the intake data are actually available, the preferred strategy for assessment would be to estimate the proportion with usual intakes below $E_{\text{R}}^{\text{normative}}$ or $E_{\text{R}}^{\text{basal}}$. This does not depend on any assumption about variability of intake, and only on minimal assumptions about the variability of requirement (namely, that the distribution of requirements is approximately symmetrical and that requirements and intakes are essentially independent of one another).

It has been repeatedly noted in this report that "populations" should be stratified to yield relatively homogeneous groups (e.g. by age group, sex, physiological characteristics) and that it may also be highly desirable to stratify populations by locally important sociodemographic characteristics. Such stratification procedures may be undertaken for two different reasons. Firstly, within the context of this report, it is advocated that stratification be used to obtain a reasonable match between requirement estimates and group characteristics. Stratification for age and sex is mandatory. However, if the nature of the diet (factors affecting availability) differs in major ways between identifiable cultural groups and these groups are large in size, it would be desirable to stratify on this basis as well (again to obtain an appropriate match between the availability assumed in the adjusted requirement estimate and that in the diets consumed by the subgroup). Conversely, if the cultural groups are small and can be considered to be randomly distributed through the larger population, the assumption of an average availability based on the typical mix of foods consumed, without prior stratification by cultural group or diet type, is reasonable. A second reason for stratification may be to divide the population into groupings that have practical meaning in terms of the actions that might be taken (which groups in the population are really at risk?).

As long as the sampling ratios for each stratum are known, and there is assurance that the samples drawn are representative of that stratum (adequate sample size, randomized selection procedures), a total population estimate can always be generated (e.g. as a weighted mean prevalence). It must be recognized, however, that as the number of strata increases, there is likely to be a requirement for a larger total sample size. In the design of practical surveys, the gains and losses of precision must be balanced against the logistic realities and costs of running a large field study. There is no simple formula.

5. Usual intakes of individuals, groups and populations

All requirement estimates, minimal and maximal population mean intake estimates and intake distribution estimates specified in this report refer to *usual* intakes. This is not a well defined concept but, in general terms, the *usual intake* of an individual refers to his or her average intake over moderate periods of time (*1, 2, 6–9*). This is important both conceptually and practically. Conceptually, the inference is that requirement estimates do not relate to the intake on each individual day. It is implicitly assumed that the human body is able to compensate for modest variation in day-to-day intakes. At the basal level of requirements, this capability may be reduced, and major or prolonged downward deviations in intake below the requirement level might have functional effects. Sensitivity to the duration of periods of low intake can be expected to differ from one element to another and at different stages of physiological development. For example, young growing children respond rapidly to periods of low zinc intake and recover rapidly when repleted; responses to changes in copper, selenium or iodine intake appear to be much slower.

The practical implication of the focus on *usual* intakes lies in the estimation of the distribution of such intakes. Observed distributions will reflect both *between-person* and *within-person* (day-to-day) variation. It is the former that is of interest since it is the variation in *usual* intakes. Collecting data over a number of days and averaging such data for each individual reduces the residual *within-person* variability, and hence the distribution of such averages is a better description of that of *usual* intakes. With repeated observations, statistical procedures may be available for estimating the partitioning of variance and adjusting the observed distribution to remove the effects of *within-person* variation (2, 6–9). Table A4 illustrates the impact of the number of days on which data are collected on the observed SD. The example presented in the table assumes normality of distributions of both *between-* and *within-person* variation. It also assumes that the CV of *within-person* variation is 25%. A CV of 25% is also taken for the *between-person* variation in keeping with the estimate of variability of usual zinc intakes.

As is also seen from Table A4, the presence of *within-person* variation does not bias the estimate of the true mean intake; however, it does affect the reliability of that estimate (as shown by the standard error of the mean).

Table A4 should be read in conjunction with Table A3, which shows the reproducibility of the estimate of CV and the mean as a function of sample size. No allowance was made for the effect of *within-person* variation.

In summary, the number of days on which data are collected is important in dealing with requirements expressed as group mean intakes, but is not as critical as in the estimation of the true *usual* intake of a particular individual. For large groups, it would be expected that the mean of 1-day intakes and the mean of multiple-day intakes would be very similar. It follows that, as long as it is not deemed essential to estimate the SD of *usual* intakes for the group, large survey databases based on single-day intakes can be accepted and utilized.

6. Interpretation of population mean intakes falling below E_{PImin}

There is always a temptation to interpret data simplistically, i.e., to see assessment in binary terms—adequate or inadequate. That would be a serious and possibly misleading error. When a group mean intake falls below E_{PImin} for normative or basal requirements, it does not mean that the entire group has an inadequate intake but simply that the prevalence of inadequate intakes in the group has begun to rise. As the group mean falls further below E_{PImin}, the prevalence of inadequate intakes and of associated functional or biochemical signs would be expected to increase.

This can be illustrated for zinc. Fig. A2 reflects the specific assumptions of this report, notably that the intake distribution is normally distributed with CV = 25%. It shows the proportion of the group expected to have intakes below $E_{PImin}^{normative}$ and E_{PImin}^{basal} for a series of distributions with means as plotted. This association must be borne in mind when examining the review of reported zinc intakes around the world presented in Chapter 22.

Table A4. Example of impact of number of days on which data are collected for each individual

No. of subjects	No. of days	Expected CV of intake[a]	Expected mean[b]	Expected standard error of mean
100	1	35.4%	100	3.5
100	3	28.9%	100	2.9
100	7	26.7%	100	2.7
1000	1	35.4%	100	1.1
1000	3	28.9%	100	0.9
1000	7	26.7%	100	0.8

[a] True *between-person* CV = 25%.
[b] True mean taken as 100.

Figure A2. Relationship between prevalence of inadequate intakes (population risk) and group mean intake for zinc in adult men

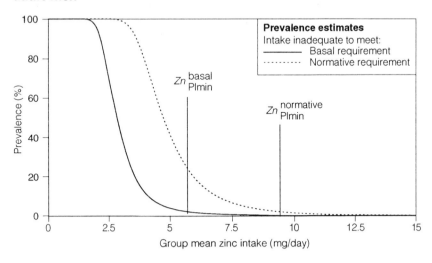

WHO 94661

The curves show the proportion of the group with intakes below Zn_R^{basal} or $Zn_R^{normative}$. This is an estimate of the proportion of individuals expected to have intakes below their own requirement. A moderate-availability diet is assumed, 35% of the zinc being available for absorption for the basal requirement and 30% for the normative requirement, together with a CV of usual intakes of 25%. A normal distribution is also assumed.

References

1. *Energy and protein requirements. Report of a Joint FAO/WHO/UNU Expert Consultation.* Geneva, World Health Organization, 1985 (WHO Technical Report Series, No. 724).

2. National Research Council Subcommittee on Criteria for Dietary Evaluation. *Nutrient adequacy: assessment using food consumption surveys.* Washington, DC, National Academy of Sciences, 1986.

3. Gregory J et al. *The dietary and nutritional survey of British adults.* London, HMSO, 1990.

4. Baghurst K et al. *The Victorian nutrition survey*, Part 2. Adelaide, Commonwealth Scientific and Industrial Research Organisation, Division of Human Nutrition, 1987: 66–67.

5. Beaton GH. New approaches to the nutritional assessment of population dietary data. In: Murphy, Rauchwarter, ed. *Proceedings of the 10th National Nutrient Data Bank Conference.* Springfield, VA, NTIS, 1985.

6. Liu K et al. Statistical methods to assess and minimize the role of intraindividual variability in obscuring the relationship between dietary lipids and serum cholesterol. *Journal of chronic diseases*, 1978, **31**: 399–418.

7. Beaton GH et al. Sources of variance in 24-hour dietary recall data: implications for nutrition study design and interpretation. *American journal of clinical nutrition*, 1979, **32**: 2556–2559.

8. Beaton GH et al. Sources of variance in 24-hour dietary recall data: implications for nutrition study design and interpretation. Carbohydrate sources, vitamins and minerals. *American journal of clinical nutrition*, 1983, **37**: 986–995.

9. Life Sciences Research Office. *Guidelines for use of dietary intake data.* Bethesda, MD, Federation of American Societies for Experimental Biology, 1986.

Index

Page numbers in **bold** indicate main discussions of a topic; those in *italics* refer to figures or tables.